Writer's
Guide to
Nursing
Periodicals

Dedicated to my parents: Laurane and Bill

Thank you to my family: Bernie, John, Bernie Jr. and Mary, the Brodt Family, and Dave and Sandy.

Writer's Guide to Nursing Periodicals

Jeanette M. Daly

Sage Publications, Inc.
International Educational and Professional Publisher
Thousand Oaks ■ London ■ New Delhi

For information:

Sage Publications, Inc.
2455 Teller Road
Thousand Oaks, California 91320
E-mail: order@sagepub.com

Sage Publications Ltd.
6 Bonhill Street
London EC2A 4PU
United Kingdom

Sage Publications India Pvt. Ltd.
M-32 Market
Greater Kailash I
New Delhi 110 048 India

Printed in the United States of America

Library of Congress Cataloging-in-Publication Data

Daly, Jeanette M.
  Writer's guide to nursing periodicals / By Jeanette M. Daly.
      p. cm.
Includes index.
  ISBN 0-7619-1491-9 (cloth) — ISBN 0-7619-1492-7 (pbk.)
  1. Nursing—Authorship—Handbooks, manuals, etc. I. Title.
RT24 .D35 2000
808′.06661—dc21   00-008048

This book is printed on acid-free paper.
00   01   02   03   04   05   06   7   6   5   4   3   2   1

Acquisition Editor: Rolf Janke
Editorial Assistant: Heidi van Middlesworth
Production Editor: Sanford Robinson
Copy Editor: Linda Gray
Editorial Assistant: Victoria Cheng
Typesetter: Danielle Dillahunt
Cover Designer: Candice Harman

Contents

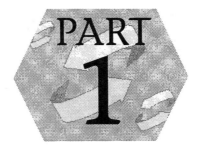

PART

1

Writing for Publication in Nursing Journals

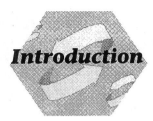

Introduction

Writer's Guide to Nursing Periodicals is a reference book that offers helpful information for writers who want to submit their work to journals in the field of nursing. This reference is a single source of the specific guidelines required by the editors of 99 nursing journals, with behind-the-scenes discussion of the editorial policies. This should be a useful tool for novice as well as professional writers and for students, scholars, and teachers of writing.

Each journal is described in a separate entry that includes the purpose or focus of the journal, manuscript submission instructions, and author guidelines for the typing and layout of the manuscript, along with the name of the journal editor or managing editor, correspondence address, journal facts, copyright information, indexing information, and sample journal titles. Key journal facts include publication schedule, circulation information, number of papers submitted each year for publication and their acceptance rate, monetary reimbursement, average turnaround time once a manuscript is submitted for a response, publishing time after a manuscript has been accepted, and the Internet address of the publisher.

The collection of nursing periodicals covered here includes journals for nurses in all practice settings and specialties in the United States. The smaller journals may serve as springboards for novice writers, whereas the larger, more prestigious journals provide outlets for well-established writers of nursing practice, education, and research.

The guide forms a basis for authors, educators, and students who are earnest about staying abreast of specialties in nursing that are expanding the arena for publication. The journals are grouped according to the following categories, which have been established for easy inspection of those journals in a specialty area: acute care, administration, advanced practice, community/home health, critical care, education, gerontology, holistic nursing, legislative issues, maternal/child care, nephrology, oncology, operative nursing, orthopedic/rehabilitative nursing, professional development, psychiatric nursing, research, skin and wound care, and specialty practices. Some journals overlap more than one area but were placed in a specific category through analysis of the purpose statement of the journal. For example, the *Journal of Pediatric Oncology Nursing* could have been placed in the maternal/child care category but instead was grouped in the oncology specialty. The number of journals in the maternal/child care category is rather large. The two specialties (maternal care and child care) were grouped together because some journals—for example, *JOGNN* or the *Journal of Obstetric, Gynecologic, and Neonatal Nursing*—overlap the two specialties.

Journals/clinics/seminars that are guest-edited or that have manuscripts solicited from authors and published in a single- or double-topic format have been excluded from this publication. Examples include *AACN Clinical Issues: Advanced Practice in Acute and Critical Care; Nurse Practitioner Forum; Nursing Clinics of North America; Primary Care Practice;* and

Seminars for Nurse Managers. Newsletters and updates such as *Home Infusion Therapy Management* and *Perianesthesia and Ambulatory Surgery Nursing Update* have also been omitted.

In the field of nursing, the range and quantity of publications is increasing dramatically, and identifying the specific publication to target for submission is an extremely important step. Nursing writers will find this collection of guidelines extremely useful in making a decision about which journal is best suited for their work. After identifying the area of interest for a promising manuscript, an author should review the information provided here for each journal in that area. For example, for a paper titled "Psychotropic Medication Reduction for Residents in Long-Term Care," an author should review the section on gerontology, where two journals are listed: *Geriatric Nursing* and *Journal of Gerontological Nursing.* After the review, an author may want to send a query letter to both journals or send the manuscript to only one of the journals, following the manuscript preparation guidelines provided here.

Definition of Terms

Blind review: Neither reviewers nor author(s) know each other's identity when a manuscript is reviewed for publication. After review, comments from the reviewers are returned anonymously to the author(s).

Copyright: This is a statutory privilege extended to creators of works fixed in a tangible medium of expression.

Keypoints or key words: These single words or small groups of words that summarize or highlight the essence of a paper are used for indexing.

Peer review: A manuscript is reviewed by two or three reviewers in the topic specialty who comment on its quality and appropriateness.

Proofreading marks: These belong to an established system of marking a manuscript to correct errors on proof pages (see Appendix F at the end of Part 1).

Query letter: This letter, sent to a journal editor, describes the manuscript so that the editor can determine if that manuscript would be of interest to the journal.

Refereed: Submitted manuscripts are reviewed by experts who judge the merit of the manuscript.

Rejection letter: This letter is sent to an author declining acceptance of the manuscript for publication.

Nurses Writing for Publication

Nurses, who are a prime source of valuable health information, need to translate their experience and research into manuscripts distributing this information and knowledge to others in the field. Many reasons have been suggested for writing and publishing one's work. Styles (1978) emphasizes the primary reason to publish: "because the future of the profession depends on it" (p. 29). Other reasons include the following:

- The desire to write
- To convey information/knowledge about nursing and patient care
- To describe the work of nursing
- To reach wider audiences than individual contacts
- For recognition for one's work (prestige) or a chance at fame
- To make money (profit)
- Academic pressure—to receive promotions or tenure
- The need for self-expression
- To disseminate new knowledge
- Piety
- Because writing is highly rewarding
- To teach the layperson through lay media

McCloskey and Swanson (1985) identify three motivations for publication: knowledge, reward, and change. Nursing practices will be improved by the dissemination of nursing knowledge. Bestor (1976) suggests three worthwhile reasons for publishing:

We write for the value that our observations have to others, for the added sense of professionalism that making such contributions will give us, and finally for the increasing satisfaction we will find as we get more and more involved in the process of writing down our own discoveries and giving them permanent form. (p. 23)

The reasons nurses are reluctant to publish include false modesty, lack of time, and inadequate training in writing skills. But their personal experience, observations, and analysis qualify nurses to share their knowledge.

MANUSCRIPT PREPARATION

A unique or original idea is the basis for successful publication: The implementation of a new nursing intervention, a description of a cerebral palsy patient with necrotizing fasciitis, a new flow sheet for documentation on the ambulatory care center, or successful recruitment strategies can serve as the platform for one's writing efforts. It is advisable to choose a topic or case history with which you are thoroughly familiar. The idea is the starting point.

Writing is work. You may not want to start with an elaborate piece but, rather, with something short and to the point. You can write a book review or a letter to an editor regarding a current publication in a journal. You can ask other nurses to collaborate with you on this endeavor; coauthorship with other colleagues is another way to get started writing.

Prepare for writing by carefully researching unanswered questions; checking pertinent facts, specific names, and dates; and tying up any other loose ends, such as gathering complete bibliographic information for references you plan to cite. Then you are more likely to feel comfortable, knowing that you have enough information to proceed. Write the paper in your own style, in a fashion that makes sense to you. You may or may not develop an outline to serve as a framework for writing. You may write the central or middle part of the paper, then add the beginning and summary. You may start with tables, knowing what you want the tables to illustrate, then describe the tables in text. No one way of writing a paper is perfect or absolute. No one way works for everyone.

The theme or thesis of the manuscript should be stated at the very beginning, with the body of the manuscript elaborating that thesis and the final section or paragraph summarizing the findings and conclusions of the paper. A first writing should be considered a draft and the basis for the final manuscript. Rewriting—as many as six drafts is not uncommon—is always worthwhile if the manuscript is to be well written. It is also a good idea to have another person read it for a second viewpoint. (If possible, have someone read the paper out loud to you. You'll be more likely to notice where the wording seems awkward or where a point needs clarification.) After you've shared your paper with colleagues, rewrite and share again with others. Ponder their criticisms and comments; they are invaluable to you.

Writing a manuscript need not be as difficult as many nurses claim. Instead, it can be satisfying and rewarding. The satisfaction will come from knowing that the information given will help other nurses. The reward is personal enhancement and recognition by your peers. Nursing is a caring profession, and the act of writing is a demonstration of caring, a contribution to the future of the profession, which depends on nurses sharing what they've learned through experience, observation, and analysis.

MANUSCRIPT SUBMISSION

A thought for submission might be "finding the best, most prestigious journal, with the best and largest audience for your study" (Overfield, 1981, p. 419). This is one viewpoint, but a thorough understanding of your work needs to be weighed against a review of the journals you are considering for submission of you manuscript. The number of journals has increased dramatically over the last few years, and more specialty journals are available. The prospective author must be careful to examine the journals and determine the journal most appropriate for the initial submission of the manuscript. Look closely at several issues of each journal for which you think your manuscript might be appropriate. Read several articles, noting their format and writing style. One needs to know what a journal editor expects in a manuscript. Choosing the appropriate journal will expedite the publishing process and enhance the possibility of success. Know the answers to the following questions: Is the journal peer-reviewed? Is there a wide readership? What audience will read the published manuscript and is your paper appropriate for that audience? What is the time frame for accepting or rejecting a manuscript? After a manuscript is accepted, how long will it take to be published?

Once the manuscript is ready for submission, a thorough check of requirements is beneficial. A checklist is sometimes provided by journals for review, and a sample is found in Appendix A at the end of Part 1.

REVIEW PROCESS

An idea has been generated and described in a paper. Once the author determines it is time for submission, he or she has two choices. The author can send query letters (see Appendix

B) to a number of journals or submit the manuscript with a cover letter (see Appendix C) to one journal. Regardless of the choice, the author must await the response from the editor.

It is common to wait 3 to 4 months for a response. A query letter is appropriate if no editorial response is received after this period of time. The editor should respond in about a month following the query letter.

When a manuscript is submitted to a journal editor, the policies of the publisher have to be adhered to for the review process. Some editors may simply reject the manuscript due to inappropriate content (see Appendix D). Editors may forward manuscripts for others to review. The reviewers will notify the editor of their decision.

When an editor thinks a manuscript might be acceptable, the manuscript will be sent to the editorial board or peer review board. Usually, two or three reviewers are sent copies of the manuscript. This is most often done as a blind review. The manuscript is evaluated on the scholarly merit of the work. The criteria that may be given as guidelines for the reviewers are (a) appropriate topic for the journal, (b) logical and succinct organization, (c) accuracy, and (d) appropriate methods of research. The reviewers usually have a review form for recording their evaluation according to the criteria. The review form and reviewer comments are returned to the editor.

After receiving the reviewers' evaluation forms and comments, the editor analyzes the material and makes a decision regarding acceptance of the manuscript. At this stage, based on the editorial review, the editor makes one of the following decisions: (a) to accept the manuscript for publication, (b) to accept the manuscript for publication with minor revisions, (c) to ask that the manuscript be substan-tially revised and resubmitted for review (see Appendix E for sample revision letters and acceptance letters), or (d) to reject the manuscript.

If the manuscript is accepted with revisions or substantial changes and rewriting, the anonymous reviewers' comments and editor's summary are returned to the author. These returned documents will have proofreading marks (see Appendix F) on them and will need correction. Guidelines for revision and deadline for resubmittal are sometimes included with the returned manuscript. It is advantageous to carefully take into consideration all reviewers' comments and suggestions. The author may want to have a colleague review the revised manuscript before submitting to the journal a second time. If substantial revisions and rewrites are required, usually, the manuscript is sent out for review again, often to the same reviewers.

Once a manuscript is accepted for publication, the publication date may vary from 3 months to 3 years. Some journals note the acceptance date on the article when in print. For example, a manuscript may have been accepted in January 1997 and published in February 1999. When an author has not heard from an editor after approximately 3 months, a letter requesting information on the status of the manuscript is appropriate.

SUMMARY

The review process is time-consuming, and authors need to be persistent in their endeavor to have a manuscript published. Rejections or revisions do not end a manuscript's possibilities. They are simply the beginning of required work to accomplish the task at hand—publishing one's work.

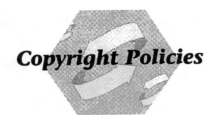

Copyright Policies

In each journal description, there is a section regarding copyright. Some journals address these topics in great detail and others minimally. Once an author has finished writing a manuscript, he or she owns the property, which is called the *copyright* if it is an original work of authorship. The Copyright Act of 1976 provides authors with protection for their work.

COPYRIGHT

Copyright involves five separate rights: (a) the right to reproduce or copy the work; (b) the right to prepare derivative works; (c) the right to distribute copies of the work to the public; (d) in the case of audiovisual works, the right to perform the work publicly; and (d) in the case of literary, musical, dramatic, and choreographic works, pantomimes and pictorial works, and graphic or sculptural works, the right to display the work publicly. The duration of copyright since January 1, 1978, is protected at the time of creation throughout the life of the author plus 50 years after the death of the author.

As an author, understanding some basics about copyrights is imperative. It is an assumption that when an article is published, the copyright belongs to the publisher. However, should the author desire to own the copyright, this is possible. At the time of submission, some journals require a signed transfer-of-copyright form prior to review; others do not ask that a copyright transfer form be completed until acceptance of a manuscript.

In some instances, an author may prefer not to grant copyright to a publisher. This is negotiated between the author and publisher. For example, if an author published the descriptive research of developing an attitude scale, the attitude scale could be copyrighted to the author.

When the manuscript is distributed as copies to the public, it is usually done so in a "for sale" mode. To determine if a manuscript is copyrighted, check for a copyright notice. Most journals have a copyright notice on the business page in the front of the journal. Most journals are copyrighted by the publisher. A few journals are copyrighted by the respective professional organizations. Some journals state that pages with a designated symbol are protected by copyright. This is so indicated in the permissions section of the journal business page.

To determine if a work is copyrighted, a search may be ordered from the copyright office. To copyright an article or other material, write to the following address: Register of Copyright, Library of Congress, Washington, DC 20559-6000. Three elements are necessary for copyright completion: (a) an application form completed in all spaces, (b) a nonrefundable $20 filing fee in check or money order payable to Register of Copyright, and (c) the deposit material.

A search may also be completed through the Copyright Clearance Center, 222 Rosewood Drive, Danvers, MA 01923. The search can be completed by the center or through the Internet at www.copyright.com where a title database for registered publication is found.

The search can be completed by title, publisher keyword, Copyright Clearance Center title ID, exact title, or standard number (ISSN or ISBN).

The application form asks for some of the following information: title of work, previous titles, publication as a contribution (to a periodical, serial, or collection), name of author, year in which creation of the work was completed, copyright claimant, previous registration, and a derivative work or compilation. The application itself is a two-page form and can be found at most public libraries. The publisher attends to preparing the copyright application, registering the work, and depositing copies at the copyright office.

The purpose of copyright is to "promote the progress of Science and Useful Arts" (American Library Association and National Education Association, 1987, p. 5). Fair use limits the author's or copyright owner's monopoly by allowing others to have reasonable use of copyright material without the consent of the author. Fair use is of importance to researchers, students, authors, and teachers. For instance, fair use allows us to watch a videotaped game of *Monday Night Football* on Sunday afternoon. It allows nurses to use nursing diagnoses when writing care plans.

The court system through case trials has set forth the parameters of fair use. Congress initially set the parameters in Section 107 of Title 17 of the U.S. Code. Fair use is not in effect when the copyright owner has given written permission for the material's use. Fair use applies when written permission has not been obtained.

One way to determine fair use is to ask if the copying of material is for "productive" or "intrinsic" purposes. Productive work might be the continuation or duplication of research for the purpose of validation. An intrinsic use might be selling critical pathways to hospitals.

PERMISSIONS

As an author, you are responsible for obtaining permission for what is not covered under that constituted as fair use. Usually, the publisher has a specific form for obtaining permissions. It is the author's responsibility to obtain *all* permissions required for his or her work. This is so for a number of reasons. A publisher may be viewed as a potential rival to another publisher, whereas the author is not seen in this light and more easily obtains the permission. In instances when permission is refused, the author can then make the decision to delete or replace the work. Last, if the borrowed work has been updated or changed compared with what is in the author's work, the author can update the material before final submission.

Permissions are essential for any of the following copyrighted material: photographs, drawings, charts, tables, any borrowed or adapted material from a publication or colleague, prose quotations of 300 words or more, poetry, or song lyrics. If an author has published previous manuscripts and wishes to include some of the material in a new article, permission from the original publisher must be obtained, if the publisher holds the copyright.

Permission request forms need to be completed by the author and sent to the copyright holder. The request form usually includes detailed information about the material to be borrowed, such as title; author; editor; publisher; copyright year; inclusive page numbers; table, figure, or illustration numbers; journal title; and volume number. Additional information required is a description of where the material will be printed, such as the title, author(s), publisher, editor, journal name, volume number, and year. If a modification of the work is being requested, the modification must be explained in detail to the copyright holder. Always keep a copy of the permission request form and a copy of the approval of such request for your files.

All permission forms should be submitted to a publisher when a manuscript is submitted for initial review. It is the author's responsibility to meet the conditions stipulated with any permissions. If a fee is required, the author and publisher negotiate for who will pay the fee. There may be specific language stipulated for use for the borrowed work, and the author is responsible to see that this is accomplished.

Authors need to identify borrowed material in their work and give appropriate credit. Specific terminology is essential to clarify if the work is "adapted," "from," or "modified." Material used from a health care institution should be so reflected in phrases such as "provided by" or "courtesy of."

Photographs with people need to have a release form signed by all individuals in the picture. In the case of minors or mentally challenged persons, the parents or guardians need to sign the release form. An example of a simple form is provided here.

Photograph Release Form

Date: _____

I hereby grant permission to reproduce my image with or without my name in any format for publication. This permission shall be for all rights.

Full name: _____

Signature: _____

Address: _____

City: _____State: _____ Zip Code: _____

Permission to photocopy is a different aspect of permissions. The Copyright Clearance Center, Inc. Transactional Reporting Service offers an efficient, cost-effective way for individuals and organizations to comply with copyright law by providing instant photocopy authorizations. Currently, the Copyright Clearance Center is able to grant permission to photocopy over 1.75 million publications, from over 9,200 copyright holders worldwide. On the business page of most journals, if the publication is registered with the center, it is so designated.

Internet Nursing Journals On-Line

Internet on-line journals are a new media format for prospective authors. Often, information for authors is available at the respective journal home page. Journals available only on the Internet are becoming prolific. Some are unique and imaginative in their presentation. The following is a sample of journals available on the Internet.

can purchase them individually or by annual subscription.

On-line Journal of Clinical Innovations

The *On-line Journal of Clinical Innovations* was born of a need reported by individuals in the clinical setting time and time again in searching the CINAHL® database. These individuals needed more than just bibliographic information; they needed information to help with clinical problems occurring right now. Their need for research information, anecdotal information, ideas, and suggestions spawned this project and led to the journal's publication. For many years, Cinahl Information Systems has encouraged research-based practice through information literacy and literature searching, and this journal is the logical next step.

The topics covered will be clinically relevant, and each article, with the exception of the knowledge utilization paper and the editorial, will be accompanied by a summary. This summary is the key link to the CINAHL bibliographic database; it is indexed and searchable as any other article would be. Never before has the published literature complemented the bibliographic database so well. The summary will provide users of the CINAHL database genuinely useful information on the spot. Generally three to four pages in length plus a full list of references from the complete article, the summaries contain information designed to stimulate thought and problem solving in the clinical setting. Readers can use the information as a starting point in developing their own programs and interventions, adapted to their own clinical situation.

To take their search for knowledge a step further, individuals can obtain the full articles from Cinahl's Website (www.cinahl.com) by choosing "Journal Articles on the Web," and

On-line Journal of Nursing Informatics

Internet: milkman.cac.psu.edu/~dxm12/
    main.html
Editors: Dee McGonigle, RNC, PhD, FACCE
    Renee Eggers, PhD

Philosophy of the Journal

The *On-line Journal of Nursing Informatics* is committed to enhancing nursing knowledge on nursing informatics for nurses working in diverse settings. The *On-line Journal of Nursing Informatics* will provide nurses with an electronic format to share findings, experience, perceptions, knowledge, and wisdom with nursing colleagues involved in all facets of nursing informatics. The *On-line Journal of Nursing Informatics* wants to exploit the power of cyberspace to create an electronic nursing informatics community that provides both virtually accessible and timely information about nursing informatics globally. The *On-line Journal of Nursing Informatics* will further enhance the speed of cyber-communications through an expedited editorial process that provides rapid turnaround and publication times. The *On-line Journal of Nursing Informatics* recognizes the importance of both the academic and practice-based perspectives in nursing informatics. Therefore, article submissions will be encouraged from all facets of nursing informatics. The *On-line Journal of Nursing Informatics* is committed to scholarly excellence. Thus, the journal will maintain a high standard for peer-review, and when necessary, the editorial staff will attempt to provide assistance to authors as a means of eliciting high-quality manuscripts suitable for publication.

Telephone Nursing Telezine

Internet: www.katsden.com/tnt/index.html
Editor: Kathi Webster, BSN, RN

Telephone nursing takes many forms. It can be an organized call center of nurses or a single nurse on the telephone. All nursing specialties do it to some extent. *Telephone triage nursing* is a term used for a well-known group within the ranks of telephone nurses.

But telephone triage is just a part of what we do. There are opportunities in areas such as special needs programs, health awareness, community outreach, university health, and case management (including disease management)—to name just a few. Telenurses may use additional monitoring devices such as the EKG or fetal monitors to enhance assessment and their practice. The Internet is also a way to reach out to patients via the telephone.

If you do a large part of your nursing practice using a telephone, you most certainly have something to contribute to and learn from the *Telephone Nursing Telezine.*

Internet Journal of Advanced Nursing Practice

Internet: www.ispub.com/journals/ijanp.htm
Editor: Susan D. Ruppert, PhD, RN, CCRN, CS, NP-C, FCCM

Online Journal of Knowledge Synthesis for Nursing

Internet: www.stti.iupui.edu/library/ojksn

Published by Sigma Theta Tau International, Honor Society of Nursing, the *Online*

Journal of Knowledge Synthesis for Nursing is an electronic journal that makes current research findings available for the immediate use of clinical nurses, academicians, and researchers. The journal provides critical reviews of research literature to guide nursing practice and research.

Urology Nurses Online

Urology Nurses Online of the *Digital Urology Journal* welcomes original didactic or research articles relevant to nurses practicing in the area of urology.

Editorial Office: Urology Nurses Online of the Digital Urology Journal, 300 Longwood Avenue, Hunnewell 3, Boston, MA 02115; telephone: (617) 355-6169; fax: (617) 355-6587; e-mail for *Digital Urology Journal:* urology@tiac.net; e-mail for *Urology Nurses Online:* e-mail mail@duv.com
Internet: www.duj.com/unohome.html

REFERENCES

American Library Association and National Education Association. (1987). *The copyright primer for librarians and educators.* Chicago: American Library Association.

Bestor, D. K. (1976, May-June). Writing an article for publication: Part two. *Nurse Practitioner,* pp. 21-23.

McCloskey, J. C., & Swanson, E. (1985). Publishing in practice journals: A responsibility of the researcher. *CNR, 12*(3), 1-4.

Overfield, T. (1981). Publish or perish: How to accomplish the former and avoid the latter. *Western Journal of Nursing Research, 3*(4), 417-420.

Styles, M. M. (1978). Why publish? *Image, 10*(2), 28-32.

SUGGESTED READINGS

Carroll-Johnson, R. M. (1995). Then or now? Reflections on 20 years of publishing. *Oncology Nursing Forum, 22*(3), 467.

Covington, C. (1994). Editorial: The speed of write in nursing: An X ray of hope? *Issues in Comprehensive Pediatric Nursing, 17*(4), iii-v.

Frisch, N. (1996). Writing for publication. *Nursing Diagnosis, 7*(3), 95-96.

Gilles, D. A., Kleinschmidt, K., & Holm, K. (1986). Writing for the popular press: A professional nursing responsibility. *Heart & Lung, 15*(1), 55-56.

Goldstein, N. (1996). *Stylebook and libel manual.* New York: Addison-Wesley.

Haller, K. B. (1995, July-August). The road a manuscript travels. *JOGNN,* p. 491.

Hayes, P. (1995). Authors, editors, and the world of computers. *Clinical Nursing Research, 4*(1), 3-5.

Hutchinson, D. (1999). *The Internet workbook for health professionals.* Sacramento, CA: New Wind.

McConnell, E. A. (1995). Journal and publishing characteristics for 42 nursing publications outside the United States. *Image: Journal of Nursing Scholarship, 27*(3), 225-229.

Stern, P. N. (1995). Getting published: View from the editor's/author's desk. *Health Care for Women International, 16*(1), v-viii.

Swanson, E., & McCloskey, J. C. (1982). The manuscript review process of nursing journals. *Image, 14*(3), 72-77.

Swanson, E., & McCloskey, J. (1986). Publishing opportunities for nurses. *Nursing Outlook, 34*(5), 227-235.

Wood, J. (1996). *How to write attention-grabbing query & cover letters.* Cincinnati, OH: Writer's Digest Books.

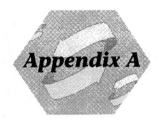

GENERIC CHECKLIST FOR
FINAL MANUSCRIPT SUBMISSION

_____ Letter of submission/cover letter
_____ Original and XX photocopies of manuscript
_____ Postcard self-addressed, stamped to acknowledge receipt of manuscript
_____ Envelope, large, self-addressed, stamped for return of manuscript

Title page
_____ Title of article
_____ Full name(s), academic degree(s), and affiliations of author(s)
_____ Author biographical sketch
_____ Author to whom correspondence and reprint requests are to be sent
_____ Corresponding author's address: business and home
_____ Corresponding author's telephone numbers: business, fax, and home
_____ Acknowledgments

Abstract
_____ Title included or omitted
_____ Purpose, methodology, results, conclusions
_____ Word count completed
_____ Key words listed

Text
_____ Pages numbered
_____ Running head
_____ Margins as required
_____ Double-spaced
_____ $8\frac{1}{2} \times 11$-inch paper

References
_____ Correct style
_____ Counted, number limitation calculated
_____ Complete
_____ Current

Illustrations
_____ Tables
_____ Figures
_____ Legends
_____ Photographs

Permissions
_____ Permission to reproduce published material or cite unpublished data
_____ Informed consent for patient photographs
_____ Copyright transfer letter

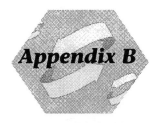

SAMPLE QUERY LETTER

Date

Mary Deean, RN, PhD, FAAN
1111 New Street
Anytown, IA 66666

Dear Dr. Deean:

Two colleagues and myself have completed a survey of 500 staff nurses in long-term care throughout the United States. We asked about their knowledge and information needs regarding long-term care federal rules and regulations. A manuscript titled "Nurses Knowledge and Information Needs Regarding Long-Term Care Federal Regulations" is in process.

The manuscript details the results of a survey sent to staff nurses in long-term care settings throughout the United States. The survey met rigorous review standards before use and had a return response rate of 44%. Interesting findings are noted. Overall, it was found that staff nurses are very knowledgeable regarding long-term care rules and regulations. Would you be interested in reviewing this manuscript? This manuscript is not under review by any other journal and is being submitted exclusively to you.

Thank you for your time and support in this endeavor. I look forward to your response.

Sincerely yours,

The Author

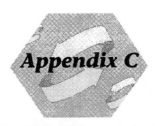

SAMPLE COVER LETTER

Date

Mary Deean, RN, PhD, FAAN
1111 New Street
Anytown, IA 66666

Dear Dr. Deean:

Enclosed is a manuscript titled "Nurses Attitudes and Knowledge Needs Regarding Long-Term Care and Federal Regulations." An original and three copies are enclosed for your consideration for publication in the journal, *Journal of Nursing Care*. There are three coauthors of this manuscript, and I am the corresponding author.

The manuscript details the results of a survey sent to staff nurses in long-term care settings throughout the United States. The survey met rigorous review standards before use and had a return response rate of 44%. Interesting findings are noted. Overall, it was found that staff nurses are very knowledgeable regarding long-term care rules and regulations.

Thank you for your time and support in this endeavor. I look forward to your response.

Sincerely yours,

The Author

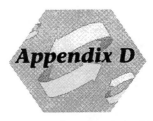

SAMPLE REJECTION LETTER

Date

Jane Doe, RN, PhD
1000 Main Street
Anywhere, IA 10000

RE: Manuscript Number 12-288-97

Dear Dr. Doe:

I am returning your manuscript, "Rural Health Care Provider's Educational Needs Regarding AIDS," without review. The article is not appropriate for the journal. We are interested in articles about this disease, its treatment, the preparation of providers for treating AIDS, and other aspects of the rural health care delivery system that bring substantial new knowledge to the field. This article represents a useful assessment of how your continuing education system can be structured for the convenience of Iowa providers. Unfortunately, the assessment does not develop information that will be of substantial benefit beyond your program.

We would be interested in articles that are more generalizable and applicable to other systems and places and that present more detail concerning the state of knowledge about the treatment of AIDS disease.

Sincerely,

Editor

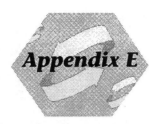

Appendix E

SAMPLE ACCEPTANCE LETTER

Date

Jane Doe, RN, PhD
1000 Main Street
Anywhere, IA 10000

RE: 68-1
TITLE: Information Resources and Knowledge Needs of Nurses Regarding AIDS

Dear Dr. Doe:

Please be advised that the above article has been accepted as edited for publication in the *Journal of Nursing.* The reviewers note the need to clarify if the word "rural" is accurate. Additional comments are included in the manuscript.

If this article was computer-generated, please send us a copy of the revision on disk that is IBM compatible or DOS or ASCII formatted. Please be sure to include a revised hard copy.

In addition, please provide three "key points" to accompany your article. These statements should summarize the main points of your article.

Page proofs will be faxed to you prior to publication. Please provide us with your fax number if available.

Sincerely,

Managing Editor

SAMPLE REVISION LETTERS

Date

Jane Doe, RN, PhD
1000 Main Street
Anywhere, IA 10000

RE: 98-0000022
TITLE: Information Resources and Knowledge Needs of Staff Nurses in Long-Term Care

Dear Dr. Doe:

Thank you for the above manuscript that you submitted for consideration in the *Journal of Nursing.*

Before a final decision can be made, some revision is necessary. To assist you to this end, we have provided some specific editing and comments (enclosed). Additional suggestions include the following:

1. Omit all tables except #6.
2. Condense/shorten abstract.
3. Discuss questionnaire characteristics.
4. Use both *n* and % in findings.
5. Incorporate assertions in introduction with implications and findings in conclusions.
6. Include recent references if possible.

Please send us four copies of the revised manuscript along with the "edited" manuscript. If you would like us to acknowledge receipt of your revision, please enclose a self-addressed, postage-paid postcard.

We will keep your file open for six months. Should you require additional time or have any questions, please call. Thank you for your interest in the journal, and we hope to hear from you soon.

Sincerely,

Executive Editor

Date

Jane Doe, RN, PhD
1000 Main Street
Anywhere, IA 10000

RE: MS98-077

Dear Dr. Doe:

The initial review of your manuscript, "Information Resources and Knowledge Needs of Staff Nurses in Long-Term Care," is complete. The reviewers thought this was an interesting manuscript that would be of interest to *Journal of Nursing* readers, but they also believe that revisions and a re-review are necessary before a publication decision can be made. I am enclosing two copies of the manuscript and the reviewers' comments for your review. I encourage you to consider their suggestions and revise the manuscript. When I receive your revised manuscript, I will send it to the same reviewers for re-review. At that time, based on the comments from the second review, I will make a publication decision.

When you resubmit your revised manuscript, you will need to return the following to me: 1) the two edited copies of the manuscript (the ones I am returning to you) and the reviewer's comments, 2) three printed copies of the revised manuscript, 3) a letter describing the changes made in the manuscript (this will be sent to the reviewers with your revised manuscript), 4) a disk version of the manuscript (which must be identical to the printed copy), 5) a large business-sized envelope with sufficient postage to return the manuscript to you, and 6) the enclosed forms.

I look forward to receiving your revised manuscript. If you have any questions, please do not hesitate to contact me.

Thank you again for your interest in the *Journal of Nursing,* and I look forward to receiving your revised manuscript in the near future.

Sincerely yours,

Editor-in-Chief

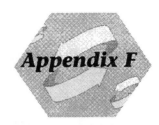

PROOFREADING MARKS

(*Iowa*)	Abbreviate		∧	Insert word
	Delete		*lc*	Lowercase
a.	Don't abbreviate		∨	Make superscript
⊐	Flush right		∧	Make subscript
⊏	Flush left		*no ¶*	No paragraph
¶	Indent for paragraph		¶	Paragraph
ᵛ	Insert apostrophe		⌒	Remove space
(:)	Insert colon		= /	Retain hyphen
⌃	Insert comma		*bf*	Set boldface
⁻ₘ	Insert dash		*ital*	Set italic type
| = |	Insert hyphen		*rom*	Set roman type
#	Insert space		*sp*	Spell it out
(|)	Insert parentheses		*tr or* ∪	Transpose
⊙	Insert period		*cap*	Uppercase
ⱽ ⱽ	Insert quotation marks		(*sixty*)	Use figure

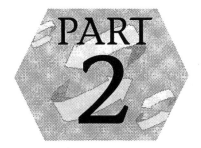

PART
2

Nursing Journal Guidelines for Authors

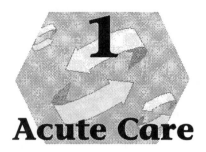

Acute Care

American Journal of Nursing

The *American Journal of Nursing* is published by Lippincott Williams & Wilkins and is the official journal of the American Nurse's Association.

JOURNAL FOCUS/ PURPOSE

The primary purpose of the *American Journal of Nursing* is to provide our readers with the most current and most useful clinical information related to their daily practice. We recognize that nurses are busy people, with little time to read. Our goal is to tell them what they need to know to become more skilled clinicians, and to do this in an accessible, easy-to-read format, enhanced by strong clinical artwork. We're also dedicated to providing our readers with the latest news about their profession, to exploring legal, ethical, and professional growth issues, and enhancing *AJN*'s reputation for nursing advocacy. By presenting a "total package," covering both clinical and professional topics, we plan to become a more viable, competitive publication. Our ultimate goal is to become the world's largest and most prestigious nursing journal.

JOURNAL FACTS

Publication schedule: monthly

Circulation: 350,000

Submitted papers per year: approximately 400

Acceptance rate: less than 50%

Monetary honorarium: honorarium paid, no rate given

Average turnaround time: 3 months

Publishing timetable: within 12 months after acceptance

Correspondence:
Lippincott Williams & Wilkins
Business Offices
227 East Washington Square
Philadelphia, PA 19106-3780
Telephone: (215) 238-4200

Or
12107 Insurance Way
Hagerstown, MD 21740
Telephone: (301) 714-2300
Fax: (301) 714-2398
Customer service: 1-800-638-3030

Internet site: www.nursingcenter.com/journals

MANUSCRIPT SUBMISSION

Manuscripts should be submitted on standard-size typing paper. Include the following on separate pages: (1) a title page with your name, your position, and the institution where you work, your home address, and home and work phone numbers; (2) a list of references used in preparing the manuscript (no more than 10, please, and none more than 5 years old); (3) a signed statement that no other publication is considering your manuscript and that it won't be submitted elsewhere until you hear from the *American Journal of Nursing.*

Put the page number and manuscript title on each page, but don't include your name. Send three copies—typed and double-spaced, using only one side of the paper—and keep a fourth for yourself. If you used a computer, please send a diskette also (IBM-PC or Mac-Write compatible); it will help in the editing process if we accept your manuscript. Manuscripts will be returned if you send a stamped, self-addressed envelope.

Send copies to:

Diana Mason, RN, PhD, FAAN
Editor in Chief, *American Journal of Nursing*
345 Hudson Street
New York, NY 10014
Telephone: 1-800-933-6525, ext. 359
E-mail: diana.mason@ajn.org

MANUSCRIPT PREPARATION GUIDELINES

Manuscripts should be typed double-spaced and accompanied by a 35-word summary.

REFEREED PUBLICATION

The *American Journal of Nursing* is a peer-reviewed journal. You will be notified that your manuscript has been received by the *American Journal of Nursing,* and if it is appropriate for the journal, it will be entered into the peer-review process. You will be informed of the editors' decision within 4 to 8 weeks, depending on the length and complexity of the manuscript.

COPYRIGHT

The content of the *American Journal of Nursing* is copyrighted by Lippincott Williams & Wilkins.

INDEXED

The *American Journal of Nursing* is indexed in *Chemical Abstracts, Cumulative Index to Nursing and Allied Health Literature, Current Contents, Hospital Literature Index, Index Medicus, International Nursing Index, International Pharmaceutical Abstracts, Nursing Abstracts, Nutritional Abstracts and Reviews, Public Affairs Information Service, Psychological Abstracts,* and *Social Sciences Index.*

SAMPLE JOURNAL ARTICLE TITLES

- "Back to Basics: Providing Effective Patient Teaching"
- "Cancer-Related Hypercalcemia: How to Spot It, How to Manage It"
- "Emergency! Crush Injury"
- "Medication Compliance in Adults With Asthma"
- "More Than a Friend: The Special Bond Between Nurses"

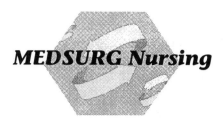

MEDSURG Nursing

M EDSURG *Nursing* is published by Jannetti Publications, Inc., and is the official journal of the Academy of Medical-Surgical Nurses (AMSN).

JOURNAL FOCUS/PURPOSE

The primary purpose of *MEDSURG Nursing* is to provide its readers with the multidisciplinary information they need to provide clinically excellent patient care and to enhance their nursing practice. *MEDSURG Nursing* supports adult health/medical-surgical nurses and advanced practice nurses as they strive for excellence in patient care, private practice, and outpatient health care settings.

JOURNAL FACTS

Publication schedule: bimonthly

Circulation: 5,000

Submitted papers per year: 50

Acceptance rate: approximately 50%

Monetary honorarium: none

Average turnaround time: 2-3 months

Publishing timetable: 6-12 months after acceptance

Correspondence:
Jannetti Publications, Inc.
East Holly Avenue
Box 56
Pitman, NJ 08071-0056
Telephone: (856) 256-2300

Internet site: www.ajj.com/jpi or
www.inurse.com/spi

MANUSCRIPT SUBMISSION

The journal accepts original articles, case studies, letters, descriptions of clinical care, and research. Query letters are welcomed, but not required. Material must be original and never published before. Material is submitted for review with the understanding that it is not being nor will it have been submitted to any other journal prior to final consideration by the journal.

Five copies of the manuscript should be submitted to the editorial office; the author retains one copy. Manuscripts not accepted for publication will not be returned to the author unless requested within 30 days of notification of rejection.

Send all articles to:
Editor
MEDSURG Nursing
East Holly Avenue
Box 56
Pitman, NJ 08071
Telephone: (856) 256-2300

Upon acceptance of the manuscript, the author will yield copyright to *MEDSURG Nursing*. Acquiring permission to reprint previously published materials is the responsibility of the author. Manuscripts accepted are subject to copyediting. The author will receive proofs for review prior to publication.

MANUSCRIPT PREPARATION GUIDELINES

Manuscripts must be typed, double-spaced on 8.5 × 11-inch white paper. Style should generally follow the *Publication Manual of the American Psychological Association* (APA). Please use the author-date method of citation within the text—(Doe, 1995) or "Doe (1995) states . . . ." With multiple authors, the first citation must list all authors; in subsequent citations, list only the last name of the first author and "et al."

Include the manuscript title, authors' names, credentials, and a biographic statement. Also include a brief abstract of 40 words or less along with an address for correspondence and day and evening phone numbers.

Double-space all typing, using 1.5- to 2-inch margins. Include the title, or short descriptor, on top of each page, but do not include the author's name. Include subheadings in the manuscript where possible. Type all subheadings flush to the left margin.

List all references in alphabetical order. Sample references are shown below:

Books:

Doe, J. R. (1993). *Skin and aging processes.* Boca Raton, FL: CRC Press.

Chapter in a Book:

Doe, J. R., & Smith, B. (1993). Aging of the human skin. In R. Jones (Ed.), *Handbook on aging* (pp. 123-234). New York: Nostrand-Rheinhold Company.

Periodical:

Jones, J. F. (1993). Skin cancer. *American Journal of Nursing, 84*(1), 1234-1456.

Figures include line drawings, photographs, diagrams, and graphs. Each figure must be numbered, and the number must correspond to a statement in the text directing the reader to see that figure. Include a separate legend sheet with double-spaced captions. The author must obtain permission for figures borrowed from another source. Photographs may be black and white, glossy, 5 × 7-inch, or color 5 × 7-inch or 35 mm slides.

The journal will accept both IBM and Macintosh format diskettes sent with manuscripts. All diskettes should be clearly labeled with the author name, manuscript title, disk type (IBM or Macintosh), file name, and word processor name and version (or file type, if ASCII). IBM diskette densities should be 1.2 MB or lower for 5.25″ and 1.44 MB or lower for 3.5″; Macintosh diskette density should be 1.44 MB or lower.

Most, but not all, IBM and Macintosh word processor files are acceptable for submission to the journal. When possible, all files should be saved as WordPerfect. Many spreadsheet files may also be acceptable but must be approved prior to sending. To ensure acceptability of your disk, please contact the journal office before sending any material.

Please use only common fonts (CG Times, Universe, Helvetica, Courier, etc.) and avoid complex font attributes such as outline. All graphics (tables, graphs, etc.) must be submitted in camera-ready form.

REFEREED PUBLICATION

MEDSURG Nursing is a refereed journal. All manuscripts submitted undergo review by the editor and blind reviews by the manuscript review panel and/or editorial board. Each article is evaluated on its timeliness, importance, accuracy, clarity, and applicability. Upon submission of the manuscript, the author will yield copyright to the journal, contingent on publication of the manuscript. Acquiring permission to reprint previously published material is the responsibility of the author. Manuscripts accepted are subject to copyediting. The author will receive proofs that reflect all editing prior to publication.

COPYRIGHT

Copyright by Jannetti Publications, Inc.

INDEXED

MEDSURG Nursing is indexed in *Access to Uncover, Cumulative Index to Nursing and Allied Health Literature, Nursing Abstracts, RNdex Top 100,* and *UMI* (University Microfilms International).

SAMPLE JOURNAL ARTICLE TITLES

- "Breaking the Boundaries: Collaborating to Develop a Model Ventilator Training Program"
- "Implementing a Residency Program for the Acute Care Nurse Practitioner"
- "Midlife Women and Urinary Incontinence: Causes, Lifestyles, and Treatment"
- "The Integration of a Tuberculosis Control Plan Into a Standard of Care for Tuberculosis"
- "Update on Acute Pancreatitis"

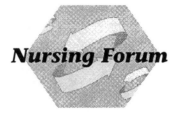

Nursing Forum

Nursing Forum is published by Nursecom, Inc.

JOURNAL FOCUS/PURPOSE

The primary purpose of *Nursing Forum* is to explore, explicate, or report issues, ideas, trends, and innovations that shape the nursing profession.

JOURNAL FACTS

Publication schedule: quarterly
Circulation: 2,300
Submitted papers per year: 50-60
Acceptance rate: 30%
Monetary honorarium: none
Average turnaround time: 6 months

Publishing timetable: 6-9 months after acceptance
Correspondence:
Nursing Forum
Nursecom, Inc.
1211 Locust Street
Philadelphia, PA 19107
Telephone: (215) 545-7222 or 1-800-242-6757
Fax: (215) 545-8107
E-mail: juall46@bellatlantic.net
Internet site: www.nursecominc.com/html/nf.html

MANUSCRIPT SUBMISSION

Send four hard copies to:
Lynda Juall Carpenito, RN, MSN
Editor, *Nursing Forum*
Nursecom, Inc.
1211 Locust Street
Philadelphia, PA 19107
Telephone: (215) 545-7222 or 1-800-242-6757

Fax: (215) 545-8107
E-mail: 74472.57@compuserve.com

Manuscripts must be accompanied by the following statement signed by the author(s):

As the author(s) of (title of article), I/we hereby transfer copyright ownership to Nursecom, Inc. if the work is published. I/we warrant that the article is original, has not been submitted to another journal, and has not been previously published. I/we warrant that I/we have participated in the development, actual writing and revising of the manuscript, and thus qualify as author(s) of this manuscript.

In addition, the author(s) is (are) responsible for the content of the original and edited manuscript, once it is approved, and for the accuracy of references, quoted material, and for any violation of copyright.

MANUSCRIPT PREPARATION GUIDELINES

All manuscripts must adhere to the following: (1) typed double-spaced, with 1-inch margins and numbered pages; (2) author's page with title of article, author(s) full name(s), academic degrees, affiliation, title(s), corresponding author's name, home address, telephone numbers (home, business, fax); (3) list references on a separate page, in American Psychological Association style; all references must be cited at least once in the text; (4) type each figure, chart, or table on a separate page (reference each in text); (5) include permissions for all artwork or use of copyrighted material; and (6) include an abstract of 75-100 words.

Photographs, line drawings, graphs, tables, and charts are encouraged if they enhance or amplify the text and are of publishable quality. Photographs of people must be accompanied by a signed statement by the individual(s) photographed or the person with the legal right to sign such a statement.

Author signatures attest they have participated in the development of the manuscript in all of the following ways: (1) conception and design or analysis and interpretation of data; (2) drafting the article or revising it critically for important intellectual content; (3) final approval of the version to be published (International Committee of Medical Journal Editors).

Authors can acknowledge colleagues, supervisors, or faculty who do not qualify for coauthorship but who have participated or supervised the project or reviewed the manuscript in an "acknowledgment."

REFEREED PUBLICATION

Nursing Forum is a refereed journal. All submissions will be acknowledged within 3 weeks of receipt. Promising manuscripts will be reviewed by at least two members of the editorial or review board. This process is anonymous, so author names should not appear on any page but the author's page (prior to title page).

Accepted manuscripts are subject to editorial revisions (punctuation, grammar, clarity). Content revisions will be done by the author. Authors will be asked to submit revisions on a disk in Word or WordPerfect.

COPYRIGHT

Copyright is by Nursecom, Inc.

INDEXED

Nursing Forum is indexed in the *Cumulative Index to Nursing and Allied Health Literature, Index Medicus, International Nursing Index, Hospital Literature Index,* and *RNdex Top 100.*

SAMPLE JOURNAL ARTICLE TITLES

- "Compliance: A Concept Analysis"
- "Reminiscence as an Intervention: Rediscovering the Essence of Nursing"
- "Spirituality and People With Potentially Fatal Diagnoses"
- "Stress Management for Nurses: Controlling the Whirlwind"

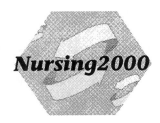

N*ursing2000* is published by Springhouse Corporation.

JOURNAL FOCUS/PURPOSE

The primary purpose of *Nursing2000* is to provide the latest information and skills for direct caregivers. *Nursing2000* focuses on the clinical, patient care side of nursing. We stress the teaching of hands-on skills and procedures, and we address legal, ethical, and professional and career issues as well.

JOURNAL FACTS

Publication schedule: monthly
Circulation: 317,890
Submitted papers per year: not available
Acceptance rate: not available
Monetary honorarium: $50-75 per page
Average turnaround time: 1-2 months
Publishing timetable: 1-3 years after acceptance
Correspondence:

Nursing2000
Editorial Department
1111 Bethlehem Pike
P.O. Box 908
Springhouse, PA 19477-0908
Telephone: (215) 646-8700
Fax: (215) 653-0826
E-mail: nursing@springnet.com
Internet site: www.springnet.com/pn/nurse99.htm

MANUSCRIPT SUBMISSION

Send all articles and topic query letters to:
Nursing2000, Editorial Department
1111 Bethlehem Pike
P.O. Box 908
Springhouse, PA 19477-0908
Fax: (215) 653-0826

Manuscripts must be accompanied by a self-addressed, stamped envelope for their return. If you don't need the manuscript back, just send a stamped, regular-size envelope for our reply. Accepting and rejecting manuscripts is a matter of editorial judgment. We try to respond to all authors in 6 to 8 weeks, depending on the length and complexity of the manuscript.

MANUSCRIPT PREPARATION GUIDELINES

If possible, send your article on computer disk (in WordPerfect or ASCII file), along with three printouts; note on the disk your file name, what program and version used, and whether you worked on a PC or a Macintosh. (If this isn't possible, submit your manuscript typed and double-spaced on standard-size typewriter paper.) Leave generous margins so editors can make notes.

Start with a cover page including your name, address, and home and work phone numbers, plus a fax number if possible. Be sure each page of your manuscript is numbered and includes the title of your article. Don't put your name on each page, as we'd have to delete it before sending your article for a blind peer review. If there are multiple authors, please designate one author to handle all contact with us.

On separate pages, please include a single copy of each of the following: a list of references you used in preparing the article (none more than 5 years old, please), a brief description of your professional education and your present employer and position (for each author)—or attach a résumé—a signed statement that no other publisher is considering your article and that you won't send it to another publisher until you hear from *Nursing2000*. (Don't submit an article to more than one publisher at a time.)

Include charts, illustrations, and photographs, if appropriate. Label and caption them clearly, and note the source if it's not your original creation. We will have illustrations redrawn by professional artists, but we welcome rough drawings that you feel would be helpful.

We require signed releases from all persons photographed. (We can supply forms if needed.)

Don't be concerned about the manuscript length—just write until you've covered your topic thoroughly, probably 12 to 15 typed pages for a long feature article. If you find your article running much longer than that, you may be covering too much.

All articles are edited to conform with our editorial style; in most cases, this entails heavy editing, rewriting, condensing, and reorganizing. However, every effort is made to retain content, and you'll get a copy of the edited version of your article for approval before publication. Contact between authors and editors is encouraged, and we work hard to make sure everyone is satisfied with the final copy.

REFEREED PUBLICATION

Manuscripts are submitted to the Editorial Review Board for evaluation and to two or more nursing authorities for a blind peer review.

COPYRIGHT

If an article is accepted, you will be sent an author's agreement, transferring all rights to your article to Springhouse Corporation, the publisher of *Nursing2000*.

INDEXED

Nursing2000 is indexed in the *Cumulative Index to Nursing and Allied Health Literature, Hospital Literature Index,* and *International Nursing Index.*

SAMPLE JOURNAL ARTICLE TITLES

- "Action Stat: Acute Pulmonary Edema"
- "Diabetes: Taking a New Look at an Old Adversary"
- "Nurse's Guide to Common Postoperative Complications"
- "Tips and Time-Savers for Pediatric Patient Care"
- "Ventricular Tachycardia"

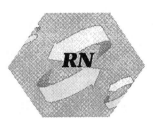

R*N* is published by Medical Economics.

Montvale, NJ 07645
Telephone: (201) 358-7300
Internet site: www.rnweb.com

JOURNAL FOCUS/PURPOSE

The primary purpose of the *RN* is to keep nurses up to date on practical, clinical, and professional developments, with heavy emphasis on information that can be applied immediately in everyday nursing practice. Subjects include nursing care and assessment in medical/surgical, critical care, and all specialty nursing areas, patient education, drugs, management topics, bedside research, and any innovations in policies or procedures that promote improved patient care.

JOURNAL FACTS

Publication schedule: monthly
Circulation: 250,000
Submitted papers per year: more than 200
Acceptance rate: greater than 45%
Monetary honorarium: $50 to $250 for the typical article
Average turnaround time: 12 weeks
Publishing timetable: 4-6 months
Correspondence:
  Clinical Editor, *RN*
  Five Paragon Drive

MANUSCRIPT SUBMISSION

Send queries and manuscripts to:
  Marianne Dekker Mattera, Editor
  RN
  Five Paragon Drive
  Montvale, NJ 07645
  E-mail: theresa-metules@medec.com

MANUSCRIPT PREPARATION GUIDELINES

All articles should be thoroughly researched. If you quote from other publications, enclose the quoted material in quotation marks and reference it. Also cite references for statistics, research findings, and information paraphrased from other publications. Citations and a complete reference list should follow American Psychological Association style.

The writing style used in *RN* is simple and direct—colloquial rather than formal, one professional talking to another. Give examples from your clinical experience to illustrate specific points. Discuss clinical techniques thoroughly, precisely, and in maximum detail.

Manuscripts should be typewritten, double-spaced, on one side of $8\frac{1}{2} \times 11$-inch paper; handwritten submissions will not be considered. Aim for 10 to 15 typewritten pages. On the first page, type your name, address, home and business telephone numbers, place of employment, current license number, state of licensure, and social security number. Number all pages. Enclose a copy of your résumé or curriculum vitae. Send us the original of your manuscript and two copies. Photos, sketches, and diagrams are a most important adjunct to text, and we give manuscripts illustrated in this manner special attention. Enclose a stamped, self-addressed envelope if you want material we do not accept returned. Usual time to evaluate a submission is 8 to 10 weeks.

Authors who use an IBM or IBM-compatible microcomputer are encouraged to send a disk as well as hard copies. The piece should be in an ASCII format or Microsoft Word format.

All manuscripts that we accept are subject to editing. Such editing may involve nothing more than putting the material into conversational language, but it can entail heavy condensing and extensive restructuring. In every instance, we take pains to preserve the author's ideas. You'll see a prepublication draft of your article before it gets into print.

REFEREED PUBLICATION

RN is a refereed journal. Feature manuscripts receive two rounds of blind peer review—one before the piece is accepted, the other before publication.

COPYRIGHT

Copyright by Medical Economics at Montvale, NJ 07645. *RN* usually buys all rights but is willing to discuss other copyright arrangements.

INDEXED

RN is indexed in the *Cumulative Index to Nursing and Allied Health Literature, Hospital Literature Index, International Nursing Index,* and *Silver Platter's RNdex Top 100.*

SAMPLE JOURNAL ARTICLE TITLES

- "A Family Guide to Nursing Homes"
- "Getting UTI Patients Back on Track"
- "Helping Families Select a Nursing Home"
- "The Infection That Eats Patients Alive"
- "When MRSA Reaches Into Long-Term Care"

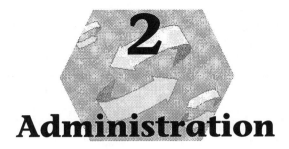

Administration

Journal of Nursing Administration

The *Journal of Nursing Administration* is published by Lippincott Williams & Wilkins.

JOURNAL FOCUS/PURPOSE

The primary purpose of the *Journal of Nursing Administration* is designed for nurse leaders in hospitals, home health care agencies, and other health care organizations. The *Journal of Nursing Administration* provides information on management and leadership development; human, material, and financial resource management; staffing and scheduling systems; staff development; research and innovations; labor-management relations; policy; legislation, regulations, and economics related to health care and program development; legal, ethical, and political issues; interdisciplinary collaboration; organization-wide projects; and professional trends.

JOURNAL FACTS

Publication schedule: 11 times per year
Circulation: 10,000
Submitted papers per year: 200
Acceptance rate: 35%

Monetary honorarium: no response
Average turnaround time: 6 weeks
Publishing timetable: 7 months after acceptance
Correspondence:
  Lippincott Williams & Wilkins
  Business Offices
  227 East Washington Square
  Philadelphia, PA 19106-3780
  Telephone: (215) 238-4200
Or
  12107 Insurance Way
  Hagerstown, MD 21740
  Telephone: (301) 714-2300
  Fax: (301) 714-2398
  Customer service: 1-800-638-3030
Internet site: www.nursingcenter.com/journals

MANUSCRIPT SUBMISSION

Send submissions to:
  Suzanne P. Smith, EdD, RN, FAAN
  Editor-in-Chief, *Journal of Nursing Administration*
  4301 32nd Street West, Suite C-12
  Bradenton, FL 34205-2748
  E-mail: drsuzsmith@aol.com

Submit three copies of the manuscript, along with a stamped, self-addressed, business-sized envelope if you want receipt of your manuscript acknowledged. If you want your original manuscript returned after the review process, enclose a self-addressed, manuscript-sized envelope with sufficient postage affixed.

All persons designated as authors should qualify for authorship. Each author should have participated significantly to the conception and design of the work and writing the manuscript to take public responsibility for it. The editor may request justification of assignment of authorship. Names of those who contributed general support or technical help may be listed in an acknowledgment.

MANUSCRIPT PREPARATION GUIDELINES

Unless otherwise stated here, prepare manuscripts according to the *American Medical Association Manual of Style* (8th ed.). While not necessary, query letters allow the editor to indicate interest in, and developmental advice on, manuscript topics.

The maximum manuscript length is 18 double-spaced pages including figures, tables, and references. As a general rule, an 18-page paper should have no more than four figures or tables. Tables and figures should be placed in the back of the manuscript after references. Tables must be numbered consecutively with arabic numbers, be double-spaced, and have a title at the top. Figures and tables must be cited in numerical order in the text.

Number pages consecutively in the upper right corner, starting with the title/author biography page. Do not justify the right margin. Do not use running headers or footers.

Subdivide the manuscript into main sections by inserting subheads in the text. Sub-

heads should be succinct, meaningful, and similar in sense and tone.

References are placed at the end of the manuscript and typed double-spaced. References are cited consecutively by number and listed in citation order in the reference list. Examples are listed below:

Journal:

> Johnson JH, Olesinski N. Program evaluation: key to success. *J Nurs Adm.* 1995;25(1):53-60.

Book:

> Flarey DL. *Redesigning Nursing Care Delivery: Transforming Our Future.* Philadelphia: JB Lippincott Co; 1994:25-35.

Each of the following should be placed on a separate page: (1) A 50- to 75-word abstract that stimulates the readers' interest in the topic and states what the readers will learn or how they will be better off after reading the article; (2) a title/author biography page. The author's biographic information includes name, credentials, position, place of employment, city, state, and e-mail address (optional). Examples: Alice M. Jones, PhD, RN, Vice President of Patient Care Services, Brown Community Hospital, New York, New York; (3) reference list; (4) acknowledgments; (5) illustrations.

Written permission must be obtained from (1) the holder of copyrighted material used in the manuscript; (2) persons mentioned in the narrative or acknowledgment; and (3) the administrators of institutions mentioned in the narrative or acknowledgment. Where permission has been granted, the author should follow any special wording stipulated by the grantor. Letters of permission must be submitted before publication of the manuscript.

REFEREED PUBLICATION

The *Journal of Nursing Administration* is a refereed journal. Published manuscripts have been reviewed, selected, and developed with the guidance of our editorial advisers. Manuscript content is assessed for relevance, accuracy, and usefulness to nurse executives and their immediate associates.

Manuscripts are reviewed with the understanding that neither the manuscript nor its essential content has been published or is under consideration by others.

The review process starts on the first day of every month. For example, February 1 is the start of the review process for all manuscripts received during January. Publication decisions and author notification occur within 8 weeks from the beginning of the review process.

COPYRIGHT

Copyright by Lippincott Williams & Wilkins.

INDEXED

The *Journal of Nursing Administration* is indexed in the *International Nursing Index, Cumulative Index to Nursing and Allied Health Literature, Nursing Abstracts, Hospital Literature Index, RNdex Top 100, Index Medicus, Current Contents/Social and Behavioral Sciences,* and the *Social Citation Index.*

SAMPLE JOURNAL ARTICLE TITLES

- "Decision-Making Activity and Influence of Nurse Executives in Top Management Teams"
- "Role Transition for Patient Care Vice Presidents: From a Single Entity to a System Focus"
- "The Professional Transitions Workshop Cornerstone of Practice"
- "Will Nursing Administration Programs Survive in the 21st Century?"
- "Work Complexity Assessment: Decision Support Data to Address Cost and Culture Issues"

Journal of Nursing Care Quality

The *Journal of Nursing Care Quality* is published by Aspen Publishers, Inc.

JOURNAL FOCUS/PURPOSE

The primary purpose of the *Journal of Nursing Care Quality* is to provide practicing nurses as well as nurses who have leadership roles in nursing care quality programs (nursing quality coordinators, coordinators in decentralized programs, chairs of quality groups, and nurse administrators) with useful information regarding the application of quality principles and concepts in the practice setting. In addition, *Journal of Nursing Care Quality*

- Provides a forum to allow scholarly discussion of "real world" implementation of quality-related activities.

- Provides articles based on observations or experimentation that add new knowledge to the field of nursing quality assurance.
- Provides analytical reviews that codify existing knowledge or throw light on the present or future roles of practitioners in the field.
- Includes evaluation studies with innovative and effective approaches to quality-related activities in the clinical setting with descriptions of the process or study used, the clinical effects of the process, and the application of the study findings to practice or resolution of the clinical issue.
- Provides studies with patient-centered as well as staff-centered outcomes that are of interest.

JOURNAL FACTS

Publication schedule: four times per year

Circulation: approximately 4,000

Submitted papers per year: approximately 75

Acceptance rate: 75%

Monetary honorarium: None

Average turnaround time: 6 weeks

Publishing timetable: approximately 6 months after acceptance

Correspondence:
Customer Services
200 Orchard Ridge Drive
Gaithersburg, MD 20878
Customer service telephone: 1-800-234-1660

Internet site: www.aspenpub.com (enter journal title in search box)

MANUSCRIPT SUBMISSION

Topics are listed on the back cover of the journal. Authors are encouraged to submit original articles that are prepared in accordance with the journal's objectives and guidelines. Articles for submission must consist of an original and two hard copies with a computer disk, preferably in Microsoft Word 6.0 or 7.0.

Evaluation studies should include a brief review of the relevant literature, the data collection tool or a sample of the tool, the tool's validity and reliability, and a brief discussion of the methodology demonstrating the soundness of the process used. Keep in mind that *JNCQ* is not a research journal. In addition, ensure absolute anonymity of the subjects (patients, nurses, or others) within the manuscript.

Manuscripts should be addressed to:

Patricia Schroeder, MSN, RN
Editor, *Journal of Nursing Care Quality*
524 BelAire Drive
Thiensville, WI 53092
Telephone: (414) 242-9262
Fax: (414) 242-0121
E-mail: pschroed@execpc.com

MANUSCRIPT PREPARATION GUIDELINES

Manuscripts should be created using Aspen's Journals Authoring Template (template is available from your journal editor or from Aspen). Manuscripts should be created on IBM-compatible (PC) equipment using Windows 95 or higher operating system. Our preferred software is Microsoft Word. Hard copy and electronic files should be submitted for all text and all artwork. All disks submitted must be new. Disks should be clearly labeled as to operating system and software application.

Manuscripts should be double-spaced (including quotations, lists, references, footnotes, figure captions, and all parts of tables).

Manuscripts should be ordered as follows: title page, abstracts, text, references, appendixes, tables, and any illustrations.

Each manuscript must include the following:

Title page, including (1) title of the article, (2) author names (with highest academic degrees) and affiliations (including titles, departments, and name and location of institutions of primary employment), and (3) any acknowledgments, credits, or disclaimers

Abstract of no more than 100 words and up to 10 key words that describe the contents of the article like those that appear in the *Cumulative Index to Nursing and Allied Health Literature (CINAHL)* or the *National Library of Medicine's Medical Subject Headings (MeSH)*

Clear indication of the placement of all tables and figures in text

Signed copyright transfer form

Completed article submission form for each contributor

Written permission for any borrowed text, tables, or figures

References must be cited in text and styled in the reference list according to the *Chicago Manual of Style,* 14th ed. (1993), with the following exceptions: They must be numbered consecutively in the order they are cited; reference numbers may be used more than once throughout an article. Page numbers should appear with the text citation following a specific quote.

References should not be created using Microsoft Word's automatic footnote/endnote feature. References should be included on a separate page at the end of the article and should be double-spaced. Note: Two authors—L. J. Tapia and E. P. Prien. Three or more authors—L. J. Tapia et al.

Here are some examples of correctly styled reference list entries:

Journals:

Author, article title, journal title, volume number, issue number or month or season of publication, year of publication, inclusive page numbers.

L. J. Tapia, S. D. Seleh, and E. P. Prien, "Interrelated Programs." *Personnel Administration* 27, no.1 (1996):25-28.

Books:

Author, book title, place of publication, publisher, year.

J. Watson, *Nursing: Human Science and Human Care* (New York: National League for Nursing, 1988).

Forthcoming works:

D. Roberts, *Health Book* (New York: Health Books, forthcoming).

Government publications:

U.S. Department of Health and Human Services, Public Health Service. *Forward Plan for Health, FY 1978-82.* DHEW Pub. No. (OS) 76-50046. Washington, D.C.: Government Printing Office, 1976.

Association as author:

American Hospital Association, *Guidelines: Contractual Relationship between Hospitals and Physicians* (Chicago: AHA, 1976).

Editor as author of book:

D. Roberts, ed., *Health Book* (Denver: Health Press, 1976), 323.

Newspapers:

A. Anders and R. Winslow, "The HMO Trend: Big, Bigger, Biggest," *The Wall Street Journal,* 30 March 1995, sec. 1A, p. 3.

Other sources:

Enough information so that material can be identified and retrieved.

Illustrations: Figures should be created using electronic software (i.e., Adobe Illustrator, Corel Draw, and Photoshop). Please save files in both the application in which they were created (i.e., Microsoft Word) and as either EPS or TIFF files. Use computer-generated lettering. Do not use screens, color, shading, or fine lines.

In lieu of original drawings and other material, a sharp, glossy, black-and-white photographic print between 5″ × 7″ and 8″ × 10″ is acceptable.

Each figure should have a label on the back indicating the number of the figure, the names of the authors, and the top of the figure. Do not write on the back of figures, mount them on cardboard, or scratch or mar them using paper clips. Do not bend figures.

Cite each figure in the text in consecutive order. If a figure has been previously published, in part or in total, acknowledge the original source and submit written permission from the copyright holder to reproduce or adapt the material.

Supply a caption for each figure, typed double-spaced on a separate sheet from the artwork. Captions should include the figure title, explanatory statements, notes, or keys as well as source and permission lines.

Provide a camera-ready copy and a separate electronic file for each piece of artwork. Do not embed art in your text file.

Tables should be on a separate page at the end of the manuscript. Number tables consecutively and supply a brief title for each. Include explanatory footnotes for all nonstandard abbreviations. Cite each table in the text in consecutive order. If you use data from another published or unpublished source, obtain permission and acknowledge fully.

Permissions: Authors are responsible for obtaining signed letters from copyright holders granting permission to reprint material being borrowed or adapted from other sources, including previously published material of your own. Authors must obtain written permission for the following material (authors are responsible for any permission fees to reprint borrowed material):

All direct quotes of 300 words or more from any full-length book

All direct quotes of 200 words or more from a periodical article

All excerpts from a newspaper article or other short piece

Any passage from a play or a song

Two or more lines of poetry

Any borrowed table, figure, or illustration being reproduced exactly or adapted to fit the needs of the subject

REFEREED PUBLICATION

Representatives of the Editorial Board conduct a blind review of manuscripts submitted for publication in the *Journal of Nursing Care Quality;* that is, all identifying names and affiliations are removed from the manuscript. The editor and board members assess manuscripts based on the following criteria: (a) The topic is consistent with the purpose of the *Journal of Nursing Care Quality;* (b) the subject of the manuscript is developed sufficiently; (c) ideas are communicated clearly, simply, and powerfully; and (d) the content is accurate and up to date.

COPYRIGHT

Copyright by Aspen Publishers, Inc.

INDEXED

The *Journal of Nursing Care Quality* is indexed in the *International Nursing Index, Cumulative Index to Nursing and Allied Health Literature, Nursing Abstracts, Hospital and Health Administration Index, Health Planning and Administration Database, RNdex Top 100,* and *Index Medicus, MEDLINE/MEDLARS.*

SAMPLE JOURNAL ARTICLE TITLES

- "A Framework for Integrated Quality Improvement"
- "Medication Self-Administration: An Outcome-Oriented, Consumer Driven Program"
- "Nurse Call Systems: Impact on Nursing Performance"
- "Outcomes Management Internet Resources"
- "Reducing High-Risk Interventions for Managing Aggression in Psychiatric Settings"

Nursing Administration Quarterly

Nursing *Administration Quarterly* is published by Aspen Publishers, Inc.

JOURNAL FOCUS/PURPOSE

The primary purpose of *Nursing Administration Quarterly* is to provide nursing administrators with practical, up-to-date information on the effective management of nursing services in all health care settings. Nursing Administration Quarterly focuses on presenting timely research, issues, and debate geared toward enhancing administrators' conceptual understanding of the administrative process and administrators' knowledge base and skills.

JOURNAL FACTS

Publication schedule: quarterly
Circulation: 7,000-10,000
Submitted papers per year: 100 plus
Acceptance rate: 75-80%
Monetary honorarium: none
Average turnaround time: 3 months
Publishing timetable: 6 months after acceptance
Correspondence:

Customer Services
200 Orchard Ridge Drive
Gaithersburg, MD 20878
Customer service telephone: 1-800-234-1660

Internet Site: www.aspenpub.com (enter journal title in search box)

MANUSCRIPT SUBMISSION

Three copies (one original, two copies, and identical version on disk) and correspondence regarding publication should be addressed to:

Barbara J. Brown, RN, EdD, FAAN, FNAP
63430 E. Desert Mesa Court
Tucson, Arizona 85739
E-mail: naqbb@aol.com

MANUSCRIPT PREPARATION GUIDELINES

Manuscripts should be created using Aspen's Journals Authoring Template (template is available from your journal editor or from Aspen). Manuscripts should be created on IBM-compatible (PC) equipment using Windows 95 or higher operating system. Our preferred software is Microsoft Word. Hard copy and electronic files should be submitted for all text and all artwork. All disks submitted must be new. Disks should be clearly labeled as to operating system and software application.

Manuscripts should be double-spaced (including quotations, lists, references, footnotes, figure captions, and all parts of tables).

Manuscripts should be ordered as follows: title page, abstracts, text, references, appendixes, tables, and any illustrations.

Each manuscript must include the following:

Title page, including (1) title of the article, (2) author names (with highest academic degrees) and affiliations (including titles, departments, and name and location of institutions of primary employment), and (3) any acknowledgments, credits, or disclaimers

Abstract of no more than 100 words and up to 10 key words that describe the contents of the article like those that appear in the *Cumulative Index to Nursing and Allied Health Literature (CINAHL)* or the *National Library of Medicine's Medical Subject Headings (MeSH)*

Clear indication of the placement of all tables and figures in text

Signed copyright transfer form

Completed article submission form for each contributor

Written permission for any borrowed text, tables, or figures

References must be cited in text and styled in the reference list according to the *Chicago Manual of Style,* 14th ed. (1993), with the following exceptions: They must be numbered consecutively in the order they are cited; reference numbers may be used more than once throughout an article. Page numbers should appear with the text citation following a specific quote.

References should not be created using Microsoft Word's automatic footnote/endnote feature. References should be included on a separate page at the end of the article and should be double-spaced.

Here are some examples of correctly styled reference list entries.

Journals:

Author, article title, journal title, volume number, issue number or month or season of publication, year of publication, inclusive page numbers.

L. J. Tapia, S. D. Seleh, and E. P. Prien, "Interrelated Programs." *Personnel Administration* 27, no.1 (1996):25-28.

Books:

Author, book title, place of publication, publisher, year.

J. Watson, *Nursing: Human Science and Human Care* (New York: National League for Nursing, 1988).

Illustrations: Figures should be created using electronic software (i.e., Adobe Illustrator, Corel Draw, and Photoshop). Please save files in both the application in which they were created (i.e., Microsoft Word) and as either EPS or TIFF files. Use computer-generated lettering. Do not use screens, color, shading, or fine lines.

In lieu of original drawings and other material, a sharp, glossy, black-and-white photographic print between 5″ × 7″ and 8″ × 10″ is acceptable.

Each figure should have a label on the back indicating the number of the figure, the names of the authors, and the top of the figure. Do not write on the back of figures, mount them on cardboard, or scratch or mar them using paper clips. Do not bend figures.

Cite each figure in the text in consecutive order. If a figure has been previously published, in part or in total, acknowledge the original source and submit written permission from the copyright holder to reproduce or adapt the material.

Supply a caption for each figure, typed double-spaced on a separate sheet from the artwork. Captions should include the figure title, explanatory statements, notes, or keys as well as source and permission lines.

Provide a camera-ready copy and a separate electronic file for each piece of artwork. Do not embed art in your text file.

Tables should be on a separate page at the end of the manuscript. Number tables consecutively and supply a brief title for each. Include explanatory footnotes for all nonstandard abbreviations. Cite each table in the text in consecutive order. If you use data from another published or unpublished source, obtain permission and acknowledge fully.

Permissions: authors are responsible for obtaining signed letters from copyright holders granting permission to reprint material being borrowed or adapted from other sources, including previously published material of your own. Authors must obtain written permission for the following material (authors are responsible for any permission fees to reprint borrowed material):

All direct quotes of 300 words or more from any full-length book

All direct quotes of 200 words or more from a periodical article

All excerpts from a newspaper article or other short piece

Any passage from a play or a song

Two or more lines of poetry

Any borrowed table, figure, or illustration being reproduced exactly or adapted to fit the needs of the subject

REFEREED PUBLICATION

Nursing Administration Quarterly is a peer-reviewed journal.

COPYRIGHT

Copyright by Aspen Publishers, Inc.

INDEXED

Nursing Administration Quarterly is indexed in *Matter of Fact, International Nursing Index, Cumulative Index to Nursing and Allied Health Literature, Nursing Abstracts, Nursing Scan in Critical Care,* and *RNdex Top 100.*

SAMPLE JOURNAL ARTICLE TITLES

- "Creative Winds of Change: Nurses Collaborating for Quality Outcomes"
- "Health Insurance Plans From the Consumer's Point of View: The Good One and the Bad One"
- "Managing Chronically Ill Older People in the Midst of the Health Care Revolution"
- "Staff Mix Models: Complementary or Substitution Roles for Nurses"
- "Understanding and Managing Change in Health Care Organizations"

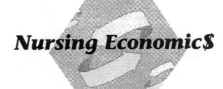

Nursing Economic$

Nursing Economic$ is published by Jannetti Publications, Inc.

JOURNAL FOCUS/PURPOSE

The primary purpose of *Nursing Economic$* is to communicate information to nurses about the business dimensions of nursing and health care.

JOURNAL FACTS

Publication schedule: bimonthly

Circulation: 6,500

Submitted papers per year: 60-80

Acceptance rate: 50%

Monetary honorarium: $20 per published page

Average turnaround time: 6-8 weeks

Publishing timetable: 2-6 months after acceptance

Correspondence:
  Nursing Economic$
  East Holly Avenue
  Box 56
  Pitman, NJ 08071-0056
  Telephone: (856) 256-2300
  Fax: (856) 589-7463

Internet Site: www.ajj.com/jpi or
  www.inurse.com/jpi

MANUSCRIPT SUBMISSION

Send an original and four copies to:
  Connie R. Curran, EdD, RN, FAAN
  Editor, *Nursing Economic$*
  East Holly Avenue, Box 56
  Pitman, NJ 08071-0056

Nursing Economic$ welcomes unsolicited manuscripts in accordance with the journal's purpose, provided they have not been previously published or accepted for publication or are under consideration for publication by another publisher. Authors are encouraged to use clear, concise, nondiscriminatory language.

MANUSCRIPT PREPARATION GUIDELINES

Manuscripts should be typewritten, double-spaced, on one side of 8.5 × 11-inch white paper; maximum length is 15 pages (3,750 words). A cover page should include the manuscript title (seven words or less, please); authors' names, credentials, and primary affiliations; and the address and telephone numbers of the primary author. This page should be followed by a substantive abstract of approximately 30 words. The manuscript title should be repeated on the first page of the text.

References, photographs, tables, and all other details of style must conform to the *Publication Manual of the American Psychological Association*. Photographs should be black-and-white, glossy 5 × 7 or 8 × 10 inches, and of crisp, clear quality. References in the text should be cited by author and date—for example (Doe & Brown, 1983)—with page numbers cited for direct quotations. The reference list at the end of the manuscript should be double-spaced, include only those references cited in the text, and be arranged alphabetically by author. See the following examples:

Journal Article:

Doe, J. R., & Brown, M. S. (1993). Writing for publication. *Nursing Economic$, 1*(2), 115-120.

Book:

Doe, J. R., & Brown, M. S. (1993). *Writing for publication.* New York: Academic Press.

REFEREED PUBLICATION

Receipt of manuscript is acknowledged by the managing editor or editorial coordinator. *Nursing Economic$* is a refereed journal; therefore, each manuscript is reviewed by members of the Manuscript Review Panel as well as the editors. Because manuscript review is blind (authors are anonymous reviewers), names of authors should appear only on the cover page. Decisions regarding acceptance for publication are based on the recommendations of the referees.

COPYRIGHT

Copyright by Jannetti Publications, Inc.

INDEXED

Nursing Economic$ is indexed in the *International Nursing Index, Cumulative Index to Nursing and Allied Health Literature, Nursing Abstracts, Hospital Literature Index, Current Contents/Social and Behavioral Sciences, Research Alert, Social Sciences, Access to Uncover, RNdex Top 100,* and *UMI* (University Microfilms International).

SAMPLE JOURNAL ARTICLE TITLES

- "Corporate Compliance: Critical to Organizational Success"
- "Cost Analysis of a Nursing Center for the Homeless"
- "Federal Funding Shapes Nursing's Future"
- "Nursing Image: Our Public Relations Responsibility"
- "The Changing Multidisciplinary Team"

Nursing Leadership Forum

Nursing *Leadership Forum* is published by Springer Publishing Company.

JOURNAL FOCUS/PURPOSE

The primary purpose of *Nursing Leadership Forum* is to present new and original content that deals with nursing leadership in any of its many guises. This may include new, insightful perspectives on prevailing practices. Reviews of extant practice or illustrations of common nursing applications are not appropriate. Leadership is considered to be exemplified in practice or administrative roles that guide the practice of others or provide leadership for patients or organizations.

JOURNAL FACTS

Publication schedule: quarterly

Circulation: just started up again after a hiatus, so circulation is being rebuilt

Submitted papers per year: 30

Acceptance rate: approximately 60%

Monetary honorarium: none

Average turnaround time: 6 months

Publishing timetable: 4-6 months after acceptance

Correspondence:
Nursing Leadership Forum
Springer Publishing Company
536 Broadway
New York, NY 10012
Telephone: (212) 431-4370
Fax: (212) 941-7842
E-mail: contactus@springerjournals.com or editorial@springerpub.com
Internet site: www.springerpub.com

MANUSCRIPT SUBMISSION

Papers that reflect influence in practice, research, or education are welcome, as are papers that provide leadership through extending and advancing the concepts and paradigms of nursing practice, including underlying ethics, ideologies, and theories.

It is expected that manuscripts sent to *Nursing Leadership Forum* are not under simultaneous review elsewhere. Material must be original and unpublished.

All correspondence concerning manuscripts should be addressed to:

Dr. Harriet R. Feldman
Editor, *Nursing Leadership Forum*
Springer Publishing Company
536 Broadway
New York, NY 10012
Telephone: (914) 773-3341
Fax: (914) 773-3480
E-mail: hfeldman@pace.edu

Nursing Leadership Forum responds to query letters or accepts completed manuscripts.

MANUSCRIPT PREPARATION GUIDELINES

Manuscripts of no more than 20 pages must be typed or word-processed, double-spaced, on $8\frac{1}{2}'' \times 11''$ nonerasable paper, following the style given in the *Publication Manual of the American Psychological Association* (4th ed.). Pages should be numbered with identifying heading given on each. Four copies of the article should be submitted, with the author retaining an additional copy. A paragraph abstract as well as a list of key words should accompany the manuscript.

Authors should be listed in the order of desired publication, along with their titles. Corresponding authors should be indicated. Addresses and phone numbers should be given for each author. Computer disks should not be sent at the time of first submission, nor should original art and/or photographs be sent; however, facsimiles of all artwork/photographs should be enclosed with the manuscript.

An edited copy of an accepted article will be sent to the author for review and correction before publication. The journal will attempt to publish accepted articles within a year of acceptance. Upon publication of an article in *Nursing Leadership Forum,* an author will receive one complimentary copy of the journal issue. Reprints are available for a fee.

REFEREED PUBLICATION

Nursing Leadership Forum is refereed, and manuscripts undergo blind review by members of the review panel. We will communicate panel decisions as rapidly as the review process permits. Upon acceptance of an article, the author will be requested to assign all rights to the journal.

COPYRIGHT

Copyright by *Nursing Leadership Forum.* Alternate arrangements may be negotiated where the author already holds a copyright for the specific material.

INDEXED

Nursing Leadership Forum is indexed in the *Cumulative Index to Nursing and Allied Health Literature, Linguistics and Language Behavior Abstracts, Sociological Abstracts,* and *Social Planning/Policy & Development Abstracts.*

SAMPLE JOURNAL ARTICLE TITLES

- "Acute Care Nurse Practitioners"
- "Consulting and Information Technology"
- "Interview With Dr. Ursula Springer"
- "Mergers: Your Role as a Nurse Executive and Leader of the System"
- "Primer for Philanthropy"

Nursing Management

Nursing Management is published by Springhouse Corporation.

JOURNAL FOCUS/PURPOSE

The primary purpose of *Nursing Management* is to provide nursing administrators with practical, up-to-date information on the effective management of nursing services for modern health care systems.

JOURNAL FACTS

Publication schedule: monthly

Circulation: 98,794

Submitted papers per year: approximately 300

Acceptance rate: 25%

Monetary honorarium: $50/article

Average turnaround time: 6 weeks

Publishing timetable: varies

Correspondence:
   Nursing Management
   Springhouse Corporation
   1111 Bethlehem Pike
   P.O. Box 908
   Springhouse, PA 19477-0908
   Telephone: (215) 646-8700, ext. 1340 or
      1-800-346-7844, ext. 1340
   Fax: (215) 653-0826
   E-mail: nursing.management@springnet.com

Internet Site: www.springnet.com/nm
   nurseman.htm

MANUSCRIPT SUBMISSION

Nursing Management considers original essays that explore, from a managerial perspective, behavioral patterns, operations, relationships, arts, sciences, technologies, fiscal (economic) matters, and political issues that concern nursing and the environments in which nurses practice. *Nursing Management* reviews only texts no longer than 15 double-spaced pages with 1-inch margins, which may be followed by pertinent references, bibliography, and exhibits. Please include a 50-word abstract. Articles must not have been previously published elsewhere nor be currently under consideration for other journals or books. Send the original and one copy of all materials.

Submit 3 copies of the articles along with a disk (indicate program/version and whether you used a Mac or an IBM-compatible computer. Briefly indicate the scope of the topic and include authors' names, current credentials, occupations, institutional affiliations, and mailing addresses. If feasible, include phone/ fax numbers for contacting authors during business hours. Clearly designate one author to whom correspondence will be addressed. If you want the manuscript returned, include an adequately stamped, self-addressed envelope.

Direct all contributions, correspondence, and questions to:

Theresa M. Steltzer, Managing Editor
Nursing Management
111 Bethlehem Pike, P.O. Box 908
Springhouse, PA 19477-0908

Nursing Management welcomes unsolicited manuscripts with disks prepared in accordance with this purpose.

MANUSCRIPT PREPARATION GUIDELINES

The Notes From the Field format has been designed as a forum for sharing the results of local/small-scale empirical studies and surveys, observations, or experiences that confirm, modify, or question prevailing policies or procedures, as well as succinct descriptions of personnel or operational techniques that have been devised and applied in particular kinds of working environments. Notes should be 500 words or less. Submit original and one copy of double-spaced pages with 1-inch margins. No references, bibliography, or exhibits are accepted for Notes. Be sure to include authors' credentials and affiliations and the mailing addresses at which interested readers may gain further information.

Career Scope is essentially the same format, and criteria from Notes are used in Career Scope. This feature focuses on a specific geographic location of the United States—for example, South Atlantic, South Central, Pacific/ Mountain, Northeast, and North Central. It appears five times yearly.

Letters to the editor of personal opinions, comments, or questions on articles or the nursing scene that are intended for publication should not exceed 250 words, must be signed, and must include the author's address. Letters are subject to technical editing.

Exhibits are any tables, charts, diagrams, sketches, maps, examples of forms, and so on that accompany article text. Use and placement of exhibits is at the discretion of editors. Exhibits must be cleared for publication through appropriate authorities, legible, and/or reasonably reproducible, and referred to specifically in text, numbered in sequence.

Observe the following styles for references. Please review references for complete citations before submissions. Be sure to spell out journal names, even the most familiar in the field. Number references consecutively in the body of the manuscript. Place reference citations at the end of articles. Cite direct quotations or authoritative statements of positions. Do not reference commonly held opinions and perceptions unless their history is the article's principal topic. Follow the standard practice for legal citations.

Examples:

1. Author, "Article," in Journal, v.:no.:pages. [Example: 30:1:27-8 or, 25:Supplement 1:69-70 or, 10:695-6]
2. Ibid. [precisely the previous citation]
3. Author, op cit., p. 697. [after intervening citations]
4. Author, Book (City: Publisher, year), p.____.
5. Author, "Article," in Jones, Edith and Mary Right, eds., Book (City: Publisher, Year), p.____.
6. Personal interview with Jane Smith, MS, RN, Director of Nursing, St. John's Hospital, January 10, 1996.
7. Source (Generator), Database (unpublished) or Database (published), depository identification (location), page or identifier.
8. Author, loc.cit. [previously cited, same pagination]

Place bibliographic data in alphabetical order. Do not cite reference materials again. Please review references for complete citations before submission. Bibliographic entries should reflect crucial resources that are fundamental to the positions taken in the article. Remember: Thoughtful selection rather than numbers characterize authoritative bibliographical work.

Examples:

Author. Book. City: Publisher. Year.

Denison, Daniel R. Corporate Culture and Organizational Effectiveness. New York: John Wiley and Sons. 1990.

Author. "Article." In_____, ed., Anthology. Second Edition. City: Publisher. Year. pp._____.

Kierkegaard, Soren. "Repetition: An Essay in Experimental Psychology." In Robert Bretall, ed., A Kierkegaard Anthology. Modern Library Edition. New York: Random House. 1946. Pp. 439-445.

Department or Bureau, Office, Section. Title. Publication numbers. Washington, D.C.: GPO, Year.

U.S. Department of Health, Education and Welfare, Office of the Assistant Secretary for Health, Public Health Service. Health–United States. HEW PHS. 78-101. Washington, D.C.: U.S. Government Printing Office. 1978.

Source [e.g., databases primary sources of materials, etc.]. Document title. Location: Depository. Identifiers [file nos., computer file nos., if available or permitted]

Nation, Carrie to Susan B. Anthony. Letters, June 15, 1888–August 10, 1890. Chicago: University of Chicago. The Friedan Collection, SBA-10.

The Nurses Consortium of SUNY. Transcripts of interview with 10 community hospital OR managers. Ithaca: Cornell Library. Sloan Business Administration Archives. SO-422.

American Hospital Association. Standard discharge data of member hospitals FY89. Chicago: American Hospital Association Office of Statistics.

Author. "Article." In Journal. v:no:pp.___.

Thompson, J. Walter. "Advertising: Negotiating Social Expectations." In The Journal of the Academy of Marketing. 1995. 14:2:120-124.

Newspaper. "Headline." Date. v:no:pp.___ (if available).

New York Times. "HCFA's Gail Wilensky." April 25, 1990. 130:115:37.

REFEREED PUBLICATION

Nursing Management is a peer-reviewed journal with a blind review process.

COPYRIGHT

Principal author is notified upon receipt of manuscript. Review process is generally about 2 months. Signed contracts transfer copyright to Springhouse Corporation, the publisher of *Nursing Management*. Actual publication date depends on a variety of factors: editorial priorities, the article's timeliness, and availability of space in the journal. Please notify the Editorial Office of changes of address and affiliation. If you want to withdraw a manuscript for publication, write to the editor of *Nursing Management* and ask for the return of your contract.

Copyright by Springhouse Corporation.

INDEXED

Nursing Management is indexed in the *International Nursing Index, Cumulative Index to Nursing and Allied Health Literature, Nursing Abstracts, Hospital Literature Index,* and *RNdex Top 100.*

SAMPLE JOURNAL ARTICLE TITLES

- "Assessment of the Need for Nursing Care"
- "Community Nursing Centers—Issues for Managed Care: Case Study 4"
- "How to Merge Telemedicine With Traditional Clinical Practice"
- "Managed Care Liability Update"
- "Sick-Child Daycare Promotes Healing and Staffing"

3

Advanced Practice

Clinical Nurse Specialist: The Journal for Advanced Nursing Practice

Clinical Nurse Specialist: The Journal for Advanced Nursing Practice is published by Lippincott Williams & Wilkins and is the official journal of the National Association of Clinical Nurse Specialists.

JOURNAL FOCUS/PURPOSE

The primary purpose of the *Clinical Nurse Specialist: The Journal for Advanced Nursing Practice* is to publish original manuscripts about issues, trends, research, and clinical innovations related to the multiple roles of the clinical nurse specialist. Objectives are to communicate innovative perspectives on advanced nursing practice and to promote cohesion and interaction between practicing clinical nurse specialists and nurses in advanced practice.

JOURNAL FACTS

Publication schedule: bimonthly
Circulation: 3,500
Submitted papers per year: 60-100
Acceptance rate: 50%
Monetary honorarium: none

Average turnaround time: approximately 12 weeks
Publishing timetable: 3-6 months after acceptance
Correspondence:
Lippincott Williams & Wilkins
Business Offices
227 East Washington Square
Philadelphia, PA 19106-3780
Telephone: (215) 238-4200
Or
12107 Insurance Way
Hagerstown, MD 21740
Telephone: (301) 714-2300
Fax: (301) 714-2398
Customer service: 1-800-638-3030
Internet Site: www.nursingcenter.com/journals

MANUSCRIPT SUBMISSION

Manuscripts are accepted for exclusive publication in the *Clinical Nurse Specialist: The Journal for Advanced Nursing Practice* journal. The editors reserve the right to accept or reject all submitted manuscripts. All accepted manuscripts become the sole property of the *Clinical Nurse Specialist.* Upon acceptance of each manuscript, it will be necessary for the editorial office to receive assignment of copyright from all authors of the manuscript.

Manuscripts should be submitted in the final, revised format. Extensive rewriting and editorial changes made by the corresponding author after the article is typeset will be charged to the respective author.

Send the original and four copies to:

Pauline C. Beecroft, PhD, RN, FAAN
17128 Colima Road, #544
Hacienda Heights, CA 91745
Telephone: (626) 964-8465
Fax: (626) 913-8667
E-mail: pbeec@telis.org

The journal is not responsible for manuscripts lost in the mail. Be sure to keep a copy of the manuscript for yourself, and we will notify you of receipt. Submit the manuscript for our sole consideration. If we reject the manuscript, all copies will be destroyed.

Authors must submit the final version of the manuscript, references, and figure legends on diskette. Identify the diskette with the name of the senior author, article title, hardware, software, and version. IBM-compatible diskettes (3½-inch) are preferred in WordPerfect 5.1, but other programs may be converted. For information, call (818) 964-8465 or e-mail pbeec@telis.org.

MANUSCRIPT PREPARATION GUIDELINES

Please include a cover letter with the name, address, and telephone number (home and work) and fax number (if available) of the author to whom all correspondence should be addressed.

All manuscripts must be typed or computer printed on white bond paper 8½ × 11 inches, with margins of 1 inch, double-spacing throughout, including separate pages for title page, abstract, text, acknowledgments, references, tables, and legends for illustrations. Type the page numbers consecutively in the upper right-hand corner of each page beginning with the title page.

All manuscripts should contain the following sections:

1. An identification page with the name, home address, phone number, fax number, and/or e-mail address (if available), position and title, and institutional affiliation, work phone number, work fax number, and/or e-mail address (if available) of each author and indicate to which author the proofs should be sent. Include the highest academic degree of each author. Do not number this page.

2. An author biographical sketch of 50 words or less for each author. Do not number this page.

3. A title page with a title that is brief, informative, and 10 words or less. Author(s) name(s) should not appear on this page. Begin page numbering here.

4. An abstract of no more than 150 words, which includes the central theme and major subdivisions of the paper. A research paper abstract should include the general purpose, methodology, results, and conclusion/application of the study. The abstract should not contain abbreviations, footnotes, or references. Include three key word descriptors for indexing purposes. Use terms from the Medical Subject Headings (MeSH®) list of Index Medicus; if suitable MeSH® terms are not yet available, use present terms.

5. Manuscripts should be no longer than 16 typed pages. Nonresearch papers should include a brief introduction to the issue or theme, followed by the body of the paper. When possible, subheadings should be used to divide areas of the manuscript. Research papers should include an introduction indicating what the study is about; a brief review of the literature; statement of the problem; a methods section describing procedures, instruments, and their reliability and validity; results; and a discussion of conclusions/application. In either case, the preferred style and format guidelines are described in "Uniform Requirements for Manuscripts Submitted to Biomedical Journals," *JAMA,* May 5, 1993, volume

269, no. 17, pp. 2282-2286. The author's name should not appear anywhere within the text of the manuscript.

6. Contributions that need acknowledging but that do not justify authorship may be acknowledged. Such persons must have given their permission to be named.

7. References should be listed at the end of the paper according to Vancouver (Uniform Requirements) style and numbered consecutively in the order in which they appear in the text. Corresponding reference numbers as superscript should be designated in the text. Journal abbreviations should follow Index Medicus. For example:

Journal article, one author:

Foreman MD. Acute confusion in the elderly. Annu Rev Nurs Res 1993;11:3-30.

Edited book:

Smith-Marker CO. Setting standards for professional nursing: the Marker model. St. Louis: Mosby 1988.

Chapter in book:

Zarit SH, Zarit JM. Cognitive impairment. In: Lewinsohn PM, Teri L, editors. Clinical geropsychiatry: new directions in assessment and treatment. New York: Pergamon 1983;38-80.

8. Type or print each tables on a separate sheet. Number tables consecutively in the order of their first citation in the text and supply a brief title for each.

9. Figures must be professionally drawn and photographed; freehand or typewritten is unacceptable. Send camera-ready-sharp glossy black-and-white photographic prints (unmounted) usually 5×7 inches but no longer than 8×10 inches. Titles and detailed explanations belong in the legends for illustrations and not on the illustrations themselves.

10. Type legends double-spaced, starting on a separate page, with arabic numbers corresponding to the illustrations or figures.

If the manuscript contains direct use of previously published material such as texts, photographs, and/or drawings, permission of the author and publisher of works must be submitted with the manuscript.

REFEREED PUBLICATION

All submitted manuscripts are reviewed by the editors and then forwarded to a minimum of two anonymous referees for blind review. Acceptance of manuscripts is based on the reviews and is the decision of the editors. All accepted manuscripts may undergo editorial revision to conform to the standards of the journal and/or improve clarity.

COPYRIGHT

Copyright by Lippincott Williams & Wilkins.

INDEXED

Clinical Nurse Specialist: The Journal for Advanced Nursing Practice is indexed in the *Cumulative Index to Nursing and Allied Health Literature, International Nursing Index, Nursing Abstracts, Nursing Citations,* and *RNdex Top 100.*

SAMPLE JOURNAL ARTICLE TITLES

- "Client Empowerment: A Nursing Challenge"
- "Diabetic Neuropathy: Pathophysiology and Prevention of Foot Ulcers"
- "Improving Nursing Practice Through Clinical Nursing Scholarship"

- "Opposition to Antitrust Legislation: Support for Medicaid and Medicare Reimbursement"

- "Process and Outcome Measures for the Multidisciplinary Collaborative Projects of a Critical Care CNS"

Journal of the American Academy of Nurse Practitioners

The *Journal of the American Academy of Nurse Practitioners* (JAANP) is published by, and is the official journal of, the American Academy of Nurse Practitioners.

JOURNAL FOCUS/PURPOSE

The primary purpose of the *Journal of the American Academy of Nurse Practitioners* is designed to serve the information needs of nurse practitioners and others with a major interest in nursing and primary health care.

JOURNAL FACTS

Publications schedule: monthly

Circulation: more than 15,000

Submitted papers per year: unavailable

Acceptance rate: 80%

Monetary honorarium: none

Average turnaround time: 3-6 months

Publishing timetable: approximately 6 months after acceptance

Correspondence:
American Academy of Nurse Practitioners
P.O. Box 12965
Austin, TX 78711
Telephone: (512) 442-4262
Fax: (512) 442-6469
E-mail: journal@aanp.org
Internet site: www.aanp.org

MANUSCRIPT SUBMISSION

We encourage submission of articles addressing clinical practice, research, education, legislation, management, and other nursing practice issues. Thought-provoking discussion pieces, letters, and abstracts of your research are also welcome.

Five copies of the manuscript should be submitted to:
The Editor
Journal of the American Academy of Nurse Practitioners
P.O. Box 12846
Austin, TX 78711
E-mail: journal@aanp.org

Authors are encouraged to send manuscripts on computer diskette to facilitate the review process.

MANUSCRIPT PREPARATION GUIDELINES

Manuscripts should be original, unpublished works submitted voluntarily for the exclusive use of the *Journal of the American Academy of Nurse Practitioners*. Manuscripts should be typed or printed on a high-quality printer, double-spaced, with reasonably wide margins. A cover sheet should carry the title of the manuscript, author name(s), address, current position, and nursing practice specialty. Author name(s) should not appear elsewhere on the manuscript. Author identification will be removed before manuscripts are assigned for review. Manuscripts should not exceed 14 pages (3,500 words); line drawings or other illustrations should be camera ready.

The fourth edition of the *Publication Manual of the American Psychological Association* provides the format for references, headings, and other matters. Titles should be short. Abbreviations should be spelled out the first time they are used (except for standard statistical symbols). Addenda and appendices are never necessary. An abstract not to exceed 100 words should be included. Tables should be typed one to a page, and relative table placement in the text should be noted with three spaces, then "Table _____ about here," then three more spaces.

Sample journal article reference:

> Pavio, A. (1975). Perceptual comparisons through the mind's eye. *Memory and Cognition, 3,* 635-647.

Sample book reference:

> Bernstein, T. M. (1965). *The careful writer: A modern guide to English usage.* New York: Atheneum.

Letters of inquiry to the editor are welcome but not required. No manuscripts or diskettes will be returned to the author. The Journal also reserves the right to edit all manuscripts to its style and space requirements and to clarify the presentations. Authors will receive article proofs to approve. Authors are responsible for checking the accuracy of the material as it appears in the proofs. Upon acceptance of the manuscript, each author will be asked to provide biographical information and a black-and-white photograph of himself or herself.

REFEREED PUBLICATION

The *Journal of the American Academy of Nurse Practitioners* is a peer-reviewed journal. Manuscripts are reviewed by at least three reviewers. Publication decisions are made on the basis of the reviews.

COPYRIGHT

Accepted manuscripts become the property of the *Journal of the American Academy of Nurse Practitioners.*

INDEXED

The *Journal of the American Academy of Nurse Practitioners* is indexed in the *Cumulative Index to Nursing and Allied Health Literature, International Nursing Index, Nursing Abstracts,* and *RNdex Top 100.*

SAMPLE JOURNAL ARTICLE TITLES

- "Dysmenorrhea"
- "Exercise Programs for Fitness and Health for Geriatrics"
- "Health Care Seminars for Adolescents: Are we Meeting Developmental Needs?"
- "Medical Reimbursement for Nurse Practioners"
- "Substance Abuse Resources on the Internet"

Nursing Case Management

Nursing Case Management is published by Lippincott Williams & Wilkins.

JOURNAL FOCUS/PURPOSE

The primary purpose of *Nursing Case Management* is dedication to the process of case management in hospitals and other health care delivery settings. The journal will feature best practices and industry benchmarks for the professional nurse case manager focused on coordination of services, management of payer issues, population and disease-specific aspects of patient care, efficient use of resources, improving the quality of care, data and outcomes analysis, and patient advocacy. The journal will provide practical, hands-on information for the day-to-day activities involved in managing the process of patient care.

JOURNAL FACTS

Publications schedule: bimonthly

Circulation: 2,500

Submitted papers per year: 75-100

Acceptance rate: 60%

Monetary honorarium: none

Average turnaround time: 3 weeks

Publishing timetable: 2-4 months after acceptance

Correspondence:
Lippincott Williams & Wilkins
Business Offices
227 East Washington Square
Philadelphia, PA 19106-3780
Telephone: (215) 238-4200

Or
12107 Insurance Way
Hagerstown, MD 21740
Telephone: (301) 714-2300
Fax: (301) 714-2398
Customer services: 1-800-638-3030
Internet Site: www.nursingcenter.com/journals

MANUSCRIPT SUBMISSION

Manuscripts should be sent to:
Diane B. Williams, RN, MSHA
Nursing Case Management
13343 NW Old Germantown Road
Portland, OR 97231
Telephone: (503) 283-8797
Fax: (503) 283-3294
E-mail: nursingcm@aol.com

An original manuscript and two copies should be submitted.

MANUSCRIPT GUIDELINES

Manuscripts should be typed double-spaced on one side of the paper with 1-inch margins. Include page numbers at either the top or bottom of the page. Three sets of high-quality illustrations should accompany the submission. It is advised that authors retain copies of submitted manuscripts. The final version of an accepted manuscript must include a version of said article on computer disk, prepared using a standard word processing program.

The title page should include the title of the article, all authors' names and academic degrees, the institution(s) each author represents, authors' current addresses (if different), a complete description of any grants supporting the research, and the complete mailing address, telephone number, fax number, and e-mail address of the corresponding and reprint request authors.

The second page of the article should contain an abstract of no more than 150 words. The abstract should describe briefly the ideas conveyed in the article.

Brief biographies (approximately 50 words each) of all authors should be included with the manuscript.

Submissions should not exceed 20 manuscript pages, excluding references, tables, and figure legends. An acknowledgments section may follow the text.

Dorland's Medical Dictionary (28th ed.) and *Merriam Webster's Collegiate Dictionary* (10th ed.) should be used as standard references. Scientific (generic) names of drugs should be used when possible. Copyright or trade names of drugs should be capitalized and placed in parentheses immediately following the name of the drug. The manufacturers of supplies and equipment cited in a manuscript should be cited in parentheses, along with the city and state or country of the manufacturer. Units of measure should be expressed in the metric system. Temperatures should be expressed in degrees Celsius.

In general, style should be patterned after the *American Medical Association Manual of Style,* 8th ed. (1989), published by the American Medical Association, 535 North Dearborn Street, Chicago, IL 60610.

Send three sets of camera-ready illustrations. Black-and-white illustrations will be reproduced without charge. The publisher reserves the right to establish a reasonable limit on the number of illustrations. Lettering should be large enough to be legible after necessary reduction. Illustrations should be numbered, and the top indicated. A separate typewritten sheet of legends for the illustrations should be supplied at the end of the manuscript.

A bibliography of numbered references in order of citation should appear double-spaced at the end of the manuscript with corresponding numbering in the text. Unpublished data, personal communications, material published only in abstract form, or papers presented at meetings should not be numbered references but should be cited parenthetically in the text (e.g., Jones SA, personal communication, April 1995; or Jones SA, presented at the 1994 Annual Meeting of the Council of Biology Editors). References should conform to the following style:

Journal article:

Johnson JK, Olesinski N. Program evaluation: Key to success. J Nurs Adm 1995;25:53-60.

Book:

Flarey DL. Redesigning Nursing Care Delivery: Transforming Our Future. Philadelphia: JB Lippincott Co;1994:25-35.

Written permission must be obtained from (1) the holder of copyrighted material used in the manuscript, (2) persons mentioned in the narrative or acknowledgment, and (3) the administrators of institutions mentioned in the narrative or acknowledgment. Where permission has been granted, the author should follow any special wording stipulated by the grantor. Letters of permission must be submitted before publication of the manuscript.

REFEREED PUBLICATION

Nursing Case Management is a peer-reviewed journal with a blind review process.

COPYRIGHT

Copyright by Lippincott Williams & Wilkins.

INDEXED

Nursing Case Management is indexed in *International Nursing Index* and *MEDLINE*.

SAMPLE JOURNAL ARTICLE TITLES

- "Comprehensive Nursing Case Management: An Advanced Practice Model"
- "Evolution of a Role to Enhance Care Coordination"
- "Measuring Comprehensive Case Management Interventions: Development of a Tool"
- "Outcomes System Implementation for Subacute Care"
- "The Practice of Professional Nurse Case Management"

Perspectives in Psychiatric Care

Perspectives in Psychiatric Care is published by Nursecom, Inc.

JOURNAL FOCUS/PURPOSE

The primary purpose of *Perspectives in Psychiatric Care* is to publish peer-reviewed manuscripts that will enhance nurse psychotherapists' ability to provide high-quality client services, whether in a private or agency/institutional setting. *Perspectives in Psychiatric Care* is for nurse psychotherapists/advanced practice psychiatric nurses.

JOURNAL FACTS

Publications schedule: quarterly
Circulation: 2,000
Submitted papers per year: 40
Acceptance rate: 75%
Monetary honorarium: none

Average turnaround time: 4 months
Publishing timetable: 3-4 months after acceptance
Correspondence:
Perspectives in Psychiatric Care
Nursecom, Inc.
1211 Locust Street
Philadelphia, PA 19107
Telephone: (215) 545-7222 or 1-800-242-6757
Fax: (215) 545-8107
E-mail: margon@compuserve.com
Internet Site: www.nursecominc.com

MANUSCRIPT SUBMISSION

Manuscripts and correspondence should be sent to:

Mary Paquette, RN, CS, PhD
6724 De Celis
Van Nuys, CA 91406
Telephone: (818) 901-9221
Fax: (425) 732-1931
E-mail: mary77@concentric.net

Send four hard copies of the manuscript to the editor. Include a stamped, self-addressed envelope for manuscript return.

Perspectives in Psychiatric Care invites original articles on clinical practice, education, research, and administration. Submissions will become the property of *Perspectives in Psychiatric Care.*

MANUSCRIPT PREPARATION GUIDELINES

Submit manuscript on typed, double-spaced pages with 1-inch margins. Include a title page with title of article, author(s) full name(s), academic degrees, affiliation(s), and title(s). Identify each page with a number in upper right corner, but not with author's name.

List references on a separate page; use American Psychological Association (APA) style. Type each figure, chart, or table on a separate page. Reference each one in the text. Write a short legend for each one. Include permissions for all artwork, as necessary, and for use of copyrighted material.

Include keywords and a structured abstract of 75-100 words. For research articles, include topic/problem, methods, findings, and conclusions. For nonresearch articles, include topic, purpose, sources (of information), and conclusions. Identify corresponding author, including home address, telephone number, and e-mail address. At time of acceptance, send your manuscript on a disk in Word or WordPerfect or e-mail manuscript to margon@compuserve. com.

All manuscripts will be edited to conform to the style of this journal. The author is responsible for the content of the original and edited manuscript, once it is approved, and for the accuracy of references, quoted material, and for any violation of copyright.

Illustrations, charts, tables: Photographs, line drawings, graphs, tables, and charts are en-couraged if they enhance or amplify the text and are of publishable quality. All need to be referenced in the text. Photographs of people must be accompanied by a signed statement by the individual(s) photographed or the person with the legal right to sign such a statement.

All submissions must be accompanied by the following statement signed by the author(s):

As the author(s) of (title of article), I/we hereby transfer copyright ownership to Nursecom, Inc. if the work is published. I/we warrant that the article is original, has not been submitted to another journal, and has not been previously published.

REFEREED PUBLICATION

All manuscripts will be reviewed by the editor and at least two members of the review panel before a decision to publish is made. Accepted manuscripts may be revised in order to conform to the standards and style of this journal.

COPYRIGHT

INDEXED

Perspectives in Psychiatric Care is indexed in the *Cumulative Index to Nursing and Allied Health Literature, Hospital Literature, Index Medicus, International Nursing Index, Psychological Abstracts,* and *RNdex Top 100.*

SAMPLE JOURNAL ARTICLE TITLES

- "A Qualitative Study of Factors Influencing Psychiatric Nursing Practice in Australian Prisons"

- "Rage and Women's Sexuality After Childhood Sexual Abuse: A Phenomenological Study"

- "The Psychotherapeutic Needs of Women Who Have Been Sexually Assaulted"

The Nurse Practitioner: The American Journal of Primary Health Care

The Nurse Practitioner: The American Journal of Primary Health Care is published by Springhouse Corporation and is the official journal of the American College of Nurse Practitioners, American Registered Nurse Practitioners United, National Association of Nurse Practitioners in Reproductive Health, New York State Coalition of Nursing Practitioners, and the Uniformed Nurse Practitioner Association.

JOURNAL FOCUS/PURPOSE

The primary purpose of The Nurse Practitioner: The American Journal of Primary Health Care is to be the leading source of practical, state-of-the-art clinical and professional information for the nurse practitioner (and other advanced practice nurses and clinicians) involved in providing primary health care to people of all ages.

JOURNAL FACTS

Publications schedule: monthly
Circulation: approximately 30,000
Submitted papers per year: 300-400
Acceptance rate: not available
Monetary honorarium: none

Average turnaround time: 6-8 weeks
Publishing timetable: 6-8 months after acceptance
Correspondence:
> The Nurse Practitioner: The American Journal of Primary Health Care
> Business Office
> Springhouse Corporation
> 1111 Bethlehem Pike
> P.O. Box 908
> Springhouse, PA 19477-0908
> Telephone: (215) 646-8700

Internet Site: www.springnet.com/np/nursepract.htm

MANUSCRIPT SUBMISSION

Prior to submitting an article and during the revision process, the author can expedite review by having the manuscript reviewed by colleagues and at least two peers who are experts on the article topic. In addition, the manuscript should follow the style outlined below.

Submit an original and two copies of all manuscripts, tables, and illustrations to:

> Linda Pearson, Editor in Chief
> The Nurse Practitioner: The American Journal of Primary Health Care
> 13424 West Virginia Dr.
> Lakewood, CO 80228
> Telephone: (303) 986-8344
> Fax: (303) 969-9517

E-mail: linda.pearson@springnet.com

Article topics particularly suited for publication include (a) the latest in research, diagnosis, or management of acute and chronic illnesses; (b) new approaches or developments in health maintenance; and (c) protocols for management of an acute or chronic symptom or condition specific to an ambulatory population.

MANUSCRIPT PREPARATION GUIDELINES

Type the manuscripts on $8\frac{1}{2}'' \times 11''$ white paper, using $1''$ margins and double-spacing throughout. While some content requires more pages, aim for a maximum of 15 double-spaced pages of text.

List the title and each author's full name, degrees, and hospital or university affiliation. At the bottom, include the exact address with zip code and phone number of the author to whom we can send communications, proofs, and reprint requests. Also include a fax number where he or she can be reached, if possible. Number the title page as page 1.

Include a factual, complete abstract of 150 to 250 words. The abstract should be informative. If research, present a statement of the problem, method of study, results, and conclusion. Avoid abbreviations and reference citations in the abstract. Type the abstract on a separate sheet, numbered page 2.

Keep the text clear and concise. Avoid jargon because it may not be familiar to some readers. Use acronyms only if they are spelled out when first cited. Note suppliers of specific instruments or drugs, giving the company name and city. Give generic names in parentheses after any trade drug names.

Type references double-spaced and listed in order of appearance in the article. Make sure that all references are complete and accurate. Identify abstracts as such.

Books:

Author: Title With Caps. City: Publisher, Year:pages.

Burke M: Care of the Frail Elderly. New York: Mosby, 1992:229-39

Multiple authors: Valenti WM, Trudell RG:

More than three authors: Valenti WM, Trudell, RG, Bentley DW, et al:

Chapter in book:

Fink DJ: Cancer detection. In: Holland JF, ed. Cancer Medicine, 3rd ed. Philadelphia: Lea and Febiger, 1993:408-31.

Article in journal:

Author: Article title with initial cap only. Journal (abbreviated) Year; Volume (issue or month): pages.

Crossley KB: Nursing home-acquired pneumonia. Semin Respir Infect 1989;4(1):164-72.

Type each table double-spaced on a separate sheet of $8\frac{1}{2}'' \times 11''$ paper. Do not use oversized paper unless absolutely necessary. Give each table a title.

Submit illustrations as high-quality, glossy, unmounted, black-and-white photographic prints. Do not send original artwork. Number illustrations consecutively and cite them in the text. Type legends double-spaced on a separate sheet of paper.

Acknowledgments should be kept brief and follow the last page of text. All grant support must be acknowledged, and grant support should follow acknowledgments to persons. If the article is based on a thesis or meeting presentation, indicate this as well.

The Short Communications section allows people with a broad variety of views to express themselves and share information with readers. The Short Communications section is divided into three sections: In Response (for author/reader dialogue), Information and Research Exchange (for sharing clinical information and research studies), and NP Dialogue (for passing along experiences, thoughts, and helpful hints). Not all sections will appear in every issue. *The Nurse Practitioner: The American Journal of Primary Health Care* does not make claims that these letters always have scientific merit. The goal is to allow a free dialogue among journal readers. A transfer of copyright is required for letters to the editor as well as for articles. All letters are subject to copyediting.

Mail only the final accepted revision of a manuscript to the editor as an electronic file. We can handle the following programs (any version) in their native format:

- IBM Compatible: Microsoft Word, Multimate, PFS Write, PFS Professional, Q&A Write, Volkswriter, WordPerfect, WordStar, WordStar 2000, XyWrite
- Macintosh (do not use Fast Save): MacWrite, Microsoft Word, WordPerfect

If your manuscript was prepared using a different word processing program, save it in ASCII files.

The publisher will handle all design considerations such as typefaces and layout. You do not need to input special typesetting codes. However, you should use your word processor's capabilities to indicate bold, underline, italic, subscript, and superscript.

A "hard return" results from tapping the keyboard's Enter key. Use a hard return only to end a paragraph or for titles, headings, list items, and so forth. Do not use your word processor's hyphenation capabilities. Use two hyphens for long dashes. In tables, use only tabs, not spaces, to align columns.

Accepted manuscripts in final, publication-ready form may be mailed to the editor-in-chief on 3.5″ diskettes. Diskettes should be accompanied by a copy of the final revision of the manuscript and any illustrations in conformity with the standard Information for Authors. Diskettes should be labeled with the author's name, article title, operating system (IBM compatible or Macintosh), format (double or high-density disk), and word processing software and version.

Authors are responsible for obtaining written permission to reproduce any material with preexisting copyright. This includes material that is extracted or closely adapted from a previously published source. Submit proof of permission granted with the final manuscript revision. Also submit letters of permission from each identifiable patient or subject in any photograph.

REFEREED PUBLICATION

The Nurse Practitioner: The American Journal of Primary Health Care is a refereed journal. The editorial staff reviews feature article manuscripts for originality, timeliness, validity, and interest to the readers. Then they send appropriate manuscripts (without author identification) to at least two members of the Editorial Board. Some revision is almost always required. Short Communications are not refereed by the Editorial Board.

Before submitting an article and during its revision, you can expedite review by having the manuscript reviewed by colleagues and at least two peers who are experts on the article topic. If a manuscript is accepted for publication, the authors must transfer the copyright. No part of the published material may be reproduced elsewhere without the written permission of the publisher.

COPYRIGHT

The names and contents are copyrighted by Springhouse Corporation.

INDEXED

The Nurse Practitioner: The American Journal of Primary Health Care is indexed in the *Cumulative Index to Nursing and Allied Health Literature, Hospital Literature Index, Index Medicus, International Nursing Index, International Pharmaceutical Abstracts, Nursing Abstracts, RNdex Top 100,* and *Socio/ Economic Bibliographic Information Base.*

SAMPLE JOURNAL ARTICLE TITLES

- "Case Report: Human Immunodeficiency Virus: Early Steps in Management"
- "Overview of Common Obstetric Bleeding Disorders"
- "Strategies for Weight Control Success in Adults"
- "The Perimenopausal Hot Flash: Epidemiology, Physiology, and Treatment"
- "Using Osteoporosis Management to Reduce Fractures in Elderly Women"

4

Community/Home Health

Home Health Care Management and Practice

Home Health Care Management and Practice is published by Aspen Publishers, Inc.

JOURNAL FOCUS/PURPOSE

The primary purpose of *Home Health Care Management and Practice* is designed to provide home health care professionals, clinical directors, and educators with an authoritative source of timely, relevant, practical information regarding current health care issues, clinical techniques, procedures, and approaches to home health care. Issues of *Home Health Care Management and Practice* can be devoted to a single topic or current practice issues. *Home Health Care Management and Practice* is clinically oriented, and the content encompasses the coordinated responsibilities of nurses, managers, educators, administrators, and other practitioners.

JOURNAL FACTS

Publication schedule: bimonthly
Circulation: 2,500

Submitted papers per year: 1,080

Acceptance rate: 85%

Monetary honorarium: none

Average turnaround time: 8 weeks

Publishing timetable: 6 months after acceptance

Correspondence:
   Customer Services
   200 Orchard Ridge Drive
   Gaithersburg, MD 20878
   Customer service telephone: 1-800-234-1660

Internet site: www.aspenpub.com (enter journal title in search box)

MANUSCRIPT SUBMISSION

Home Health Care Management and Practice is devoted to enhancing the effective coordination and delivery of home care. Because the journal's emphasis is on the practical, clinical information needed by health professionals, authors are encouraged to include checklists, guidelines, and other instruments designed to facilitate the provision of home health care services. Acceptance or rejection of an article is based on the judgment of peer reviewers.

Manuscripts and correspondence regarding publication should be addressed to the editors:

Barbara Stover Gingerich, Editor
Home Health Care Management and Practice
140 Roosevelt Avenue, Suite 107
The Goodridge Center
York, PA 17404
Telephone: (717) 812-8877

Deborah Anne Ondeck
204 Aspen Lane
Lititz, PA 17543
Telephone: (717) 627-2937

Submissions must comprise an original and three copies of a manuscript, plus an identical version on disk, to be created on IBM-compatible (PC) equipment using Microsoft Word version 6.0 or 7.0 for Windows 95 or a higher operating system. However, manuscripts created using Microsoft Word 6.0 or 7.0 for a Macintosh System 7 are acceptable. The manuscript must include the following: a completed article submission form, an original, signed copyright transfer form, an abstract of the manuscript of 100 words or less, and a brief author bio of 100 words or less.

The journal editors will review to determine the article's suitability for publication and will work with the author to ensure that articles meet the journal's needs and adhere to its standards. At the editor's discretion, selected Editorial Board members may be asked to review particular articles. The editors may recommend that an article be revised or rewritten before being accepted for publication. The author may withdraw the article or make revisions according to the editor's recommendations. If the article is revised, the new version will again be subject to review.

Authors must release copyright ownership of their manuscript at the time of its submission to the journal.

Articles that are selected for publication are edited by the editorial staff at Aspen and sent to type. Galley proofs will be sent to the author for review and approval.

MANUSCRIPT PREPARATION GUIDELINES

Manuscripts should be created using Aspen's Journals Authoring Template (template is available from your journal editor or from Aspen). Manuscripts should be created on IBM-compatible (PC) equipment using Windows 95 or higher operating system. Our preferred software is Microsoft Word. Hard copy and electronic files should be submitted for all text and all artwork. All disks submitted must be new. Disks should be clearly labeled as to operating system and software application.

Manuscripts should be double-spaced (including quotations, lists, references, footnotes, figure captions, and all parts of tables).

Manuscripts should be ordered as follows: title page, abstracts, text, references, appendixes, tables, and any illustrations.

Each manuscript must include the following:

Title page, including (1) title of the article, (2) author names (with highest academic degrees) and affiliations (including titles, departments, and name and location of institutions of primary employment), and (3) any acknowledgments, credits, or disclaimers

Abstract of no more than 100 words and up to 10 key words that describe the contents of the article like those that appear in the *Cumulative Index to Nursing and Allied Health Literature (CINAHL)* or the *National Library of Medicine's Medical Subject Headings (MeSH)*

Clear indication of the placement of all tables and figures in text

Signed copyright transfer form

Completed article submission form for each contributor

Written permission for any borrowed text, tables, or figures

References must be cited in text and styled in the reference list according to *American Medical Association Manual of Style,* 9th ed. (1998). They must be numbered consecutively in the order they are cited in the text; reference numbers may be used more than once throughout an article. Page numbers should appear with the text citation following a specific quote. References should not be created using Microsoft Word's automatic footnote/endnote feature. References should be included on a separate page at the end of the article and should be double-spaced.

References should also include citations within the text (see examples below).

Citation:

Reliability has been established previously[1,2-8,19]

Citation following a quote should include page numbers:

Jacobsen concluded that "the consequences of muscle strength . . ."[5(pp3,4)]

Reference list style for book:

1. Gregory CF, Chapman MW, Hanse ST Jr. Open fractures. In: Rockwood CA Jr, Green DP, eds. *Fractures.* Philadelphia: JB Lippincott Co; 1984: 169-218.
2. Yando R, Seitz U, Zigler E, et al. *Imitation: A Developmental Perspective.* New York: John Wiley & Sons; 1978.

Reference list style for journal (journal names should be abbreviated as shown):

3. Fielding JW, Hensinger RN, Hawkins RJ. Os Odontoideum. *J Bone Joint Surg Am.* 1980;62:376-383.

Reference list style for unpublished material:

4. Sieger M. The nature and limits of clinical medicine. In: Cassell EJ, Siegler M, eds. *Changing Values in Medicine.* Chicago: University of Chicago Press. In press.

Reference list style for dissertation and thesis:

5. Raymand CA. Uncovering Ideology: Occupational Health in the Mainstream and Advocacy Press, 1970-1982. Ithaca, NY: Cornell University; 1983. Thesis.

Illustrations: Figures should be created using electronic software (i.e., Adobe Illustrator, Corel Draw, and Photoshop). Please save files in both the application in which they were created (i.e., Microsoft Word) and as either EPS or TIFF files. Use computer-generated lettering. Do not use screens, color, shading, or fine lines.

In lieu of original drawings and other material, a sharp, glossy, black-and-white photographic print between $5'' \times 7''$ and $8'' \times 10''$ is acceptable.

Each figure should have a label on the back indicating the number of the figure, the names of the authors, and the top of the figure. Do not write on the back of figures, mount them on cardboard, or scratch or mar them using paper clips. Do not bend figures.

Cite each figure in the text in consecutive order. If a figure has been previously published, in part or in total, acknowledge the original source and submit written permission from the copyright holder to reproduce or adapt the material.

Supply a caption for each figure, typed double-spaced on a separate sheet from the artwork. Captions should include the figure title, explanatory statements, notes, or keys as well as source and permission lines.

Provide a camera-ready copy and a separate electronic file for each piece of artwork. Do not embed art in your text file.

Tables should be on a separate page at the end of the manuscript. Number tables consecutively and supply a brief title for each. Include explanatory footnotes for all nonstandard abbreviations. Cite each table in the text in consecutive order. If you use data from another published or unpublished source, obtain permission and acknowledge fully.

Permissions: Authors are responsible for obtaining signed letters from copyright holders granting permission to reprint material being borrowed or adapted from other sources, including previously published material of your own. Authors must obtain written permission for the following material (authors are responsible for any permission fees to reprint borrowed material):

All direct quotes of 300 words or more from any full-length book

All direct quotes of 200 words or more from a periodical article

All excerpts from a newspaper article or other short piece

Any passage from a play or a song

Two or more lines of poetry

Any borrowed table, figure, or illustration being reproduced exactly or adapted to fit the needs of the subject

REFEREED PUBLICATION

Home Health Care Management and Practice is a peer-reviewed journal with a blind review process.

COPYRIGHT

Copyright by Aspen Publishers, Inc.

INDEXED

Home Health Care Management and Practice is indexed in the *Cumulative Index to Nursing and Allied Health Literature, International Nursing Index,* and *IMFL (Inventory of Marriage and Family Literature).*

SAMPLE JOURNAL ARTICLE TITLES

- "Focused Nutritional Intervention in the Home Care Setting"
- "Methods for Recruiting and Evaluating Job Candidates"
- "Outsourcing: An Alternative Solution to Providing Management and Staff Development"
- "Preparing the Baccalaureate Student for Community-Focused Nursing"
- "Product Management: A Powerful Approach for Home Health Care Management"

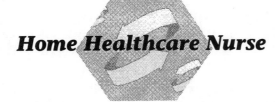

Home Healthcare Nurse

Home Healthcare Nurse is published by Lippincott Williams & Wilkins and is the official journal of the Home Healthcare Nurses Association.

JOURNAL FOCUS/PURPOSE

The primary purpose of *Home Healthcare Nurse* is to address the educational and information needs of practicing home care nurses while advancing the specialty.

JOURNAL FACTS

Publication schedule: 10 times per year

Circulation: 11,000

Submitted papers per year: 550

Acceptance rate: approximately 65%

Monetary honorarium: none

Average turnaround time: 6-8 weeks

Publishing timetable: 4-6 months after acceptance

Correspondence:
Lippincott Williams & Wilkins
Business Offices
227 East Washington Square
Philadelphia, PA 19106-3780
Telephone: (215) 238-4200

Or

12107 Insurance Way
Hagerstown, MD 21740
Telephone: (301) 714-2300
Fax: (301) 714-2398
Customer service: 1-800-638-3030

Or

Home Healthcare Nurses Association
7794 Grow Drive
Pensacola, FL 32514
Telephone: (850) 474-1066 or 1-800-558-
HHNA
E-mail: hhna@puetzamc.com

Internet Site: www.nursingcenter.com/journals or www.hhna.org

MANUSCRIPT SUBMISSION

Submit three copies of the manuscript, along with a stamped, self-addressed, business-sized envelope if you wish receipt of your manuscript acknowledged. If you want your original manuscript returned after the review process, enclose a self-addressed, manuscript-sized envelope with sufficient postage affixed.

Send to:
Carolyn J. Humphrey, MS, RN
Editor, *Home Healthcare Nurse*
3904 Therina Way
Louisville, KY 40241
Telephone: (502) 339-9005
Fax: (502) 339-0087
E-mail: chump@homehealth.win.net

Although not necessary, query letters allow the editor to indicate interest in, and give advice on, manuscript topics.

Home Healthcare Nurse publishes the following types of articles and departments:

Research papers should not exceed 12-14 double-spaced pages, plus tables, illustrations, and references. Papers reporting original research should include (1) abstract, (2) the purpose of the study, (3) clear and full description of the methodology, (4) report of results, (5) discussion, and (6) implications for practice.

A clinical manuscript describes accurately, with depth and specificity, current home care nursing practice problems as faced by the practicing nurse. Clinical articles may (1) describe implementation of a new nursing technique or clinical equipment; (2) provide current information on disease management and health problems and related care and treatment; (3) provide insight into the behavior of the patient, family, or nurse; (4) offer new solutions to old problems (helpful hints are always welcome); (5) describe current physiology and/or pathophysiology related to client management; and (6) present creative programs related to all aspects of patient care, student experiences, and material that addresses the nurse's practice, such as productivity, time management, and so on. In each of these articles, the implications for home care nursing practice must be clearly stated.

Papers may be submitted for publication to any individual departments within *Home Healthcare Nurse*. The typical length of these papers is 4-8 pages, excluding tables and references. Some department examples include the following: Client Challenge: a case scenario of a difficult client and an approach that worked; Clinicians' Forum: provides a forum for sharing ideas, insights, procedures, or programs in a broad range of categories related to clinical patient management; Home Care Today: topics that allow home care nurses to better understand the trends that affect daily practices (e.g., the impact of managed care, examples of collaborative practice between nurses and other health professionals, reimbursement trends, etc.); Relationships: nursing roles and relationships with other members of the interdisciplinary team, including working with home health aides, case managers, physicians, or other team members; Commentary: a thought piece that presents different sides of an issue, somewhat like a guest editorial—found on the last page of the journal, no more than 650 words.

Features and departments focus on practical, up-to-date approaches to everyday situations as well as analysis of how home care and health care trends affect the nurse's daily practice.

MANUSCRIPT PREPARATION GUIDELINES

Manuscripts should be typed double-spaced, on one side of $8\frac{1}{2} \times 11$-inch white paper. One-inch margins should be used throughout, and pages should be numbered consecutively in the upper right-hand corner, beginning with the title page. Do not send a disk with the original manuscript.

The title page should include (1) the title of the manuscript; (2) all authors' names, academic degrees, and institutional affiliations; (3) the complete mailing address, telephone, fax, and e-mail address (if available) of the corresponding author; and (4) acknowledgment of financial and/or other support. The title page is the only place in the manuscript where the author(s) should be identified.

The second page of the article should contain the title of the article and a brief paragraph of no more than 75 words describing the article. Submissions to departments do not require an abstract. Submissions for research and clinical articles should not exceed 14 pages, including references, tables, and figures.

All tables and figures should be placed in the back of the manuscript after the references. Tables should be numbered consecutively with arabic numbers, double-spaced, and have a title at the top. Figures and tables must be cited in numerical order in the text. Authors are encouraged to use sidebars, bulleted lists, and other strategies that make the material clearer to the reader. A complete description of any grants supporting the material should be listed. An acknowledgments section may follow the text.

Do not justify the right margins, and do not use running headers or footers. Subdivide the manuscript into main sections by inserting subheads in the text. Subheads should be succinct, meaningful, and similar in sense and tone.

Prepare manuscripts according to the *Publication Manual of the American Psychological Association* (APA, 4th ed.).

Scientific (generic) names of drugs should be used when possible. Copyright or trade names of drugs, if applicable, should be capitalized and placed in parentheses immediately following the generic name of the drug. The manufacturers of supplies and equipment cited in a manuscript should be cited in parentheses, along with the city and state or country of the manufacturer. Units of measure should be expressed in the metric system.

Three sets of high-quality illustrations (if applicable) must accompany the manuscript. All figures and tables must be provided on paper (hard copy), not on computer disk. Illustrations should be numbered, and the top should be indicated on the back of the figures. A separate typewritten sheet of legends for the illustrations should be supplied at the end of the manuscript before any tables.

A reference list should appear in alphabetical order, double-spaced at the end of the manuscript with corresponding citations in the text (APA style). Although the references will be proofread and corrected by a copy editor, it is the author's responsibility to furnish all references based on APA style. References should conform to the following style:

Journal article:

> Cale-Lawrence, J., Peploski, J., & Russell, J. C. (1995). Training needs of home healthcare nurses. *Home Healthcare Nurse, 13,* 53-61.

Book:

> Spradley, B. W., & Alexander, J. A. (1995). *Community health nursing: Concepts and practice* (4th ed.). Philadelphia: Lippincott Williams & Wilkins.

Written permission must be obtained from (1) the holders of copyrighted material used in the manuscript, for reprint or adaptation of their work; (2) persons mentioned in the narrative or acknowledgment for publication of their names; and (3) the administrators of institutions mentioned in the narrative or acknowledged, for publication of the institution's name. Where permission has been granted, the author should follow any special wording stipulated by the grantor.

REFEREED PUBLICATION

Home Healthcare Nurse is a professional, peer-reviewed, contemporary journal.

COPYRIGHT

Copyright by Lippincott Williams & Wilkins publishers.

INDEXED

Home Healthcare Nurse is indexed in the *Cumulative Index to Nursing and Allied Health Literature, MEDLINE, International Nursing Index,* and *RNdex Top 100.*

SAMPLE JOURNAL ARTICLE TITLES

- "A Time for Self-Care: Role of the Home Healthcare Nurse"
- "Basic Musculoskeletal Assessment: A Guide for the Home Health Nurse"
- "Joint Commission Infection Control Requirements"
- "Mental Health Services in the Home: A Balance of Sophistication and Caring"
- "Tips for Using OASIS Now"

Home Healthcare Nurse Manager

Home *Healthcare Nurse Manager* is published by Lippincott Williams & Wilkins.

JOURNAL FOCUS/PURPOSE

The primary purpose of *Home Healthcare Nurse Manager* is to provide home care managers with strategies and approaches to successfully respond to changes in the home care industry and to grow in their own professional development.

JOURNAL FACTS

Publication schedule: bimonthly
Circulation: 2,000
Submitted papers per year: 225
Acceptance rate: 75%
Monetary honorarium: none
Average turnaround time: 6-8 weeks
Publishing timetable: 4-6 months after acceptance
Correspondence:
    Lippincott Williams & Wilkins
    Business Offices
    227 East Washington Square
    Philadelphia, PA 19106-3780
    Telephone: (215) 238-4200
Or
    12107 Insurance Way
    Hagerstown, MD 21740
    Telephone: (301) 714-2300
    Fax: (301) 714-2398
    Customer service: 1-800-638-3030
Internet Site: www.nursingcenter.com/journals

MANUSCRIPT SUBMISSION

Submit three copies of the manuscript, along with a stamped, self-addressed, business-sized envelope. If you want the entire manuscript returned after the review process, enclose a self-addressed, manuscript-sized envelope with sufficient postage affixed. Do not send a disk with the initial submission.

All manuscripts and correspondence should be sent to:

    Carolyn J. Humphrey, MS, RN
    Editor, *Home Healthcare Nurse Manager*
    3904 Therina Way
    Louisville, KY 40241
    Telephone: (502) 339-9005
    Fax: (502) 339-0087

E-mail: chump@homehealth.win.net

While not necessary, query letters allow the editor to indicate interest in, and give advice on, manuscript topics. Manuscripts should be voluntary contributions submitted for the exclusive attention of *Home Healthcare Nurse Manager.*

Submissions are limited to shorter manuscripts (2-6 pages) with only one or two longer ones (10-12 pages) included in each issue. The editor will work with authors to determine the best placement for material, based on its focus.

Manuscripts that deal with performance improvement, staff development, legal issues, risk management, ethical subjects, human resources, the use of technology, and regulatory and accreditation compliance strategies are most welcome. Career development, professional trends, financial management, and analysis of how legislation affects the management of a home health organization are also highly desired. Case examples of home care situations and programs that have been tested should be used whenever possible.

MANUSCRIPT PREPARATION GUIDELINES

The *Publication Manual of the American Psychological Association* (APA), 4th ed., provides the format for all references, headings, and other matter. Tables and figures should follow the reference list. Authors are encouraged to use graphs, figures, tables, photo/slides (color), and other visual mechanisms that clarify the manuscript. Tables should be typed one to a page and relative placement of tables noted in text.

Manuscripts should be printed on a letter-quality printer and double-spaced. A face sheet for one of the copies should include (1) title;

(2) all author(s) names, academic degrees, and affiliations; and (3) the complete mailing address, phone and fax number at both work and home, and e-mail, if available, of the corresponding author. Author names should not appear on the manuscript. Do not use running headers. Manuscripts can range from 2 to 12 pages, including tables.

REFEREED PUBLICATION

Home Healthcare Nurse Manager is a peer-reviewed publication with a blind review.

COPYRIGHT

Copyright by Lippincott Williams & Wilkins Publishers.

INDEXED

Home Healthcare Nurse Manager is indexed in the *Cumulative Index to Nursing and Allied Health Literature, MEDLINE, International Nursing Index,* and *RNdex Top 100.*

SAMPLE JOURNAL ARTICLE TITLES

- "Development of an Infection Surveillance Project for Home Healthcare"
- "Education and Training for Home Care Information Systems Part II: A Roadmap for an Effective Program"
- "Making the Transition From Clinician to Manager"
- "Management Strategies for Implementing OASIS"
- "Regency Home Care Pediatric Safety Checklist"

Journal of Community Health Nursing

The *Journal of Community Health Nursing* is published by Lawrence Erlbaum Associates, Publishers.

JOURNAL FOCUS/PURPOSE

The primary purpose of the *Journal of Community Health Nursing* is to focus on health care issues relevant to all aspects of community practice—schools, homes, visiting nursing services, clinics, hospices, education, and public health administration. Well-researched articles provide practical and up-to-date information to aid the nurse who must frequently make decisions and solve problems without the backup support systems available in the hospital. The journal is a forum for community health professionals to share their experience and expertise with others in the field.

JOURNAL FACTS

Publication schedule: quarterly
Circulation: 1,100

Submitted papers per year: not available

Acceptance rate: 60-65%

Monetary honorarium: none

Average turnaround time: 3 months

Publishing timetable: 3 months after acceptance

Correspondence:
Lawrence Erlbaum Associates, Inc.
10 Industrial Avenue
Mahwah, NJ 07430-2262
Telephone: (201) 236-9500

Internet Site: www.erlbaum.com

MANUSCRIPT SUBMISSION

Submit three (3) high-quality manuscript printouts to:

Arlene Cairns and Alice Schroeder, Editors
Journal of Community Health Nursing
354 Marlboro Road
Wood-Ridge, NJ 07075

All manuscripts submitted will be acknowledged promptly. Authors should keep a copy of their manuscripts to guard against loss. All manuscripts submitted become the exclusive property of the *Journal of Community Health Nursing*.

In a cover letter, include the contact author's address and telephone and fax numbers and state that the manuscript includes only original material that has not been previously published and that is not under review for publication elsewhere.

After manuscripts are accepted, authors are asked to (a) submit a disk containing two files (word processor and ASCII versions of the manuscript); (b) make sure the content of the files exactly matches that of the printed, accepted, finalized manuscript (provide revised printout if necessary); (c) submit camera-ready figures; and (d) sign and return a copyright transfer agreement. It is the responsibility of the contact author to ascertain that all coauthors approve the accepted manuscript and concur with its publication in the journal.

Files of accepted manuscripts are copyedited and typeset into page proofs. Authors read proofs to correct errors and to answer editors' queries. Authors may order reprints of their articles when they receive proofs.

MANUSCRIPT PREPARATION GUIDELINES

Prepare manuscripts according to the *Publication Manual of the American Psychological Association* (4th ed., 1994, APA, 750 First Street NE, Washington, DC 20002-4242). Follow "Guidelines to Reduce Bias in Language." Use 1½-inch margins. Type all components double-spaced and in the following order: title page (p. 1), abstract and key words (p. 2), text (including quotes), acknowledgments, references, appendices, footnotes, tables, and figure captions. On the cover page, type article title, author name(s) and affiliation(s), running head (abbreviated title), and name and address of the person to whom requests should be addressed. Research articles should include an abstract of no more than 150 words. Type author notes and acknowledgments at the end of the article (just before the reference section). Attach photocopies of all figures. To facilitate anonymous review, only the cover page should include the author's name. Careful effort should be made by the authors to see that the manuscript itself contains no clues to their identities.

Authors are responsible for all statements made in their work and for obtaining permission from copyright owners to reprint or adapt a table or figure or to reprint a quotation of 500 words or more. Authors should write to original author(s) and publisher to request nonexclusive world rights in all languages to use the material in the article and in future editions. Provide copies of all permission and credit lines.

REFEREED PUBLICATION

All manuscripts are reviewed by the editors. Specific articles are referred to appropriate members of the Editorial Board. Manuscripts are then reviewed by several members of our editorial staff. Acceptance of an article depends on several points: the depth to which a subject is developed, the current importance of the subject, and the appropriateness of the subject for community health nursing. Included with each manuscript should be a complete and accurate list of every source—book, magazine, or other—that was used in writing the article.

COPYRIGHT

Copyright by Lawrence Erlbaum Associates, Inc.

INDEXED

The *Journal of Community Health Nursing* is indexed in *Applied Social Sciences Index &* *Abstracts, Cambridge Scientific Abstracts, Cumulative Index to Nursing and Allied Health Literature, EMBASE/Excerpta Medica, Health and Safety Science Abstracts, Index Medicus, MEDLINE, Inventory of Marriage and Family Literature, PsycINFO/Psychological Abstracts, RNdex Top 100, SilverPlatter Information, Sociological Abstracts, Risk Abstracts,* and *Wise for Medicine.*

SAMPLE JOURNAL ARTICLE TITLES

- "A Community-Based Nursing Approach to the Prevention of Otitis Media"
- "Community Health Nurses' Knowledge of Lyme Disease: Implications for Surveillance and Community Education"
- "Poor Women Living With HIV: Self-Identified Needs"
- "Program Evaluation Application of a Comprehensive Model for a Community-Based Respite Program"
- "The Role of the Community Health Nurse in the Provision of Care to Youth Gangs"

Public Health Nursing

Public Health Nursing is published by Blackwell Science, Inc.

JOURNAL FOCUS/PURPOSE

The primary purpose of *Public Health Nursing* is to provide a vehicle by which the discourse of a broad diversity of the latest and very best information, with a focus on public health, is made possible. This forum allows the distribution of a wide range of cutting-edge knowledge relating to research, evaluation studies, program evaluation and reports, education and scholarship, and conceptual and practice issues, including appropriate applications of our science, deemed to be of interest to our readers.

JOURNAL FACTS

Publication schedule: bimonthly
Circulation: 1,650

Submitted papers per year: 125

Acceptance rate: 50%

Monetary honorarium: none

Average turnaround time: 3-6 months

Publishing timetable: 3-6 months after acceptance

Correspondence:
Blackwell Science, Inc.
350 Main Street
Malden, MA 02148
E-mail: phnjournal@juno.com

Internet Site: www.blacksci.co.uk

MANUSCRIPT SUBMISSION

Submit three copies of the manuscript—the original and two duplicates—plus all artwork to:

Katherine J. Young Graham, PhD, FAAN
Editor, *Public Health Nursing*
P.O. Box 549
Mukilteo, WA 98275
Telephone: (206) 290-3048

Manuscripts will be considered for publication in the form of original research and evaluation studies, program evaluation, analytic or methodological papers, and letters.

Submission of a paper implies that it reports unpublished work, except in abstract form, and is not being submitted simultaneously to another publication. Accepted manuscripts become the sole property of *Public Health Nursing* and may not be published elsewhere without consent from the publisher.

Material accepted for publication is copyedited and typeset. Proofs are sent to contributors for final review. Contributors are responsible for the entire content of the copyedited article. Extensive changes to the proofs other than printer's errors, will be charged to the contributors and could delay publication.

Proofs must be returned within 3 days of receipt; late return may cause a delay in publishing the article.

MANUSCRIPT PREPARATION GUIDELINES

The entire manuscript should be typed double-spaced using 1½-inch margins on standard white heavy-duty bond. Do not use erasable paper. Submit the original typescript and two high-quality photocopies of all elements of the manuscript. Keep a copy of the manuscript for your reference.

Place senior author's name in the upper right-hand corner of the first page; then number pages consecutively in this order: title page, abstract, text, references, tables, figure legends. Include original figures in a protective folder along with the manuscript.

On the title page, provide the complete title and a brief title (not to exceed 45 letters and spaces) for use as a running head. List each contributor's name, academic degrees, and institutional affiliation. Provide the name, address, and telephone number of the contributor responsible for the manuscript and proofs. This is the person to whom reprints will be sent.

The abstract may have up to 200 words. It should summarize the problems presented and describe the studies undertaken, results, and conclusion.

The text of the manuscript should be in the following sequence: introduction, text, acknowledgments, references, tables, and figure legends. Type footnotes (double-spaced) on the bottom of the page on which they are mentioned. Cite all tables and figures in the text, numbering them sequentially as they are cited.

References must follow the author-date method, in which the last name of the author and the year of publication are inserted in parentheses in the text at an appropriate point. If a work has two authors, cite both names in every reference. If a work has more than two authors, cite all authors at the first reference, then only the first author and "et al." for all following references. The citation of a specific page, chapter, or figure should be made with the reference in the text, not in the reference list.

The reference list should appear alphabetically by main author's last name and conform to the style used by the *Publication Manual of the American Psychological Association,* latest edition. Journal titles are not abbreviated, and the initial letter of all major words are capitalized. Book and journal titles, and volume numbers, are underlined and will appear in italics when typeset. For article, chapter, and book titles, only the initial letter of the first word is capitalized, except for proper names, and other common usage. All references must be verified by the author(s).

Sample references follow. Pay special attention to the punctuation.

Journals: List all authors.

Lewis, B. R., & Bradbury, Y. (1982). The role of the nursing profession in hospital accident and emergency departments. *Journal of Advanced Nursing, 7,* 211-221.

Books and monographs:

Personal author:

Varney, H. (1987). *Nurse-midwifery* (2nd ed.). Boston: Blackwell Scientific Publications.

Corporate author:

The Geological Society. (1978). *List of serial publications held in the library of the Geological Society.* London, Oxford: Blackwell Scientific Publications.

Editor, compiler, chairman, as author:

Kneedler, J. A., & Dodge, G. H. (Eds.). (1987). *Perioperative patient care: The nursing perspective* (2nd ed.). Boston: Blackwell Scientific Publications.

Nahm, H. E. (1985). History of nursing—a century of change. In J. C. McCloskey & H. K. Grace (Eds.), *Current issues in nursing* (2nd ed., pp. 14-26). Boston: Blackwell Scientific Publications.

Tables should be typed double-spaced on separate sheets and numbered consecutively within the text. Tables and text should not duplicate each other. If possible, hold tables to one standard manuscript page; if the table continues past one page, repeat all heads and the stub (left-hand column). Explain all abbreviations in a footnote. Provide a number and title for each table.

Each figure must have a corresponding legend that must be typed double-spaced, on a separate sheet of paper. Do not attach the legends to the figures. Each legend must be numbered with an arabic numeral to correspond to the illustration as it appears in the text. Explain all symbols, arrows, numbers, or letters used in the figure and provide information on scale and/or magnification. For photomicrographs, include information on the method of staining.

Note that the original and two copies of all illustrations must be submitted. Illustrations should be submitted unmounted. Do not trim or write on the back; do not use paper clips. Attach a gummed label to the back of each illustration giving the figure number, author's name, and an arrow to indicate the top of the figure.

Have artwork drawn by an experienced illustrator. Labels and callouts should be done by preset type or template letters, not by hand. The labels should be legible when the figure is reduced to column width. The publisher does not reconstruct artwork. Black-and-white photostats (5″ × 7″) of drawn materials should be supplied, not the illustrator's original art.

For halftones (photographs, photomicrographs), clear black-and-white prints must be submitted. For photographs of recognizable subjects, submit a signed release form from the patient authorizing publication. Photomicrographs must have internal scale markers.

Indicate crop marks on tracing paper overlays. Arrows, indicators, or letters can be applied using a professional graphic transfer product (such as Chartpak). Consider clarity after reduction.

Cite each figure in the text by its number. Figures should be numbered consecutively as they appear in the text. If a figure has been previously published, permission must be received in writing for its use regardless of authorship or publisher. Acknowledgment of the original source must be included in the legend.

Give all measurements in metric units. Use generic names of drugs. Adhere to acceptable English usage and syntax; avoid jargon, euphemistic phrasing, and obscure terms. Standard abbreviations, units, and acronyms are allowed. The first time an abbreviation or acronym is used, it should be preceded by the full name for which it stands.

REFEREED PUBLICATION

All articles submitted to *Public Health Nursing* are subject to review by experienced referees. The editors and Editorial Board judge manuscripts suitable for publication, and decisions by the editors are final.

COPYRIGHT

Copyright on all published articles is held by Blackwell Science, Inc.

INDEXED

Public Health Nursing is indexed in the *Cumulative Index to Nursing and Allied Health Literature, Current Contents/Social and Behavioral Sciences, Index Medicus, MEDLINE, Nursing Abstracts, Research Alert, RNdex Top 100, Social Sciences Citation Index,* and *Social SciSearch.*

SAMPLE JOURNAL ARTICLE TITLES

- "Adolescent Pregnancy and Loneliness"
- "Effect of Parity and Weaning Practices on Breastfeeding Duration"
- "Family Ritual Facilitates Adaptation to Parenthood"
- "Giving Voice to Elderly People: Community-Based Breastfeeding Duration"
- "Severity of Abuse and Reports of Abuse Ending"

5

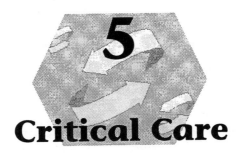

Critical Care

American Journal of Critical Care

American Journal of Critical Care is published by the American Association of Critical-Care Nurses and is the official journal of the American Association of Critical-Care Nurses.

JOURNAL FOCUS/PURPOSE

The primary purpose of the *American Journal of Critical Care* is to provide the latest research in critical care, as well as guidelines for clinical practice.

JOURNAL FACTS

Publication schedule: bimonthly
Circulation: 69,000
Submitted papers per year: 225
Acceptance rate: 30%
Monetary honorarium: none
Average turnaround time: 2 months
Publishing timetable: 6 months after acceptance
Correspondence:
Editorial Office, AACN Critical Care Journals
101 Columbia
Aliso Viejo, CA 92656-1491
Telephone: 1-800-809-CARE or (949) 362-2000
Fax: (949) 362-2049
Internet site: www.aacn.org

MANUSCRIPT SUBMISSION

Manuscripts for publication in the *American Journal of Critical Care* should be prepared in the form and style described in these guidelines.

Authors from west of the Mississippi River submitting manuscripts should send an original and three copies to:

Kathleen Dracup, RN, DNSc
School of Nursing, University of California at Los Angeles
Factor Building, P.O. Box 956918
Los Angeles, CA 90095
Telephone: (310) 206-2644
Fax: (310) 794-7482
E-mail: AJCC@sonnet.ucla.edu

Authors from east of the Mississippi River submitting manuscripts should send an original and three copies to:

Christopher W. Bryan-Brown, MD
Department of Anesthesiology, Montefiore Medical Center
111 E. 210th Street
Bronx, NY 10467-2490

Telephone: (718) 920-4175
Fax: (718) 881-2245
E-mail: cbbajcc@aol.com

The editors invite the submission of original manuscripts describing investigations, advances, or observations from all specialties concerned with care of the critically ill patient. Papers that are the result of or that promote collaborative practice and research are particularly welcome. Manuscripts will be accepted for consideration on the understanding that they have not been published or submitted elsewhere and are submitted solely to the *American Journal of Critical Care.* This restriction does not apply to published abstracts.

Submissions are usually acknowledged within 2 weeks of receipt in the editorial offices. If you do not receive acknowledgment in a timely fashion, please contact the editor concerned. The Journal cannot accept responsibility for lost or mislaid manuscripts; keep original copies in your possession.

The following types of manuscripts are published. Please note the text length guidelines for each type of paper.

- Clinical studies (1,500-4,000 words)
- Basic research studies (1,500-4,000 words)
- Preliminary or short communications (500-1,500 words)
- Case reports (500-1,500 words)
- Reports on new apparatus and techniques
- Clinical and basic science reviews, including historical material (1,500-4,000 words)
- Editorials
- Letters to the editors (250-500 words)
- Book reviews

Once a manuscript is accepted, the author will be required to submit it on IBM-compatible or Macintosh diskette. Instructions on the submission of electronic manuscripts are available from the editorial offices on request.

With each manuscript submitted, please include a cover letter with the following copyright transfer statement signed and dated by each author:

MANUSCRIPT PREPARATION GUIDELINES

The contents of the manuscript should be laid out in the manner of the "Uniform Requirements for Manuscripts Submitted to Biomedical Journals" (N Engl J Med 1991;324: 424-428).

The title page is page 1 and should contain the following:

- Title of manuscript. This should be short and to the point to facilitate indexing.
- Running title (usually two to five words).
- The authors' full names in preferred publishing order, with degrees, credentials, ranks, and affiliations.
- The name, address, telephone (home and office), and fax numbers (if available) of the author to whom all correspondence and reprint requests should be addressed.
- The institution(s) in which the work was performed.

- Key words.
- Grant or other financial support used in the study.

Page 2 is the abstract. Abstracts are not required for preliminary or short communications and case reports. Abstracts for review articles need not be structured. Clinical and basic research studies and meta-analyses must have structured abstracts of not more than 250 words (Haynes RB, Mulrovv CD, Huth EJ, Altman DG, Gardner MJ. "More informative abstracts revisited." Ann Intern Med 1990;113:69-76). Abstracts should be written in the third person. Abstracts for clinical studies should have the following subheadings: Background, Objectives, Methods, Results, and Conclusions.

For laboratory studies and new apparatus and techniques, a shorter form is requested (Relman AS. "New information for authors and readers." N Engl J Med 1990;323:356). Abstracts should have the following subheadings: Background, Methods, Results, and Conclusions.

When human experimentation is being reported, a statement must be included to confirm that the work was done in accordance with the appropriate institutional review body and carried out with the ethical standards set forth in the Helsinki Declaration of 1975. When laboratory animals are used as experimental subjects, provide a statement that the work was carried out according to the National Research Council's protocol for, or any national law on, the care and use of laboratory animals.

References should start on a separate page following the text. They must be numbered consecutively by their order of appearance in the text. In the text, designate reference numbers either as superscript or on the line in parentheses. Do not use footnote function. Abbreviate journal titles as found in Index Medicus. If in doubt as to the correct abbreviation, cite the complete journal name. Please follow the format and punctuation shown in the following examples. Do not use periods in abbreviations of journal titles. List all authors, but if the number exceeds six, give the first three followed by et al.

Journal article:

Mihn F, Halperin B. Noninvasive detection of profound arterial desaturation using a pulse oximetry device. Anesthesiology. 1985;62:85-87.

Book chapter:

Schiffman JD. Immunology of influenza. In: Cane MB, ed. Viruses and Influenza. Orlando, Fla: Academic Press; 1990:191-196.

Book:

Avery GB. Neonatology: Pathophysiology and Management of the Neonate. 3rd ed. Philadelphia, Pa: JB Lippincott; 1987:77-80.

Each table must be numbered (consecutively in the order mentioned in the text) and titled. Each column within a table should have a heading. Abbreviations must be explained in the legend. Please do not type more than one table on a page.

For illustrations, black-and-white line art and photographs of good quality will be considered. Submit one original and three copies of unmounted, untrimmed black-and-white glossy prints. The back of each print should note the figure number, last name of the first author, and orientation of the figure (top/left/right). Write this information on an adhesive label and place the label on the back of the print. Color artwork should be submitted as slides or transparencies. Include the name of the photographer, if applicable. For computer-generated graphics, please supply original files in Photoshop 3.0, Adobe Illustrator 5.5, or QuarkXpress 3.32 (or earlier versions of these programs). Contact the editorial office for further information at 1-800-809-CARE or (949)

362-2000. In clinical photographs in which the patient could be recognized, the manuscript must be accompanied by a statement signed by the patient or the patient's guardian granting permission to publish the photograph for educational purposes. If permission is not obtained, the photograph will be cropped accordingly to ensure that the patient's identity is not disclosed. Include signed consent release from owner of photo or artist if different from author.

If any material in the manuscript is from a prior copyrighted publication, the manuscript must be accompanied by a letter of permission to reproduce the material from the copyright holder. For photos and artwork, please contact the Journal's office at 1-800-899-1712 for the release form. Figure legends should begin on a new manuscript page, after the tables. They should be typed double-spaced in consecutive order.

Letters to the editors raising points of current interest or commenting on articles published in the *American Journal of Critical Care* are welcome. The editors reserve the right to accept, reject, or excerpt letters without changing the views expressed by the writer. The author of an original article will be given the opportunity to respond to published comments. Letters should be sent to Dr. Dracup.

Books and monographs will be reviewed as space allows. All books received will be listed and selected titles reviewed. Books for review should be sent to Dr. Bryan-Brown.

Accepted manuscripts become the property of the American Association of Critical-Care Nurses (AACN) and may not be published without the written permission of the AACN. All accepted manuscripts are subject to editing. Authors will be asked to review galleys prior to publication.

For drug names, use complete generic names only. The trade name of a drug may be cited in parentheses the first time the generic name appears.

Units of measurements as length, height, weight, and volume should be reported in metric units or their decimal multiples. Temperatures should be given in degrees Celsius. Physiologic measurements should be reported in the metric system, with the International System of Units (SI) reported parenthetically after each value.

Avoid nonstandard abbreviations. Do not use abbreviations in the title or abstract. The full term for which an abbreviation or symbol is being used should precede its first use, unless it is a standard unit of measurement. When many abbreviations are being used, they should be listed in table form for insertion into a box at the beginning of the text.

REFEREED PUBLICATION

All materials submitted are subject to peer review. Two or more authorities will be asked to judge the validity, originality, and significance of the work presented, and whether subject matter is suitable for publication. Although the initial review process is usually completed within 2 months, delays are sometimes unavoidable. After the manuscript has been reviewed, the author will be informed whether it has been accepted for publication, rejected, or requires revision. Only one copy of the manuscript will be resumed to the author.

COPYRIGHT

Copyright held by the American Association of Critical-Care Nurses.

INDEXED

The *American Journal of Critical Care* is indexed in the *Cumulative Index to Nursing and Allied Health Literature, Index Medicus, MEDLINE,* and *SilverPlatter Information.*

SAMPLE JOURNAL ARTICLE TITLES

- "Effects of Injectate Volume on Thermodilution Measurements of Cardiac Output in Patients With Low Ventricular Ejection Fraction"

- "Endotracheal Tube Narrowing After Closed-System Suctioning: Prevalence and Risk Factors"
- "Preoperative ICU Tours: Are They Helpful?"
- "Psychosocial Factors and Survival in the Cardiac Arrhythmia Suppression Trial (CAST): A Reexamination"
- "The Impact of Routine Chest Radiography on ICU Management Decisions: An Observational Study"

Critical Care Nurse

Critical Care Nurse is published by InnoVision Communication, a division of the American Association of Critical-Care Nurses and is an official journal of the American Association of Critical-Care Nurses.

JOURNAL FOCUS/PURPOSE

The primary purpose of *Critical Care Nurse* is to provide information relevant to critical care nursing practice. A secondary purpose is to provide content useful to critical care nursing education and management.

JOURNAL FACTS

Publication schedule: bimonthly

Circulation: approximately 72,000

Submitted papers per year: not available

Acceptance rate: approximately 50% to 60% (after revisions)

Monetary honorarium: none

Average turnaround time: 6 months

Publishing timetable: 3 months after acceptance

Correspondence:

Editorial Office
AACN Critical Care Journals
101 Columbia
Aliso Viejo, CA 92656-1491
Telephone: 1-800-809-CARE or (949) 362-2000
Fax: (949) 362-2049
E-mail: critnurse@aol.com

Internet site: www.aacn.org

MANUSCRIPT SUBMISSION

Critical care nurses are invited to submit articles for consideration. Clinical topics must apply directly to the care of critically ill patients and their families, with case presentations and clinical tips especially welcome.

Send articles to:

Grif Alspach, RN, MSN, EdD, FAAN
Editor, *Critical Care Nurse*
PO Box 6680
Annapolis, MD 21401-0680

Submissions are usually acknowledged within 2 weeks of receipt in the editorial office. If you do not receive acknowledgment in a timely fashion, please write to the editor. *Critical Care Nurse* accepts no responsibility for lost or mislaid materials, so authors are advised to keep copies in their possession. All articles are subject to peer review and copy editing. Submit four complete copies.

Please include a cover letter with the name, address, telephone number (home and work), and fax number (if available) of the author to whom all correspondence should be addressed.

On a separate sheet, include the following signed and dated copyright transfer statement:

> The undersigned author transfers all copyright ownership of the manuscript [insert title of manuscript] to the American Association of Critical-Care Nurses, in the event the work is accepted for publication in *Critical Care Nurse*. Permission to publish is also given for all subsequent use, including reprints, electronic media, audiovisual, and any other subsidiary print rights worldwide of said article. The author will have the right to use this material, provided permission is requested in writing from the publisher. The undersigned author affirms that this material is original, is not under consideration by another publication, and has not been previously published. I sign for and accept responsibility for releasing this material on behalf of any and all co-authors.

MANUSCRIPT PREPARATION GUIDELINES

The title page should contain the following: title of article, which should be to the point and reflect the substance of the article, and the authors' full names, with degrees, credentials, and institutional affiliations.

Feature articles should generally not exceed 15 pages, excluding references, tables, and figures.

References should be double-spaced at the end of the text. Number them consecutively by their order of appearance in the text and designate reference numbers as superscripts in the text. Do not use footnote function in WordPerfect. If a source lists more than six authors, list only three, followed by "et al." Follow the *American Medical Association Manual of Style,* 9th ed. (1998) for format and punctuation, as shown below.

For journals:

Last name and initials (without periods) of authors, title of article (capitalize only the first word, proper names, and abbreviations normally capitalized; no quotation marks), journal title (underline and use Index Medicus abbreviations), year of publication, volume, inclusive page numbers.

1. Reed FD, Watson NP. Nursing care of the patient with cardiomyopathy. *Am J Nurs.* 1985;4:121-124.

For books:

Last name and initials of authors, title of book (underline and capitalize all significant words), edition number (if after first edition), last name and initials of editor if any, city and state of publication, publisher, year of publication, page numbers (only if specifically cited).

2. Carlson ATC. *Critical Care Nursing Process.* 3rd ed. Boston, Mass: Beacon Hill Press; 1985:245-252.

For book chapters:

Last name and initials of authors, title of chapter, "In:" followed by last name and initials of editors, "ed.," title of book (as above), etc.

3. Schiffman JD. Immunology of influenza. In: Cane MB, ed. *Viruses and Influenza.* Orlando, Fla: Academic Press; 1990:191-196.

Tables must be titled and numbered consecutively (Table 1, Table 2) in the order mentioned in the text. Give each column a heading and explain abbreviations in the legend.

Figures of black-and-white line art and photographs of good quality will be considered. Color artwork should be submitted as slides or transparencies. For computer-generated graphics, please supply original files in Photoshop 3.0, Adobe Illustrator 5.5, or QuarkXpress 3.32 (or earlier versions of these programs). Contact the editorial office for further information 1-800-809-CARE or (949) 362-2000. Include signed consent/release forms from all identifiable individuals. If permission from subjects is not obtained, photographs will be cropped appropriately. Include the name of photographer or illustrator for credit line. Include signed consent/release from owner of photo or artist if different from author.

If any material in the article is from a prior copyrighted publication, include a letter of permission to reproduce the material from both the author and the copyright holder.

All accepted articles are subject to editing to conform to the format and style of *Critical Care Nurse,* as well as journalistic standards for clarity and grammar.

All material must be double-spaced, on white paper, with margins of at least 1 inch on all sides. Number all pages sequentially, including references, tables, and figures. For drug names, use generic names only. The trade name of a particular drug may be cited in parentheses the first time the generic name appears.

For units of measurement, report all physiologic measurements using the metric system. Use metric units or decimal multiples for length, height, weight, and volume. Show temperature in degrees Celsius and blood pressure in millimeters of mercury.

Avoid nonstandard abbreviations. Use the full term for an abbreviation or symbol on first reference, unless it is a standard unit of measure.

If the manuscript is accepted for publication, author will be required to send article on an IBM-compatible or Macintosh diskette.

REFEREED PUBLICATION

All articles are subject to peer review and copyediting.

COPYRIGHT

Copyright by the American Association of Critical-Care Nurses.

INDEXED

Critical Care Nurse is indexed in the *Cumulative Index to Nursing and Allied Health Literature, International Nursing Index, MEDLINE, NurseSearch, Nursing Abstracts, RNdex Top 100,* and *UMI (University Microfilms International) Article Clearinghouse.*

SAMPLE JOURNAL ARTICLE TITLES

- "A Research-Based Sibling Visitation Program for the Neonatal ICU"
- "Adult Respiratory Distress Syndrome After Near Drowning"
- "Breaking Down the Walls: Critical Care at Home and on the Road"
- "Psychosocial and Functional Outcomes in Women After Coronary Artery Bypass Surgery"
- "Women and Heart Disease: The Issues"

Critical Care Nursing Quarterly

Critical Care Nursing Quarterly is published by Aspen Publishers, Inc.

JOURNAL FOCUS/PURPOSE

The primary purpose of *Critical Care Nursing Quarterly* is to serve as a resource for continuing education and the clinical practice of critical care. Each issue addresses a timely topic of vital importance to nurses directly involved in the management of critically ill patients and their families and will be suitable for use as a supplementary text as well as a journal and reference work.

JOURNAL FACTS

Publication schedule: quarterly

Circulation: international

Submitted papers per year: approximately 75

Acceptance rate: approximately 80%

Monetary honorarium: none

Average turnaround time: 4 weeks

Publishing timetable: 3 months after acceptance

Correspondence:
Customer Services
200 Orchard Ridge Drive
Gaithersburg, MD 20878
Customer service telephone: 1-800-234-1660

Internet site: www.aspenpub.com (enter journal title in search box)

MANUSCRIPT SUBMISSION

The content of *Critical Care Nursing Quarterly* is topical and consists of articles written by various members of the intensive care professional team. Although the content of the issue is designed for direct application to clinical nursing practice, basic research is included when it is deemed essential to support a comprehensive presentation of a subject. Material from management, legal, behavioral, and other supporting sciences will be judiciously selected too in order to enhance certain topics.

To be considered for publication in this journal, articles should reflect the contemporary needs of clinicians and be prepared in accordance with the "Aspen Author's Manuscript Checklist for Journals."

Manuscripts (an original and three copies and a disk containing an exact version of the original hard copy) should be addressed to:

Janet Barber, Editor
Critical Care Nursing Quarterly
9383 E County Road 500 S
Greensburg, IN 47240-8138
E-mail: dlduval@seidata.com or
janet.barber@hill-rom.com

Invited papers: Manuscripts (one original and three copies) and a disk containing an exact version of the original hard copy of *invited* articles should be submitted to the *editor* (no later than the date indicated by the editor). A completed Article Submission Form and an original Copyright Release must accompany the submission. If the article is not accepted for publication, the copyright assignment will automatically return to the author.

Authors must release copyright ownership to their manuscript at the time of its submission to the journal. This form must accompany the manuscript before processing for publication can begin. It is understood that articles submitted to be published in the journal will not be submitted to any other publication.

Completed article submission form for each contributor

Written permission for any borrowed text, tables, or figures

MANUSCRIPT PREPARATION GUIDELINES

Manuscripts should be created using Aspen's Journals Authoring Template (template is available from your journal editor or from Aspen). Manuscripts should be created on IBM-compatible (PC) equipment using Windows 95 or higher operating system. Our preferred software is Microsoft Word. Hard copy and electronic files should be submitted for all text and all artwork. All disks submitted must be new. Disks should be clearly labeled as to operating system and software application.

Manuscripts should be double-spaced (including quotations, lists, references, footnotes, figure captions, and all parts of tables).

Manuscripts should be ordered as follows: title page, abstracts, text, references, appendixes, tables, and any illustrations.

Each manuscript must include the following:

Title page, including (1) title of the article, (2) author names (with highest academic degrees) and affiliations (including titles, departments, and name and location of institutions of primary employment), and (3) any acknowledgments, credits, or disclaimers

Abstract of 200 words or fewer describing the main points of the article. If it is a research article, prepare a structured abstract describing (1) what was observed or investigated, (2) the subjects and methods, and (3) the results and conclusions. Also include up to 10 key words that describe the contents of the article like those that appear in the *Cumulative Index to Nursing and Allied Health Literature (CINAHL)* or the *National Library of Medicine's Medical Subject Headings* (MeSH).

Clear indication of the placement of all tables and figures in text

Signed copyright transfer form

References must be cited in text and styled in the reference list according to the *American Medical Association Manual of Style*, 9th ed. (1998). References should not be created using Microsoft Word's automatic footnote/ endnote feature. References should be included on a separate page at the end of the article and should be double-spaced. References should be numbered consecutively in the order they are cited; reference numbers can be used more than once throughout an article. Page numbers should appear with the text citation following a specific quote.

Here are some examples of correctly styled reference entries:

Journals:

Author, article title, journal, year, volume, inclusive pages.

Doe J. Allied medical education. *JAMA.* 1975;23:170-184.

Doe J. Drug use during high school. *Am J Public Health.* 1976;64(5):12-22.

Books:

Author, book title, place of publication, publisher, year.

Farber SD. *Neurorehabilitation: A Multisensory Approach.* Philadelphia, Pa: Saunders; 1982.

Winawar S, Lipkin M. Proliferative abnormalities in the gastrointestinal tract. In: Card WI, Creamer B, eds. *Modern Trends in Gastroenterology.* 4th ed. London, England: Butterworth & Co; 1970.

For multiple authors in journals and books:

If six or fewer list all authors, and if more than six list the first three followed by et al.

Illustrations: Figures should be created using electronic software (i.e., Adobe Illustrator, Corel Draw, and Photoshop). Please save files in both the application in which they were created (i.e., Microsoft Word) and as either EPS or TIFF files. Use computer-generated lettering. Do not use screens, color, shading, or fine lines.

In lieu of original drawings and other material, a sharp, glossy, black-and-white photographic print between 5″ × 7″ and 8″ × 10″ is acceptable.

Each figure should have a label on the back indicating the number of the figure, the names of the authors, and the top of the figure. Do not write on the back of figures, mount them on cardboard, or scratch or mar them using paper clips. Do not bend figures.

Cite each figure in the text in consecutive order. If a figure has been previously published, in part or in total, acknowledge the original source and submit written permission from the copyright holder to reproduce or adapt the material. Include a source line. Type "Source: Author" on figures that you created. This will help Aspen identify the status of each figure.

Supply a caption for each figure, typed double-spaced on a separate sheet from the artwork. Captions should include the figure title, explanatory statements, notes, or keys as well as source and permission lines.

Provide a camera-ready copy and a separate electronic file for each piece of artwork. Do not embed art in your text file.

Tables should be on a separate page at the end of the manuscript. Number tables consecutively and supply a brief title for each. Include explanatory footnotes for all nonstandard abbreviations. For footnotes, use the following symbols, in this sequence: *, †, ‡, §, ‖, **, ††, etc. Cite each table in the text in consecutive order. If you use data from another published or unpublished source, obtain permission and acknowledge fully. Include a source line. Type "Source: Author" on tables that you created.

Permissions: Authors are responsible for obtaining signed letters from copyright holders granting permission to reprint material being borrowed or adapted from other sources, including previously published material of your own. Authors must obtain written permission for the following material (authors are responsible for any permission fees to reprint borrowed material):

All direct quotes of 300 words or more from any full-length book

All direct quotes of 200 words or more from a periodical article

All excerpts from a newspaper article or other short piece

Any passage from a play or a song

Two or more lines of poetry

Any borrowed table, figure, or illustration being reproduced exactly or adapted to fit the needs of the subject

REFEREED PUBLICATION

Critical Care Nursing Quarterly is a peer-reviewed journal with a blind review process.

COPYRIGHT

Copyright by Aspen Publishers, Inc.

INDEXED

Critical Care Nursing Quarterly is indexed in *Biological Abstracts, Cumulative Index to Nursing and Allied Health Literature, EMBASE (Excerpta Medica), Family Studies Database, Health Planning and Administration Database, Hospital and Health Administration Index, International Nursing Index, Nursing Scan in Critical Care, MEDLINE, Nursing Abstracts,* and *RNdex Top 100.*

SAMPLE JOURNAL ARTICLE TITLES

- "Current Trends in Ventilation of the Pediatric Patient"
- "Gastric Tonometry: Early Warning of Tissue Hypoperfusion"

- "New Trends in Thermometry for the Patient in the ICU"
- "Pediatric Traumatic Brain Injury"
- "Wound and Skin Care for the PICU"

Dimensions of Critical Care Nursing

Dimensions of Critical Care Nursing is published by Springhouse Corporation.

JOURNAL FOCUS/PURPOSE

The primary purpose of *Dimensions of Critical Care Nursing* is for critical care nursing, and its articles to reflect the critical care nurse's responsibilities and actions. *Dimensions of Critical Care Nursing* provides articles on advanced critical care nursing for experienced critical care nurses, CCRNs, nurse educators, managers, and clinical nurse specialists.

JOURNAL FACTS

Publication schedule: bimonthly

Circulation: not available

Submitted papers per year: 80

Acceptance rate: 50%

Monetary honorarium: none

Average turnaround time: 2 months

Publishing timetable: 10-12 months after acceptance

Correspondence:
Dimensions of Critical Care Nursing
Springhouse Corporation

1111 Bethlehem Pike
P.O. Box 908
Springhouse, PA 19477-0908
Telephone: (215) 646-8700
Fax: (215) 653-0826
E-mail: jan.enger@springnet.com

Internet site: www.springnet.com/criticalcare/dccn99.htm

MANUSCRIPT SUBMISSION

Address all questions and submission to:
Editor, *Dimensions of Critical Care Nursing*
Springhouse Corporation
1111 Bethlehem Pike, P.O. Box 908
Springhouse, PA 19477-0908

Please include your return address and both work and home phone numbers in all correspondence.

Submit the manuscript to *Dimensions of Critical Care Nursing* for sole consideration. Please send the original manuscript and three copies, plus keep a copy for yourself. Include a large self-addressed, stamped envelope, to speed return of the manuscript after review.

We will notify you of receipt of your manuscript. If it is not accepted, we will tell you the reasons why not and make specific suggestions for revision.

Dimensions of Critical Care Nursing uses a state-of-the-art, computer typesetting system. In the final step after acceptance, all final manuscripts must be submitted on computer disk. More information will be sent to authors at the time of acceptance.

Accepted manuscripts will be edited to conform with *Dimensions of Critical Care Nursing* format and style.

MANUSCRIPT PREPARATION GUIDELINES

Please use normal manuscript style, including double spacing of all lines in the manuscript, including references. Use wide margins and dark ink. Have all text in the front, and place all illustrations, one per page in the back. Spell out all abbreviations the first time they are used in the text and add unit names to all data or values.

Please follow these style points: (1) main subheads are in bold at the left margin, the next level of subheads are italic at the left margin, and any further level subheads, if needed, are indented into the paragraph in italics; (2) paragraphs are indented with a tab (not multiple spaces); (3) reference numbers in text are in superscript; (4) use plain type with no other "hidden codes" beyond those listed above. Do not use tab position changes, line space changes, font changes, underline, or any other hidden code changes within your text, because they interfere with the typesetter codes. (5) Type tables using the computer program's table feature. Don't use graphical text boxes, as they don't convert.

Include only those references actually used in the paper. Include references after all dosages, adverse effects, or other medical information and to reference studies or publications on which your manuscript is based. In the text,

use superscript numbers in consecutive order. Use the same number each time you cite the reference; do not use "ibid." or "op. cit." Accuracy and completeness of references is your responsibility.

For the reference list, *Dimensions of Critical Care Nursing* uses a modified *American Medical Association Manual of Style* format. Here's an example of the format for a journal article, followed by one for a book:

1. Artinian N. Selecting a model to guide family assessment. *Dimensions of Critical Care Nursing.* 1994;13(1):4-12.
2. Urden L, et al. *Essentials of Critical Care Nursing.* St. Louis, MO: Mosby-Year Book Inc; 1992:23-26.

Number each table or figure. Tables are illustrations that include words or numbers only. Figures include line drawings, pictures, or any material that cannot be typed. Add a comment in the text where the illustration should appear, such as "Figure 1 goes here." Then place the actual table or figure at the end of the manuscript. Include a caption for all figures and tables. On the back of all figures, very lightly done so as to leave no imprint on the face, identify each illustration with number, author's name, and an arrow pointing to the top.

Attach the following front pages to your manuscript:

1. Title page: List the article title and all authors' names with credentials.
2. Author page: List the contact author you've designated, address, and work and home phone numbers plus fax and e-mail if available. For all authors, list name, degrees/credentials, present position and employer, plus an additional sentence for any additional experience related to the topic of the article. This information will be used to compile "About the Authors," which will appear at the end of your article. We will address all correspondence to the designated contact author.

3. Abstract page: Include a two- or three-sentence paragraph that will capture reader's interest and that tells the main nursing focus of the paper.

For using, reproducing, or adapting charts, research tools, or any copyrighted material, get permission from the copyright holder before submitting the manuscript to DCCN. Get permission "to photograph and use the photograph in a professional publication" for all people in a picture. After you have received permission, add the credit line with copyright notation to the caption for the figure. Send the editor a copy of all permissions. Check all product and company names for accuracy. Getting permissions and checking accuracy of all material and references is your responsibility.

REFEREED PUBLICATION

Dimensions of Critical Care Nursing is a peer-reviewed, refereed journal with evaluation of all submitted manuscripts by several nurse-colleague reviewers.

COPYRIGHT

Copyright by Hall Johnson Communications, Inc.

INDEXED

Dimensions of Critical Care Nursing is indexed in the *Cumulative Index to Nursing and Allied Health Literature, International Nursing Index,* and *Nursing Abstracts.*

SAMPLE JOURNAL ARTICLE TITLES

- "Avoiding Respiratory Excursions: Obtaining Reliable Pulmonary Capillary Wedge Pressures"
- "Developing an Intensive Care Continuum: Incorporating Rehabilitation Services in Critical Care"
- "Low Cardiac Output Following Cardiac Surgery: Critical Thinking Steps"
- "Monitoring Patients With Acute Congestive Heart Failure"
- "Pediatric Pacemakers for Patients With Complete Heart Block"

Heart & Lung: The Journal of Acute and Critical Care

H*eart & Lung: The Journal of Acute and Critical Care* is published by Mosby, Inc.

JOURNAL FOCUS/PURPOSE

The primary purpose of *Heart & Lung: The Journal of Acute and Critical Care* is to publish articles describing investigations, advances, or observations regarding the care of the critically ill patient.

JOURNAL FACTS

Publication schedule: bimonthly
Circulation: approximately 5,000
Submitted papers per year: approximately 100

Acceptance rate: 60-65%

Monetary honorarium: none

Average turnaround time: unavailable

Publishing timetable: 3-6 months after acceptance

Correspondence:
Business Office
Mosby, Inc.
11830 Westline Industrial Drive
St. Louis, MO 63146-3318
Telephone: 1-800-453-4351
Fax: (314) 432-1158
E-mail: periodical.service@mosby.com

Internet site: www.mosby.com

MANUSCRIPT SUBMISSION

Heart & Lung: The Journal of Acute and Critical Care invites original articles describing investigations, advances, or observations regarding the care of the critically ill patient.

Manuscripts should be submitted to:
Kathleen S. Stone, PhD, RN, FAAN
Editor, *Heart & Lung*
Ohio State University, College of Nursing
1585 Neil Avenue
Columbus, OH 43210-1289

Most of the provisions of the Copyright Act of 1976 became effective on Jan. 1, 1978. Therefore, all manuscripts must be accompanied by the following written statement, signed by one author:

The undersigned author transfers all copyright ownership of the manuscript (title of article) to Mosby, Inc. in the event the work is published. The undersigned author warrants that the article is original, is not under consideration by another journal, and has not been previously published. I sign for and accept responsibility for releasing this material on behalf of any and all co-authors.

Authors will be consulted, when possible, regarding republication of their material.

MANUSCRIPT PREPARATION GUIDELINES

Manuscripts must be typewritten on one side of the paper only, with double spacing and liberal margins. The original and three copies of the manuscript are required along with four sets of figures and tables. Each article must be accompanied by an abstract (summary) not exceeding 150 words typed double-spaced on a separate sheet of paper. If unusual abbreviations cannot be avoided, use the expanded form when first mentioned and abbreviate thereafter. Standard chemical or nonproprietary pharmaceutical nomenclature should be used. Metric units and the centigrade scale are preferred. Manuscripts should be limited to 12 to 15 pages. Each page must be numbered. Once a manuscript is accepted, the final version of the manuscript may be submitted on diskette along with four copies of the printout. The author accepts responsibility for the submitted diskette's exactly matching the printout of the final version of the manuscript. Guidelines for submission of accepted manuscript on diskette will be sent to the author by the editorial office.

Original drawings or graphs must be drawn in black India ink. Typewritten or freehand lettering is not acceptable. All lettering must be done professionally and should be in proportion to the drawing, graph, or photograph. Do not send original artwork, X-ray films, or ECG tracings. Glossy print photographs, 3 × 4 inches (minimum) to 5 × 7 inches (maximum), with good black-and-white contrast or color balance are preferred. Any special instructions regarding sizing should be clearly noted. Electrocardiograms are notoriously difficult to reproduce adequately. ECG paper smudges easily, so great care must be exercised in the preparation of a glossy print. Unless a dysrhythmia is to be illustrated, one or two complexes should be photographed showing only those leads necessary to document the conclusions. A longer strip of a particularly illustrative lead may be used for dysrhythmias. All illustrations must be numbered and cited in the text. Typed legends must accompany each illustration and be listed on a separate page. Each illustration should have the following information lightly penciled on the back or typed on a gummed label affixed to the back of the figure: figure number, title of manuscript, and an arrow indicating the top of the figure. Do not use paper clips to secure illustrations because they can damage the surface. Place illustrations in a separate envelope and mail with the text. A letter of permission must accompany all photographs of persons when there is a possibility of identification. Illustrations will be returned only if requested by the author. Special arrangements must be made with the editors for color plates, elaborate tables, or extra illustrations.

Figures may be submitted in electronic format. All images should be at least 5″ wide. Images should be provided as EPS or TIFF files on Zip disk, CD, floppy, Jaz, or 3.5 MO. Macintosh or PC is acceptable. Graphics software such as Photoshop and Illustrator, not presentation software such as PowerPoint, CorelDraw, or Harvard Graphics, should be used in the creation of the art. Gray scale images should be at least 300 DPI (dots per inch) with a proof. Combination of gray scale and line art should be at least 1,200 DPI with a proof. Line art should be at least 1,200 DPI with a proof. Please include hardware and software information, in addition to the file names, with the disk.

Tables should be self-explanatory and should supplement, not duplicate, the text. Tables must be numbered consecutively and mentioned in the text, and each must have a title. Each table must be typed with double spacing on a separate sheet.

References must be cited consecutively in the text as superscript numerals. If the same reference is cited more than once, the original numeral is used. References should be typed double-spaced, on a separate sheet in numeric order.

Journal articles:

References to journal articles must contain, in order, the following information: authors' names (last names, initials); title of article (initial capital and lowercase, no quotation marks); journal name abbreviated as in Cumulated Index Medicus; and year of publication, volume number, and inclusive page numbers.

Batsone GF, Hinks L, Whitefoot R, Farral M, James LA, Lai LY, et al. Hormonal changes after thermal injury. J Endocrinol 1976;68:38-9.

Books:

References to books must include names of authors, book title (not italicized), volume number (if any), edition number (if any), city of publication, and, if applicable, pages cited.

Johanson BC, Dungca CU, Hoffmeister D, Wells SJ. Standards of critical care. 2nd ed. St. Louis: CV Mosby, 1985. p. 10, 12, 484-6.

For books with editors listed:

Banyai AL, Gordon BL, editors. Advances in cardiopulmonary disease. Chicago: Year Book Medical Publishers, 1989.

Luisada AA. Bedside diagnosis of dysrhythmias. In: Banyai AL, Gordon BL, editors. Advances in cardiopulmonary disease. Chicago: Year Book Medical Publishers, 1989:37-92.

Personal communication should not be included in the list of references but may be cited in the text in parentheses.

Manuscripts become the permanent property of *Heart & Lung: The Journal of Acute and Critical Care* and may not be published elsewhere without written permission from the author and journal publisher. All accepted manuscripts are subject to manuscript editing.

Animal experimentation must observe the "Guiding Principles in the Care and Use of Animals" published in the *Guide to Authors* of the American Physiological Society and be approved by the appropriate Animal Care Committee.

REFEREED PUBLICATION

All articles are subject to expert review and are accepted for publication with the understanding that they are contributed solely to *Heart & Lung: The Journal of Acute and Critical Care.*

COPYRIGHT

Copyright by Mosby, Inc.

INDEXED

Heart & Lung: The Journal of Acute and Critical Care is indexed in the *Cumulative Index to Nursing and Allied Health Literature, Current Contents/Clinical Medicine, Excerpta Medica, Index Medicus, International Nursing Index, Nursing Abstracts, MEDLINE,* and *Science Citation Index.*

SAMPLE JOURNAL ARTICLE TITLES

- "Atrial Infarction: A Clinical and Electrocardiographic Case Report"
- "Lung Volume Reduction: An Overview"
- "Perceptions of Patients With Cardiovascular Disease About the Causes of Coronary Artery Disease"
- "Perceived Learning Needs of Patients With Coronary Artery Disease Using a Questionnaire Assessment Tool"
- "Vascular Complications of Coronary Interventions"

Journal of Cardiovascular Nursing

The *Journal of Cardiovascular Nursing* is published by Aspen Publishers, Inc.

ments. The journal also publishes articles on innovations in practice and clinical questions.

JOURNAL FOCUS/PURPOSE

The primary purpose of the *Journal of Cardiovascular Nursing* is to foster expert clinical practice of cardiovascular nurses. Each topical issue addresses the physiological, psychological, and social responses of cardiovascular patients and families in a variety of environ-

JOURNAL FACTS

Publication schedule: quarterly

Circulation: approximately 2,800

Submitted papers per year: 40-45

Acceptance rate: 72%

Monetary honorarium: none

Average turnaround time: 6-8 weeks

Publishing timetable: approximately 3-4 months after acceptance

Correspondence:
Customer Services
200 Orchard Ridge Drive
Gaithersburg, MD 20878
Customer service telephone: 1-800-234-1660

Internet site: www.aspenpub.com (enter journal title in search box)

MANUSCRIPT SUBMISSION

Invited articles: JCN is a topic-oriented journal. Issue editors are engaged to design the journal contents and solicit authors. The number of invited manuscripts in an issue will usually be from four to six. An original and three copies of invited papers should be sent to the journal editor or directly to the issue editor where appropriate.

Unsolicited articles: Authors are encouraged to submit (1) original articles, based on observations or experimentation, that add new knowledge to the field of cardiovascular nursing and (2) analytical reviews that codify existing knowledge or throw light on the present and future roles of specialists in the field. The literature of nursing and related disciplines should be reviewed for the purpose of preparing complete and definitive manuscripts. The decision to accept or reject an article will be based on the judgment of peer reviewers. All unsolicited articles should be written to contribute to upcoming topics.

Before submitting an article, authors are requested to call either Barbara J. Riegel at (858) 594-6173 (O) or Debra K. Moser at (614) 292-4746 (O), depending on who is coordinating the issue to which the article pertains. This information is provided on the upcoming issues list available from Aspen Publishers, Inc.

After the article has been discussed, manuscripts (an original and three copies) and correspondence regarding publications should be addressed to the appropriate journal editor:

Barbara Riegel, DNSc, RN, CS, FAAN
15578 Raptor Road
Poway, CA 92064

Debra K. Moser, DNSc, RN
The Ohio State University, College of Nursing
1585 Neil Avenue
Columbus, OH 43210-1289

Please send a stamped, self-addressed postcard for acknowledgment of receipt.

MANUSCRIPT PREPARATION GUIDELINES

Manuscripts should be created using Aspen's Journals Authoring Template (template is available from your journal editor or from Aspen). Manuscripts should be created on IBM-compatible (PC) equipment using Windows 95 or higher operating system. Our preferred software is Microsoft Word. Hard copy and electronic files should be submitted for all text and all artwork. All disks submitted must be new. Disks should be clearly labeled as to operating system and software application.

Manuscripts should be double-spaced (including quotations, lists, references, footnotes, figure captions, and all parts of tables).

Manuscripts should be ordered as follows: title page, abstracts, text, references, appendixes, tables, and any illustrations.

Each manuscript must include the following:

Title page, including (1) title of the article, (2) author names (with highest academic degrees) and affiliations (including titles, departments, and name and location of institutions of primary employment), and (3) any acknowledgments, credits, or disclaimers

Abstract of 200 words or fewer describing the main points of the article. If it is a research article, prepare a structured abstract describing (1)

what was observed or investigated, (2) the subjects and methods, and (3) the results and conclusions. Also include up to 10 key words that describe the contents of the article like those that appear in the *Cumulative Index to Nursing and Allied Health Literature (CINAHL)* or the *National Library of Medicine's Medical Subject Headings* (MeSH).

Clear indication of the placement of all tables and figures in text

Signed copyright transfer form

Completed article submission form for each contributor

Written permission for any borrowed text, tables, or figures

References must be cited in text and styled in the reference list according to the *American Medical Association Manual of Style,* 9th ed. (1998). References should not be created using Microsoft Word's automatic footnote/endnote feature. References should be included on a separate page at the end of the article and should be double-spaced. References should be numbered consecutively in the order they are cited; reference numbers can be used more than once throughout an article. Page numbers should appear with the text citation following a specific quote.

Here are some examples of correctly styled reference entries:

Journals:

Author, article title, journal, year, volume, inclusive pages.

Doe J. Allied medical education. *JAMA.* 1975;23:170-184.

Doe J. Drug use during high school. *Am J Public Health.* 1976;64(5):12-22.

Books:

Author, book title, place of publication, publisher, year.

Farber SD. *Neurorehabilitation: A Multisensory Approach.* Philadelphia, Pa: Saunders; 1982.

Winawar S, Lipkin M. Proliferative abnormalities in the gastrointestinal tract. In: Card WI, Creamer B, eds. *Modern Trends in Gastroenterology.* 4th ed. London, England: Butterworth & Co; 1970.

For multiple authors in journals and books:

If six or fewer list all authors, and if more than six list the first three followed by et al.

Illustrations: Figures should be created using electronic software (i.e., Adobe Illustrator, Corel Draw, and Photoshop). Please save files in both the application in which they were created (i.e., Microsoft Word) and as either EPS or TIFF files. Use computer-generated lettering. Do not use screens, color, shading, or fine lines.

In lieu of original drawings and other material, a sharp, glossy, black-and-white photographic print between 5″ × 7″ and 8″ × 10″ is acceptable.

Each figure should have a label on the back indicating the number of the figure, the names of the authors, and the top of the figure. Do not write on the back of figures, mount them on cardboard, or scratch or mar them using paper clips. Do not bend figures.

Cite each figure in the text in consecutive order. If a figure has been previously published, in part or in total, acknowledge the original source and submit written permission from the copyright holder to reproduce or adapt the material. Include a source line. Type "Source: Author" on figures that you created. This will help Aspen identify the status of each figure.

Supply a caption for each figure, typed double-spaced on a separate sheet from the artwork. Captions should include the figure title, explanatory statements, notes, or keys as well as source and permission lines.

Provide a camera-ready copy and a separate electronic file for each piece of artwork. Do not embed art in your text file.

Tables should be on a separate page at the end of the manuscript. Number tables consecutively and supply a brief title for each. Include explanatory footnotes for all nonstandard abbreviations. For footnotes, use the following symbols, in this sequence: *, †, ‡, §, ||, **, ††, etc. Cite each table in the text in consecutive order. If you use data from another published or unpublished source, obtain permission and acknowledge fully. Include a source line. Type "Source: Author" on tables that you created.

Permissions: Authors are responsible for obtaining signed letters from copyright holders granting permission to reprint material being borrowed or adapted from other sources, including previously published material of your own. Authors must obtain written permission for the following material (authors are responsible for any permission fees to reprint borrowed material):

All direct quotes of 300 words or more from any full-length book

All direct quotes of 200 words or more from a periodical article

All excerpts from a newspaper article or other short piece

Any passage from a play or a song

Two or more lines of poetry

Any borrowed table, figure, or illustration being reproduced exactly or adapted to fit the needs of the subject

Drug names: The generic (nonproprietary) name of a drug should be used throughout a manuscript. Use the complete name of a drug, including the salt or ester (e.g., tetracy-

cline hydrochloride) at first mention and elsewhere in contexts involving dosage. When no generic name exists for a drug, give the chemical name or formula or description of the names of the active ingredients.

REFEREED PUBLICATION

Journal of Cardiovascular Nursing is a peer-reviewed journal with a blind review process.

COPYRIGHT

Copyright by Aspen Publishers, Inc.

INDEXED

The *Journal of Cardiovascular Nursing* is indexed in the *Cumulative Index to Nursing and Allied Health Literature, Index Medicus, MEDLINE/MEDLARS, International Nursing Index, Nursing Abstracts, Nursing Scan in Critical Care,* and *RNdex Top 100.*

SAMPLE JOURNAL ARTICLE TITLES

- "Cardiovascular Clinical Specialist: Insights and Inspirations"
- "Discoverer, Teacher, Friend: A Tribute to Marguerite Kinney"
- "Dysrhythmia Update: Differential Diagnosis of Supraventricular Tachycardia in an Elderly Man"
- "The Value of Mentors and Facilitators in the Pursuit of Excellence"
- "Use of Antimicrobial Agents in Patients With Cardiovascular Infection"

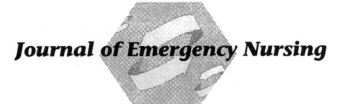

Journal of Emergency Nursing

The *Journal of Emergency Nursing* is published by Mosby, Inc., and is the official journal of the Emergency Nurses Association.

JOURNAL FOCUS/PURPOSE

The primary purpose of the *Journal of Emergency Nursing* is to contribute to the education and professional advancement of emergency nurses.

JOURNAL FACTS

Publication schedule: bimonthly

Circulation: approximately 29,000

Submitted papers per year: approximately 275

Acceptance rate: approximately 30%

Monetary honorarium: none

Average turnaround time: 8-12 weeks

Publishing timetable: approximately 4 months after acceptance

Correspondence:
Business Office
Mosby, Inc.
11830 Westline Industrial Drive
St. Louis, MO 63146-3318
Telephone: 1-800-453-4351
Fax: (314) 432-1158
E-mail: periodical.service@mosby.com

Internet site: www.ena.org

MANUSCRIPT SUBMISSION

Please submit all manuscripts to the following address:

Gail Pisarcik Lenehan, EdD, RN

Editor, *Journal of Emergency Nursing*
216 Higgins Road
Park Ridge, IL 60068-5736
Telephone: (847) 698-9400 or 1-800-900-9659
Fax: (847) 698-9407
E-mail: glenehan@ena.org

In accordance with the Copyright Act of 1976, which became effective January 1, 1978, the following statement signed by the senior or corresponding author must accompany manuscripts:

The undersigned author transfers all copyright ownership of the manuscript entitled (title of article) to the Emergency Nurses Association in the event the work is published. The undersigned author warrants that the article is original, is not under consideration by another journal, and has not been previously published. I sign for and accept responsibility for releasing this material on behalf of any and all co-authors.

MANUSCRIPT PREPARATION GUIDELINES

The *Journal of Emergency Nursing* welcomes articles relating to the broad field of emergency care nursing as well as articles concerning providers of emergency care. Special consideration will be given to manuscripts from clinical nurses and ED nurse managers.

Manuscripts are reviewed by editorial board members and selected experts in appropriate specialties with the understanding that the work is original and is contributed exclusively to the Journal. Authors will be notified on receipt of their manuscripts. The review process customarily requires 8 weeks, though there are exceptions. Inquiry calls after 8 weeks to ask about the decision are welcomed. Acceptance is based on originality of ideas, significance for emergency nursing, validity, and adherence to the prescribed submission requirements. Some degree of manuscript revision of content and style should be expected with all manuscripts.

The Journal requires all authors to acknowledge, on the title page of their manuscript, all funding sources that supported their work, as well as all institutional or corporate affiliations of all the authors. Authors are also required to disclose to the editor, in a covering letter at the time of submission of their manuscript, any commercial associations that could pose a conflict of interest or create a bias. These include consultant arrangements, honoraria, patent licensing arrangements, or payments for conducting or publicizing a study. If the article is accepted for publication, the editor will determine how any conflict of interest should be disclosed. Authors are expected to fulfill the requirements of their employer's publication policy before submitting their manuscript.

The original and five copies of manuscripts and supporting material should be submitted to the editor or appropriate section editor. One complete copy should be retained by the author. Manuscripts must be typed double-spaced (including references and tables) on $8\frac{1}{2}$ × 11-inch paper with $1\frac{1}{4}$-inch margins. Typeface must be 12 points or larger. Clinical articles should be limited to 6 to 8 typewritten pages. The manuscript should be numbered in the upper right-hand corner. Submission by disk is preferred and encouraged. Once a manuscript is accepted, the final version of the manuscript should, if possible, be submitted on diskette along with two copies of the printout. The author accepts responsibility for the submitted diskette's exactly matching the printout of the final version of the manuscript. Guidelines for submission of accepted manuscripts on diskette will be sent to the author by the editorial office.

The title page should include the title, full name(s) of author(s), academic degrees, city, and state. The corresponding author should be designated; include home address, business and home phone numbers, fax number, and e-mail address. At the bottom of the page, give the author's position and institutional affiliation.

Each article requires an abstract, the style of which varies according to the type of article. Studies require a structured abstract roughly based on the *IMRAD* style. The format should be as follows: introduction, methods, results, and discussion. Structured abstracts should not exceed 200 words and will be presented with the article. All other clinical articles use a standard abstract format, not to exceed 50 words in length. These abstracts are adapted to appear in the table of contents. All abstracts should be typed double-spaced on a separate sheet of paper.

Standard abbreviations should be used consistently throughout the article. Unusual or coined abbreviations should be spelled out at first mention and followed in parentheses by the abbreviation. The policy of the Journal is to abbreviate the term *emergency department* when it modifies a word (e.g., "ED procedure") and to spell it out when it is used as a noun (e.g., "in the emergency department"). The term *emergency nurse* should be used.

The generic name of a drug should be used instead of the proprietary name whenever possible. If it is necessary to use a trade name for a drug, it should be capitalized and inserted parenthetically after the generic name when first mentioned. Product names should be treated similarly, and the manufacturer's full name, city, and state should be cited in a footnote or in parentheses in the text.

Weights and measurements should be expressed in metric units and temperature in degrees centigrade, followed with Fahrenheit degrees in parentheses.

References should be to the original sources of information in most instances. A maximum of 15 citations should be adequate for clinical articles. Number references sequentially in order of their mention in the text, and type the reference list double-spaced at the end of the text. Bibliographies will not be published. Accuracy of references is the responsibility of the author. References should start on a separate page. Our reference style follows the Vancouver style of citation. Examples are shown below. More detailed information is available from the editorial office.

For standard journal articles, list all authors when seven or less; when more than seven, list six plus et al.:

You CH, Lee KY, Chey RY, Menguy R. Electrogastrographic study of patients with unexplained nausea, bloating, and vomiting. Gastroenterology 1980;79:311-4.

Format for books:

Weinstein L, Swartz MN. Pathogenic properties of invading microorganisms. In: Sodeman WA Jr, Sodeman WA, editors. Pathologic physiology: mechanisms of disease. Philadelphia: Saunders, 1974, p. 457-72.

Tables should be typed double-spaced on separate sheets of paper. They should be numbered in order of their mention in the text. Be sure that a title is included for each table and that full credit is given (in the form of a footnote to the table) to the original source of previously published material.

Send one complete set of illustrations. Number figures consecutively in order of their mention in the text. Mark lightly in grease or soft-lead pencil on the back of the illustration the figure number and name of the first author. Indicate orientation by marking the top edge. Drawings or graphs should be prepared in black India ink or typographic (press-apply) lettering; typewritten and freehand lettering are unacceptable. Do not send original artwork, X-ray films, or EKG strips. Black-and-white glossy prints, 3 × 4 inches (minimum) or larger, are preferred. Consistency in size of illustrations within the article is strongly preferred. Any special instructions regarding sizing should be clearly noted. It is preferable to omit figures rather than submit inadequate ones. Do not mount illustrations or mar the surface with clips or staples. Illustrations will not be returned unless requested. Legends must accompany each figure. Type legends separately and include after the references. If an illustration was previously published, the legend must give full credit to the original source.

Figures may be submitted in electronic format. All images should be at least 5 inches wide. Images should be provided as EPS or TIFF files on Zip disk, CD, floppy, Jaz, or 3.5 MO. Macintosh or PC platform is acceptable. Graphics software such as Photoshop and Illustrator, not presentation software such as PowerPoint, CorelDraw, or Harvard Graphics, should be used in the creation of the art. Gray scale images should be at least 300 DPI (dots per inch) with a proof. Gray scale line art should be at least 1,200 DPI with a proof. Please include hardware and software information, in addition to file names and fonts, with the disk.

Individual reprints of an article may be obtained from the author.

Authors are not routinely advised of specific reasons for the rejection of their manuscripts, but this information can be shared with individual authors by request.

Direct quotations, tables, and illustrations that have appeared in copyrighted material must be accompanied by written permission for their use from the copyright owner and original author and complete source information cited. Photographs of identifiable persons, whether patients or staff, must be accompanied by signed releases, such as the following: "I hereby give [author's name] permission to use the photograph of [subject's name] in the *Journal of Emergency Nursing.*"

REFEREED PUBLICATION

The *Journal of Emergency Nursing* is a peer-reviewed journal with a blind review process.

COPYRIGHT

Author(s) will be consulted, whenever possible, regarding republication of material. Since articles published in the Journal are copyrighted by Emergency Nurses Association, authors who wish to republish their work in part or whole elsewhere must request permission to do so.

INDEXED

The *Journal of Emergency Nursing* is indexed in the *Cumulative Index to Nursing and Allied Health Literature, Nursing Abstracts,* and *International Nursing Index.*

SAMPLE JOURNAL ARTICLE TITLES

- "Assessing Security in the Emergency Department: An Overview"
- "ED Physician House Staff Response to Training on Domestic Violence"
- "Latex Allergy: A Review"
- "Latex Allergy: Accessing Information on the Internet"
- "The Prehospital 12-lead EKG: Starting Outside the Emergency Department"

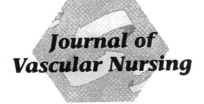

JOURNAL FOCUS/PURPOSE

The primary purpose of the *Journal of Vascular Nursing* is to provide nurses and other health care professionals with information to foster expert clinical practice in vascular nursing.

The *Journal of Vascular Nursing* is published by Mosby, Inc., and is the official journal of the Society for Vascular Nursing.

JOURNAL FACTS

Publication schedule: quarterly

Circulation: 1,400

Submitted papers per year: 20-25

Acceptance rate: 75-85%

Monetary honorarium: none

Average turnaround time: 6-8 weeks

Publishing timetable: 3-12 months after acceptance

Correspondence:
Business Office
Mosby, Inc.
11830 Westline Industrial Drive

St. Louis, MO 63146-3318
Telephone: 1-800-453-4351
Fax: (314) 432-1158
E-mail: periodical.service@mosby.com
Internet site: www.mosby.com

MANUSCRIPT SUBMISSION

As the official publication of the Society for Vascular Nursing, the Journal will publish, after editorial review, selected papers presented at the annual meeting of the society, as well as original articles from members and nonmembers.

Readers interested in submitting original manuscripts for possible publication should send the manuscript to:

Victoria A. Fahey, RN, MSN, CVN
1550 Lake Shore Dr., No. 4A
Chicago, IL 60610
Telephone: (312) 908-4975
E-mail: vfoley@nmh.org

Or to:

Janice D. Nunnelee, PhD, RN, CS/ANP, CVN
West County Family Practice
14377 Woodlake, No. 300
Chesterfield, MO 63107
Telephone: (314) 434-3333

Statements and opinions expressed in the *Journal of Vascular Nursing* are those of the author(s) and do not necessarily reflect those of the editors, the publisher, or the Society for Vascular Nursing; the editors, the publisher, and the society disclaim any responsibility or liability for such material. Neither the editors, the publisher, nor the society guarantees, warrants, or endorses any product or service advertised in this publication, and they do not guarantee any claim made by the manufacturer of such product or service.

As a result of the Copyright Act of 1976, which became effective on January 1, 1978,

the following statement, signed by one author, must accompany each manuscript submitted:

> The undersigned author transfers all copyright ownership of the manuscript (title of manuscript) to the Society for Vascular Nursing in the event the work is published. The undersigned author warrants that the article is original, is not under consideration by another journal, and has not been previously published. I sign for and accept responsibility for releasing this material on behalf of any and all co-authors. (Signature)

Manuscripts accepted for publication become the sole property of the Journal and may not be published in whole or in part without written consent of the publisher. Authors will be consulted, when possible, regarding republication of their material.

MANUSCRIPT PREPARATION GUIDELINES

A cover letter should identify the name, address, daytime telephone number, and fax number of the author(s).

An original and three clear photocopies of all typewritten material (including text, references, legends, and tables) and one set of glossy black-and-white 5 × 7-inch prints of photographs or line drawings must be submitted along with the aforementioned copyright transfer and cover letter.

All manuscripts, including text, references, legends, and tables, must be typed double-spaced on one side only of $8\frac{1}{2} \times 11$-inch paper with $1\frac{1}{2}$- to 2-inch margins. The pages must be numbered consecutively in the upper right-hand corner beginning with the title page, followed by text, references, legends, and tables. The length of the manuscript, including all supporting material, must not exceed 20 double-spaced typewritten pages. Once a manuscript is accepted, the final version should be submitted on diskette along with four copies of the printout. The author accepts responsibility for the submitted diskette's exactly matching the printout of the final version of the manuscript. Guidelines for submission of accepted manuscript on diskette will be sent to the author by the editorial office.

The following order of items should appear on the title page: title of manuscript, full name of each author along with highest earned academic degree and institutional affiliation, the name and address of the primary (corresponding) author, the name and address of the author who will receive reprint requests, acknowledgment of any grant support or other financial assistance received, and if the paper has been previously presented, the meeting name, date, and place where presented.

A one-paragraph abstract (double-spaced) of the manuscript should be included. This will be published with the manuscript.

All text material must be typed double-spaced. Manuscripts are subject to editing to conform to the Journal's standards. Generic drug names should be used whenever possible. Names of devices or products other than drugs must be accompanied by the name and city/state of the manufacturer. All standard abbreviations should be spelled out when the term is first mentioned, followed by the abbreviation in parentheses; nonstandard abbreviations should be avoided.

References should be cited selectively. All references should be verified and cited consecutively in the text as superscript numerals. The reference list must be typed double-spaced on a separate page in numeric order. A reference to an article in press must include the author name(s), title of article, and name of journal. A reference to a book in press must include all information with the exception of the year of publication and page numbers. Reference format should conform to that set forth in "Uniform Requirements for Manuscripts Submitted to Biomedical Journals" (Vancouver style) (1994). Abbreviations of journal names should conform to those in *Index Medicus*. If there are six or fewer authors or editors, cite all; if there are seven or more authors or editors, cite the first six with "et al." If the journal is paged sequentially throughout the volume, the issue number should not be cited; if the journal is not paged sequentially throughout the volume, then both the issue number and the volume number should be cited. Note the following examples:

Journal:

> Robinson LC. Chronic arterial occlusive disease of the lower extremities. J Vasc Nurs 1991;9:28.

Book:

> Hallet JW, Brewster DC, Darling RC. Patient care in vascular surgery. Boston: Little, Brown; 1987:31-5.

Chapter in book:

> Doyle JE. Renovascular hypertension. In Fahey VA, Editor. Vascular nursing. Philadelphia: WB Saunders, 1994, p. 368-90.
> Thesis:
> Munro P. Nursing and politics [thesis]. Berkeley (CA): University of California, 1989. 140 p.

Number illustrations consecutively in the order of text mention. On adhesive-backed labels, type the figure number, article title, and name of first author; indicate the top. Do not mount the illustrations on cardboard. Original drawings or graphs should be prepared in black India ink or typographic (press-apply) lettering. Typewritten or freehand lettering is unacceptable. All lettering must be professionally done and should be in proportion to the drawing, graph, or photograph. Do not send original artwork or X-ray films. Glossy print photographs 5 × 7 inches (maximum), with good black-and-white contrast are preferred. Consistency in size within the article is strongly preferred. Type legends double-spaced on a separate sheet of paper. Illustrations will be returned only if requested by the author.

Tables should be self-explanatory and not duplicate the text. Number tables consecutively in Roman numerals according to the order of text citation. Provide a brief title for each table.

Single reprints may be obtained from the author. Reprint order forms will be sent to authors as articles are published.

Written permission of the copyright holder and author for figures, tables, or quotation (200 words or more) taken from copyrighted material must accompany the submitted manuscript. The credit line should appear in the figure legend, as a footnote to the table, or as a footnote to the text, and should be worded according to the copyright holder's specifications. Subject or guardian consent must accompany any photograph that shows a recognizable likeness of a subject.

REFEREED PUBLICATION

Manuscripts are reviewed by the Editorial Board for accuracy, clarity, and significance to the practice of vascular nursing. The review process takes approximately 3 months. Accepted manuscripts are subject to copyediting to conform to the Journal's standards. Editing changes and recommendations are subject to author approval on galley proofs before publication.

COPYRIGHT

Copyright by the Society for Vascular Nursing, Inc.

INDEXED

The *Journal of Vascular Nursing* is indexed in the *Cumulative Index to Nursing and Allied Health Literature, International Nursing Index, Nursing Abstracts,* and *MEDLINE.*

SAMPLE JOURNAL ARTICLE TITLES

- "Marfan's Syndrome: A Family Affair"
- "Quality of Life After Lower-Extremity Revascularization"
- "Surveillance of Vascular Incisions: Outcomes of a Four Year Unit-Based Quality-Improvement Program"
- "Using Arm Vein as an Alternative Conduit for Lower-Extremity Bypass"
- "Vascular Nurse Practitioner: Development of an Innovative Role for the 21st Century"

Progress in Cardiovascular Nursing

Progress in Cardiovascular Nursing is published by Le Jacq Communications, Inc., and is the official journal of the American Society of Cardiovascular Nursing.

JOURNAL FOCUS/PURPOSE

The primary purpose of *Progress in Cardiovascular Nursing* is to provide a scholarly forum for communicating clinical practice and research. The journal reflects current practice of cardiovascular nursing in a wide range of environments, from prevention/rehabilitation to acute and chronic care, with an emphasis on new trends, innovations, and research as applicable in the clinical setting.

JOURNAL FACTS

Publication schedule: quarterly

Circulation: 4,000

Submitted papers per year: approximately 20

Acceptance rate: 85%

Monetary honorarium: none

Average turnaround time: 6-12 weeks

Publishing timetable: 6-12 months after acceptance

Correspondence:
Le Jacq Communications, Inc.
777 West Putnam Avenue
Greenwich, CT 06830
Telephone: (203) 531-0450
Fax: (203) 531-1713

Internet site: not available

MANUSCRIPT SUBMISSION

We invite authors to submit original or review articles or reports concerned with cardiovascular nursing implications pertaining to specific segments of the profession (i.e., CCU, cardiac catheterization lab, clinic, cardiologist office, cardiac rehabilitation, chest pain center, acute care, heart failure, lipid, and obesity clinics, etc.). Each manuscript submitted will consider what is useful to the cardiovascular nurse from a "how to" practical/clinical perspective.

Address all submission to:
Editor, *Progress in Cardiovascular Nursing*
777 West Putnam Avenue
Greenwich, CT 06830

A cover letter signed by all authors should identify the contact person, listing his or her address, telephone, and fax number. Any submissions without art may be e-mailed to managingeditor@lejacq.com.

Submit an original manuscript with three sets of original figures and four copies of the complete manuscript. Use standard-sized paper and double-space throughout. The author should retain a copy as manuscripts will not be returned.

Please send a copy of the manuscript on a 3.5″ DS, HD disk (in Macintosh; Microsoft Word 6.0.1 or less; or IBM: WordPerfect for Windows 5.1 or less).

MANUSCRIPT PREPARATION GUIDELINES

Articles should not exceed 5,000 words (roughly 20 double-spaced typewritten pages) and approximately 50 references. Please supply a word count (not including abstract or references).

Refer to drugs and devices generically. Do not use abbreviations in the title, and when used in the text provide the full name on first use with abbreviation in brackets.

The title page should include the full name, highest academic degree, and university or hospital affiliation of each author. Designate a name, address, and telephone number for reprint requests. Also includes a running title not exceeding 45 letters and spaces.

An abstract of 150 words or less should cover the main point of the review or report, statement of the issue or research question, methods and results of investigation, conclusions from the body of research or specific investigation, recommendations for practice, and questions requiring further study. Abstract should be on a separate page following the title page.

List references according to *American Medical Association (AMA) Manual of Style* (8th ed.), in the order in which they are cited in the text. References first cited in tables and figure legends must be numbered so that they will be in sequence with references cited in the text. Authors are responsible for the completeness and accuracy of all cited references. In text, tables, and figure legends, identify a reference with a superscript arabic numeral. Personal communications and unpublished data should be included within the text of the manuscript, not as references.

Examples of Reference Formats:

1. Seizer A, Langston M, Ruggeroll C, et al. Clinical syndrome of variant angina with normal coronary arteriogram. *N Engl J Med*. 1976;295:1343-1351.
2. Thom TJ. Cardiovascular disease mortality among United States women. In: Eaker ED, Packard B, Wenger NK, et al. (eds). *Coronary Heart Disease in Women*. New York: Haymarket Doyma; 1987:33-41.

Double-space tables and provide title for each. Number them in order of their citation in the text. Define table abbreviations at the bottom of the table. Cite data from studies according to numbered references. Provide tables on separate sheet of paper.

We welcome illustrations and figures. Submit (1) high-quality, glossy, unmounted black-and-white photographs; (2) black-and-white slides; or (3) professionally designed original artwork.

Number each illustration consecutively and cite in the text. Each photograph should have a gummed label on the back containing the figure number, title of manuscript, name of senior author, and an arrow indicating the top of the figure. Do not write on the back of the photograph. Include a complete, typed legend for each illustration. Acknowledge all illustrations and tables taken from other publications, and submit written permission to reprint from the original publishers. Obtaining permission to reprint is the responsibility of the author.

Page proofs must be returned within 7 days of receipt unless otherwise stated; late return may cause a delay in publication of an article. Please check text, tables, legends, and references carefully.

We include forms for ordering reprints with the author's copy of the issue in which his or her paper is published. Reprints must be prepaid in full before an order will be processed.

REFEREED PUBLICATION

Manuscripts submitted are peer-reviewed and publication cannot be guaranteed. Manuscripts are submitted with the understanding that they have not been published previously and are not under consideration by another publication. Manuscripts that are accepted are subject to copyediting by our staff; the author receives a copyedited draft for approval before publication. We make every attempt to provide rapid review and publication.

COPYRIGHT

Copyright by Le Jacq Communications, Inc.

INDEXED

Progress in Cardiovascular Nursing is indexed in the *Cumulative Index to Nursing & Allied Health, Index Medicus, International Nursing Index,* and *RNdex Top 100.*

SAMPLE JOURNAL ARTICLE TITLES

- "Heart Failure: Living With Uncertainty"
- "Learning How to Perform a 12-Lead ECG Using Virtual Reality"
- "Post Procedural Interventional Cardiology Patients on the Progressive Care Unit"
- "Update on the Treatment of Heart Failure"
- "When, How, and Why of Advance Directives"

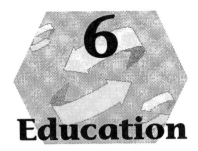

Education

Imprint

Imprint is published by the National Student Nurses' Association and is the official journal for the National Student Nurses' Association.

New York, NY 10019
Telephone: (212) 581-2211
Fax: (212) 581-2368
E-mail: NSNA@NSNA.ORG
Internet site: www.nsna.org

JOURNAL FOCUS/PURPOSE

The primary purpose of *Imprint* is to disseminate association news and articles of student opinion on current issues or trends in nursing and nursing education. Features include reports on national legislation affecting health, articles on programs and projects in which association members are involved, and help in career planning.

JOURNAL FACTS

Publication schedule: five times per year
Circulation: 48,000
Submitted papers per year: 100
Acceptance rate: 25%
Monetary honorarium: none
Average turnaround time: 2 months
Publishing timetable: 12 months after acceptance
Correspondence:
   Imprint
   National Student Nurses' Association, Inc.
   555 W. 57th Street

MANUSCRIPT SUBMISSION

Two copies of the manuscripts should be submitted to:

   Carolyn Jaffe, Managing Editor, *Imprint*
   National Student Nurses' Association, Inc.
   555 W. 57th Street
   New York, NY 10019
   E-mail: cardine@nsna.org

Once your article is submitted, you will receive an acknowledgment card from us. Reading and evaluating articles takes time, so please be patient. We will notify you of our decision as soon as possible.

MANUSCRIPT PREPARATION GUIDELINES

All manuscripts should be typed, double-spaced, on only one side of the paper, with a 1-inch margin on all sides. Recommended length for features and general articles is 1,500-2,000 words. Submissions for columns, such as "Issues," "Image," and "Reflections," should be between 800-1,000 words. The author's name should appear at the right-hand top of each page, and all pages should be numbered consecutively. Manuscripts should be submitted on computer disk (3.5) along with a hard copy. National Student Nurses' Association uses Microsoft Word for Windows. All accepted manuscripts become the property of National Student Nurses' Association and cannot be reproduced elsewhere without the permission of National Student Nurses' Association.

Information not drawn from personal experience—that is, factual information, ideas, and interpretations attributed to other individuals—must be documented. They are cited in the references. All references should appear in the text with superscript numbers, in the order they appear in the text. They should be listed at the end of the article on a separate page labeled "References," also in numerical order. References include quotations from another author (which should appear in quotations, exactly as they were written) or facts from a book or magazine article.

Book:

> *Name of the author(s), name of book (<u>underscored</u>), place of publication, publisher, date of publication, and page(s) of citation.*

> Zinsser, W. K. <u>On Writing Well</u>. New York, Harper & Row, pp. 47-50.

Chapter in a book:

> Gadow, Sally, Nursing and the Humanities: an approach to humanistic issues in health care. In: Bandman, E. L. K. and Bandman, Bertram, eds., <u>Bioethics and Human Rights</u>. Boston, Little Brown, 1978, pp. 305-312.

Magazine:

> *Author or authors. Title or article (no quotation marks, first word started with capital). Volume number, issue number, pages cited, month, and year of issue.*

> Robb, S. R. and others. Advocacy for the ages. AJN 79:10:1736-1738, Oct. 1979.

All books and magazine articles used but not cited should be placed in a bibliography on a separate page labeled "Bibliography." The same information needed for references should be included, except for page numbers, unless from a magazine or specific book chapter.

Footnotes are used to add or explain an item in the text, such as a personal communication. A footnote can also be used for a citation if there is only one citation in your article. In this case, include the same information as with the references. Footnotes should be numbered consecutively, should appear slightly above the line, and should not be enclosed in parentheses.

Photos accompanying the article can be black and white or color and should be in good condition, with identifying captions on the back, as well as who the photo should be returned to.

REFEREED PUBLICATION

Articles are not peer-reviewed for this journal.

COPYRIGHT

Copyright by the National Student Nurses Association, Inc.

INDEXED

Imprint is indexed in *International Nursing Index*.

SAMPLE JOURNAL ARTICLE TITLES

- "Community-Based Nursing Education at Northeastern University"
- "Community Health Nursing: A Challenging Career"
- "Facing Today's Job Market"
- "Graduate Education in Nursing: An Update"
- "School Nursing"

Journal of Continuing Education in Nursing

The *Journal of Continuing Education in Nursing: Continued Competence for the Future* is published by SLACK Incorporated.

JOURNAL FOCUS/PURPOSE

The primary purpose of the *Journal of Continuing Education in Nursing: Continued Competence for the Future* is to contribute to developing the body of knowledge, theory, and methods in continuing education and staff development in nursing by doing the following:

1. Disseminating relevant and critical perspectives pertinent to the practice of continuing education and staff development in nursing
2. Evaluating the impact that issues in health care nursing and education have on continuing education and staff development in nursing
3. Reporting on educational approaches proven effective in meeting some of the learning needs of nurses in practice
4. Reporting research findings resulting from studies conducted in the field of continuing education and staff development in nursing
5. Analyzing career development issues related to continuing education and staff development in nursing

JOURNAL FACTS

Publication schedule: bimonthly
Circulation: approximately 3,200
Submitted papers per year: average 60
Acceptance rate: approximately 84%
Monetary honorarium: none
Average turnaround time: 2-3 months
Publishing timetable: approximately 12-18 months after acceptance
Correspondence:
Managing Editor
Journal of Continuing Education in Nursing
SLACK Incorporated
6900 Grove Road
Thorofare, NJ 08086-9447
Telephone: (856) 848-1000 or 1-800-257-8290
Fax: (856) 853-5991
Internet site: www.slackinc.com/jcen.htm

MANUSCRIPT SUBMISSION

Submit an original and four photocopies, typed on one side only of standard-size white bond paper to:

Managing Editor, *Journal of Continuing Education in Nursing*
SLACK Incorporated
6900 Grove Road
Thorofare, NJ 08086-9447

Manuscripts will be considered for publication with the understanding that they are original contributions that have not been published previously and are not under consideration by another publication. The editor is Patricia S. Yoder-Wise, RN, C, EdD, CNAA, FAAN, Dean, School of Nursing, Texas Tech University, Health Sciences Center, Lubbock, Texas.

Manuscripts must be accompanied by a letter of copyright transmittal containing the following language in order to be reviewed for possible publication:

MANUSCRIPT PREPARATION GUIDELINES

Manuscripts should focus on any area of continuing education or staff development as referenced in the journal's Statement of Purpose. Research articles must include appropriate analysis tables. Manuscripts can range from 6 to 15 pages in length. Articles must conform to the following guidelines.

Typing should be double-spaced throughout the manuscript, including title page, acknowledgments, abstract, text, references, figure legends, and tables. Dot matrix printing is unacceptable unless it is letter quality.

Title page should include the title of the manuscript; author information should be listed on a separate page and include author's name, highest academic degree, nursing licensure and certification designations, present position and institution's name and city, correspondence address, and telephone and fax numbers. If there are multiple authors, list in the order names should appear if manuscript is published.

Include an abstract of approximately 100 words with a focus on findings and conclusions. Identify the key words that literature searches would use to locate your manuscript if it were published.

The journal follows the style guidelines delineated in the *Publication Manual of the American Psychological Association,* 4th ed. (1994). References must conform to APA style. The author must assume responsibility for the accuracy of references.

Tables should be placed at the end of the manuscript, one to a page. Figures, charts, and illustrations should be placed at the end of the manuscript, one to a page, black and white only, camera ready; glossy black-and-white photographs may be used if appropriate.

If academic, hospital, or business affiliations are given or referred to in the manuscript, it is the responsibility of the author to obtain permission from the proper authorities to use the names of such. It is also the author's responsibility to obtain written permission to reprint previously published information, charts, tables, and the like.

Manuscripts should include a self-addressed postage-paid postcard with the title of the manuscript, to be returned to the author as acknowledgment of receipt.

Extensive reviews of the literature are discouraged. Research projects with limited sample size, nonsignificant findings, and similar limitations should be converted to a nonresearch format in order to share the ideas(s) for further research.

REFEREED PUBLICATION

Manuscripts meeting the above guidelines go through the classic peer review process common to most respected professional journals. Anonymously, peers review each manuscript and approve or disapprove based on merit and clarity of presentation. This process reinforces not only the integrity of the *Journal of Continuing Education in Nursing* but also the profession through the dissemination of professional knowledge.

Manuscripts are not returned to authors after review unless authors request it in their submission letter and provide a postage-paid, self-addressed envelope. Otherwise, manuscripts are destroyed in the editorial office.

It is the policy of the *Journal of Continuing Education in Nursing* to provide complimentary copies of the journal to authors on publication.

COPYRIGHT

Contents copyrighted by SLACK Incorporated.

INDEXED

The *Journal of Continuing Education in Nursing* is indexed in *Education Index* and *RNdex Top 100*.

SAMPLE JOURNAL ARTICLE TITLES

- "Accelerated Professional Development and Peer Consultation: Two Strategies for Continuing Professional Education for Nurses"
- "Computer Conferencing in Graduate Nursing Education: Perceptions of Students and Faculty"
- "The Environmental-Skills-Delivery Model: A Heuristic Tool for Planning Staff Development in the New Millennium"
- "Transculture/Reflection on Clinical Teaching Using an Experiential Teaching-Learning Model"
- "Using Focus Group Methodology in Nursing"

Journal for Nurses in Staff Development

The *Journal for Nurses in Staff Development (JNSD)* is published by Lippincott Williams & Wilkins and is the official journal of the National Staff Development Organization.

JOURNAL FOCUS/PURPOSE

The primary purpose of the *Journal for Nurses in Staff Development* is to provide specifically for staff development and inservice educators as a specialized source of information on (1) planning, implementing, and evaluating staff development and inservice educa-

tional activities; (2) administration of staff development or inservice education departments; (3) research; (4) technological and other innovations; and (5) issues in staff development and/or inservice education that have an impact on the field. Manuscripts on patient education also are welcome.

JOURNAL FACTS

Publication schedule: bimonthly
Circulation: 5,000
Submitted papers per year: not available

Acceptance rate: 85%

Monetary honorarium: none

Average turnaround time: 1 month

Publishing timetable: 2-3 months after acceptance

Correspondence:
  Lippincott Williams & Wilkins
  Business Offices
  227 East Washington Square
  Philadelphia, PA 19106-3780
  Telephone: (215) 238-4200

Or
  12107 Insurance Way
  Hagerstown, MD 21740
  Telephone: (301) 714-2300
  Fax: (301) 714-2398
  Customer service: 1-800-638-3030

Internet site: www.nursingcenter.com/journals

MANUSCRIPT SUBMISSION

Manuscripts are considered for publication with the understanding that they are being submitted only to this journal. Do not use registered or certified mail. All manuscripts are acknowledged.

Submit the original and two copies to:
  Belinda E. Puetz, PhD, RN
  Editor, *Journal for Nurses in Staff
    Development*
  437 Twin Bay Drive
  Pensacola, FL 32534-1350
  E-mail: bepuetz@aol.com

One author should be designated as correspondent in the cover letter. The journal is not responsible in the event that a manuscript is lost. Authors should retain a copy of their manuscript.

Authors are encouraged to submit abstracts or outlines of potential articles. Feedback and advice about the topic and its development will be provided. The *Journal for Nurses in Staff Development* editorial staff is especially interested in manuscripts that present innovative ideas and suggestions. Manuscripts are carefully screened for professional content and potential value to the literature. The selection of manuscripts for publication is based primarily on these reviews and recommendations and on long-range editorial plans based on current and future needs and interests of staff development and inservice educators.

MANUSCRIPT PREPARATION GUIDELINES

Leave ample margins and use double spacing throughout (including tables, figures, and references). Do not justify text. (Justified text has even right-hand margins.)

Number the pages at the upper right from the first page of the text proper to the end of the references. The preferred length of a manuscript is 12 to 16 pages, including figures, tables, and references.

Along with the manuscript, please send the following:

- An abstract of your article (approximately 50-75 words) that gives an overview of the article and clearly states the specific benefits of the article for staff development and inservice educators.

- An author biography. Include full name followed by suitable abbreviations for both professional licenses and the highest earned degree in sequence as follows: orders, religious first; academic degrees earned in course; honorary degrees in order of bestowal; professional or occupational title and current position.
  Example: Marci J. Smith, M.S.N., R.N., is Director of Staff Development at Memorial Hospital, Anytown, U.S.A.

- A title page. Include the title of the article and the author's name as it should appear in the journal. Author identification should appear only on the title page of the manuscript. Do not include author information on any other manuscript pages.

To subdivide the article into main sections, insert subheads in the text as guides to the reader. Subheads should be kept short, succinct, and meaningful, and they should be similar in sense and tone.

Use the *Publication Manual of the American Psychological Association,* 4th ed. (1994), for style and format guidelines. Note especially the APA format for references, tables, and figures. Contact the editorial staff with questions about manuscript format prior to submission.

It is the author's responsibility to request any permission required for the use of material owned by others, such as any copyrighted material that is complete in itself: tables, charts, forms, figures. All letters of permission should be submitted with the manuscript. Where permission has been granted, the author should, within reason, follow any special wording stipulated by the grantor.

REFEREED PUBLICATION

All manuscripts are reviewed by members of the Editorial Board. These are blind reviews.

COPYRIGHT

Copyright by Lippincott Williams & Wilkins.

INDEXED

The *Journal for Nurses in Staff Development* is indexed in the *International Nursing Index, Cumulative Index to Nursing and Allied Health Literature, Nursing Abstracts,* and *Hospital Literature.*

SAMPLE JOURNAL ARTICLE TITLES

- "Designing a Competency-Based Nursing Practice Model in a Multicultural Setting"
- "Elder Abuse: Implications for Staff Development"
- "Lessons Learned in Implementing a Staff Education Program in Pain Management in the Acute Care Setting"
- "Patient Teaching for Older Adults and Families in the Long-Term Care Setting"
- "The Development of Culturally Appropriate Health Education Materials"

Journal of Nursing Education

The *Journal of Nursing Education* is published by SLACK Incorporated.

other scholarly works involving and influencing nursing education.

JOURNAL FOCUS/PURPOSE

The primary purpose of the *Journal of Nursing Education* is to publish research and

JOURNAL FACTS

Publication schedule: nine times per year
Circulation: approximately 4,000

Submitted papers per year: average 250

Acceptance rate: approximately 30%

Monetary honorarium: none

Average turnaround time: approximately 3-4 months

Publishing timetable: 2-3 years after acceptance

Correspondence:
> *Journal of Nursing Education*
> Business Office
> SLACK Incorporated
> 6900 Grove Road
> Thorofare, NJ 08086-9447
> Telephone: (856) 848-1000 or 1-800-257-8290
> Fax: (856) 853-5991
> E-mail: jne@slackinc.com

Internet site: www.slackinc.com/jne.htm

MANUSCRIPT SUBMISSION

Manuscripts should be addressed to:

> Executive Editor, *Journal of Nursing Education*
> SLACK Incorporated
> 6900 Grove Road
> Thorofare, NJ 08086-9447

Manuscripts will be considered for publication on the condition that they are submitted solely to the *Journal of Nursing Education.*

Manuscripts must be submitted in quadruplicate, one original and three copies, and typed in upper- and lowercase with double spacing between the lines. Because all manuscripts are reviewed without the reviewer's knowledge of the author's name or institution, the author's name, academic degree(s), present position, address, and telephone number should be provided on a separate sheet attached to the manuscript.

Manuscripts should include a self-addressed, postage-paid postcard with the title of the manuscript, to be returned to the author as acknowledgment of receipt. Manuscripts will not be returned to authors after review and will be destroyed in the editorial office. To have manuscripts returned, authors must request it in their submission letter and provide a postage-paid self-addressed envelope.

The *Journal of Nursing Education* limits accepted manuscripts to aspects of nursing education related to undergraduate and graduate program in schools of nursing. Inservice education, continuing nursing education, patient teaching, and clinical topics not related to teaching-learning in schools of nursing are more appropriate for other journals.

The Editorial Board will evaluate manuscripts based on the following criteria:

1. The importance of the topic to nursing education; the applicability of the ideas/research findings to other institutions
2. Readability; concise, logical ordering of ideas
3. Sound rationale for ideas; include critique of background for study, if research; discuss the development of original ideas and the soundness of argument for other works
4. Adequate documentation; citation of recent and relevant literature
5. Appropriateness of research methods or other approach to inquiry, including critique of design, sample, instruments, procedures, if research
6. Accuracy of content; soundness of conclusion

Following review by the Editorial Board, authors will receive a letter indicating the manuscript's acceptance, rejection, or suggestions for revision.

Manuscripts must include a signed copy of the following statement:

> In consideration of SLACK Incorporated's taking action in reviewing and editing my (our) submitted manuscript, (title), the author(s) undersigned hereby transfers, assigns or otherwise conveys copyright ownership to SLACK, Incorporated. The copyright so conveyed includes any and all subsidiary forms of publication, such as electronic media. The author(s) declares

that the manuscript contains no matter that is, to the best of the author's knowledge, libelous, unlawful, or that infringes upon any U.S. copyright.

If academic, hospital, or business affiliations are given or referred to in the manuscript, it is the responsibility of the author to obtain permission from the proper authorities to use the names of such.

MANUSCRIPT PREPARATION GUIDELINES

The *Journal of Nursing Education* follows the *Publication Manual of the American Psychological Association,* 4th ed. (1994), for references. Manuscripts must be typed using dark, clear, and readable typeface. Manuscripts printed on a computer must be in 10- or 12-point font. A typeface made up from dots or one that is unusual in appearance is not acceptable and will be returned to the author.

Two types of articles appear in the Journal—major articles and briefs. Major articles are (1) fully documented reports of studies on nursing education; (2) integrative reviews of literature that contribute to the advancement of knowledge about nursing education or to new applications of existing knowledge to teaching practices; (3) philosophical investigations in nursing education; or (4) political analyses of issues that influence nursing education. Reports of studies involving human subjects must indicate provisions for protection of their rights. An abstract of the article of approximately 150 words must accompany the manuscript. Major articles are generally limited to 15 narrative pages and should contain only those tables needed to clarify the presentation.

Briefs provide the opportunity for sharing new ideas. Research briefs are reports of small-scale studies (e.g., pilot work, research conducted in one setting) that may serve to either stimulate further investigation or alert other investigators of work in progress. Educational innovations describe new approaches in teaching, curriculum, or evaluation that have not yet been systematically tested but that have the potential of stimulating investigations, points of view about issues in nursing education, and other areas of interest to nursing faculty members. Briefs must be limited to eight pages and contain no tables or figures.

REFEREED PUBLICATION

All manuscripts considered go through the classic peer review procedure common to the most respected professional journals. Your anonymous peers approve or disapprove your manuscripts based on merit and clarity of presentation. This process, we believe, reinforces not only the integrity of the Journal but also your professional knowledge.

COPYRIGHT

Copyright by SLACK Incorporated.

INDEXED

The *Journal of Nursing Education* is indexed in the *Cumulative Index to Nursing and Allied Health Literature, Hospital Literature Index, Index Medicus, International Nursing Index, Nursing Abstracts, Nursing Citation Index, RNdex Top 100 Database,* and *Science Citation Index—Abridged Edition.*

SAMPLE JOURNAL ARTICLE TITLES

- "Changing Conceptions of Measurement Validity"
- "Decision-Making Task Complexity: Model Development and Initial Testing"

- "Nursing Education: Focus on Flexibility"
- "LPN-BSN: Education for a Reformed Health Care System"

- "Rehabilitation Needs and Experiential Learning"

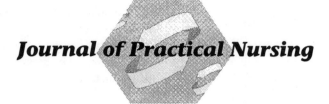

Journal of Practical Nursing

The *Journal of Practical Nursing* is published by the National Association for Practical Nurse Education and Service, Inc., and is the official journal of the National Association for Practical Nurse Education and Service.

JOURNAL FOCUS/PURPOSE

The primary purpose of the *Journal of Practical Nursing* is to keep licensed practical/vocational nurses up to date on their profession with articles about association news, infection control, nursing law, and legislation and regulations affecting LP/VNs.

JOURNAL FACTS

Publication schedule: quarterly

Circulation: approximately 8,000

Submitted papers per year: approximately 150

Acceptance rate: approximately 32%

Monetary honorarium: none

Average turnaround time: 1-2 months

Publishing timetable: 3 months after acceptance

Correspondence:
National Association for Practical Nurse Education and Service, Inc.
1400 Spring Street, Suite 310
Silver Spring, MD 20910
Telephone: (301) 588-2491
Fax: (301) 588-2839
E-mail: napnes@bellatlantic.net
Internet site: www.aoa.dhhs.gov.aoa/dir/130.html/

MANUSCRIPT SUBMISSION

Submit articles to:

Helen M. Larsen, Executive Editor
Journal of Practical Nursing
1400 Spring Street, Suite 330
Silver Spring, MD 20910

The author grants the *Journal of Practical Nursing* the right to edit, abridge, condense, and publish the article. The author also grants the *Journal of Practical Nursing* the right to determine the title, headings, and subheadings for the article, as well as the captions, illustrations, and supplementary material, if any, to accompany the article.

Prior to publication, the edited article may be sent to the author for approval if there have been substantial editorial revisions to the original manuscript and if the schedule permits. It will be sent to the address listed by the author at the bottom of this page (office address). It is the author's responsibility to inform the *Journal of Practical Nursing* if his or her address changes.

If the author would like any revisions to the edited manuscript, he or she must return the edited manuscript with clearly written revisions to the *Journal of Practical Nursing* within 14 days of the date when we mailed the article. These revisions by the author are advisory, and the editor is not required to make the suggested changes. If the edited manuscript is not returned within the 14-day period, the *Journal of*

Practical Nursing will assume the author's approval.

The author agrees that the article has not been accepted by any other nursing magazine and that he or she will not submit this article or a very similar article to any other magazine for at least 1 year after publication. Furthermore, the author attests that this is an original work and has not been published elsewhere under a different byline. Nothing in this agreement shall constitute a guarantee that the author's article will in fact be published in the *Journal of Practical Nursing*. Only a separate, official written communication by the editor can establish definite publishing agreements.

As a professional journal published by a nonprofit association, the *Journal of Practical Nursing* usually does not pay for articles published. If an author wishes to be considered for payment, he or she should inquire prior to publication and should not sign the required form.

MANUSCRIPT PREPARATION GUIDELINES

None available.

REFEREED PUBLICATION

Journal of Practical Nursing does not have a peer-review process.

COPYRIGHT

Copyright of the published article is owned by the National Association for Practical Nurse Education and Service, Inc.

INDEXED

The *Journal of Practical Nursing* is indexed in the *Cumulative Index to Nursing and Allied Health Literature* and *Silver Platter.*

SAMPLE JOURNAL ARTICLE TITLES

- "Chronic Cancer Pain"
- "Gamma Knife: The Treatment That Saved My Husband's Life"
- "Health Professionals Focus on Prevention of Medication Errors"
- "Skin Disease Lowers Self-Perception"
- "Smoking and Hypertension"

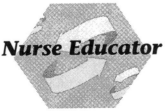

Nurse Educator

N*urse Educator* is published by Lippincott Williams & Wilkins.

JOURNAL FOCUS/PURPOSE

The primary purpose of *Nurse Educator* is to provide information on both the theories and practice of nursing education, including educational philosophy, policies, and procedures; organizational, program, curriculum, and course development; instructional methods and materials; testing and measurement; research; faculty development; and administration.

JOURNAL FACTS

Publication schedule: bimonthly
Circulation: 4,000

Submitted papers per year: 200

Acceptance rate: 20%

Monetary honorarium: none

Average turnaround time: 6 weeks

Publishing timetable: 9 months after acceptance

Correspondence:
> Lippincott Williams & Wilkins
> Business Offices
> 227 East Washington Square
> Philadelphia, PA 19106-3780
> Telephone: (215) 238-4200

Or
> 12107 Insurance Way
> Hagerstown, MD 21740
> Telephone: (301) 714-2300
> Fax: (301) 714-2398
> Customer service: 1-800-638-3030

Internet site: www.nursingcenter.com/journals

MANUSCRIPT SUBMISSION

Submit three copies of the manuscript, along with a stamped, self-addressed, business-sized envelope if you want receipt of your manuscript acknowledged. If you want your original manuscript returned after the review process, enclose a self-addressed manuscript-sized envelope with sufficient postage affixed.

Address correspondence to:
> Suzanne P. Smith, EdD, RN, FAAN
> Editor-in-Chief, *Nurse Educator*
> 4301 32nd Street West, Suite C12
> Bradenton, FL 34205-2748
> E-mail: drsuzsmith@aol.com

MANUSCRIPT PREPARATION GUIDELINES

All persons designated as authors should qualify for authorship. Each author should have contributed significantly to the conception and design of the work and writing the manuscript to take public responsibility for it.

The editor may request justification of assignment of authorship. Names of those who contributed general support or technical help may be listed in an acknowledgment, placed after the narrative and before the references.

Unless otherwise stated here, prepare manuscripts according to the *American Medical Association (AMA) Manual of Style* (8th ed.). Although not necessary, query letters allow the editor to indicate interest in, and developmental advice on, manuscript topics.

The maximum manuscript length is 15 pages, including figures, tables, and references. As a general rule, a 15-page paper should have no more than three figures or tables.

Tables and figures should be placed in the back of the manuscript after references. Tables must be numbered consecutively with arabic numbers, be double-spaced, and have a title at the top. Figures and tables must be cited in numerical order in the text.

Number pages consecutively in the upper right corner starting with the title/author biography page. Do not justify the right margin. Do not use running headers or footers.

Subdivide the manuscript into main sections by inserting subheads in the text. Subheads should be succinct, meaningful, and similar in sense and tone.

References are placed at the end of the manuscript and typed double-spaced. References are cited consecutively by number and listed in citation order in the reference list. Whenever a reference is repeated in text, it uses the same reference number each time.

Each of the following should be placed on a separate page: (1) a 50-75 word abstract that stimulates readers' interest in the topic and states what readers will learn or how they will be better off after reading the article; (2) a title/author biography page. The authors' biographic information includes name, credentials, position, place of employment, city, state, and e-mail address (optional). EXAM-

PLE: Alice M. Jones, PhD, RN, Professor, Community University, Milwaukee, Wisconsin; (3) reference list; (4) acknowledgments; (5) illustrations.

Written permission must be obtained from (1) the holder of copyrighted material used in the manuscript, (2) persons mentioned in the narrative or acknowledgment, and (3) the administrators of institutions mentioned in the narrative or acknowledgment. Where permission has been granted, the author should follow any special wording stipulated by the grantor. Letters of permission must he submitted before publication of the manuscript.

REFEREED PUBLICATION

Nurse Educator is a refereed journal. Published manuscripts have been reviewed, selected, and developed with the guidance of our editorial advisers. Manuscript content is assessed for relevance, accuracy, and usefulness to faculty and administrators. Manuscripts are reviewed with the understanding that neither the manuscript nor its essential content has been published or is under consideration by others.

The review process starts on the first day of every month. For example, February 1 is the start of the review process for all manuscripts received during January. Publication decisions and author notification occur within 8 weeks from the beginning of the review process.

COPYRIGHT

Copyright by Lippincott Williams & Wilkins.

INDEXED

Nurse Educator is indexed in the *Current Index to Journals in Education, Cumulative Index to Nursing and Allied Health Literature, Hospital Literature Index, International Nursing Index,* and *RNdex Top 100.*

SAMPLE JOURNAL ARTICLE TITLES

- "Developing and Scoring Essay Tests"
- "Nursing Students' Experience Bathing Patients for the First Time"
- "Preparing Advanced Practice Nurses for Clinical Decision Making in Specialty Practice"
- "The Iowa Articulation Story: Collaboration Works"
- "Unleashing the Power of Memory: The Mighty Mnemonic"

Nursing and Health Care Perspectives

Nursing and Health Care Perspectives is published by the National League for Nursing and is the official journal of the National League for Nursing.

JOURNAL FOCUS/PURPOSE

Nursing and Health Care Perspectives seeks articles that support nurse educators by providing a forum for the exchange of information and ideas regarding innovative educational initiatives. Manuscripts will be evaluated according to consistency with sound educational programming and/or research methodology. The overarching goal is to support the National League for Nursing mission, to advance "quality nursing education that prepares the nursing workforce to meet the needs of diverse populations in an ever-changing health care environment." Articles should reflect the art and science of nursing and/or nursing education.

JOURNAL FACTS

Publication schedule: bimonthly

Circulation: approximately 11,000

Submitted papers per year: not available

Acceptance rate: not available

Monetary honorarium: none

Average turnaround time: 3 months

Publishing timetable: 9 months after acceptance

Correspondence:
  National League for Nursing
  61 Broadway
  New York, NY 10006
  Telephone: 1-800-669-1656 or (212) 363-5555
  Fax: (212) 989-0393

Internet site: www.nln.org/journal/index.htm or www.nln.org

MANUSCRIPT SUBMISSION

Manuscripts and all other correspondence should be directed to:

  The Editor, *Nursing and Health Care Perspectives*
  National League for Nursing
  61 Broadway
  New York, NY 10006

Manuscripts should be mailed flat, unstapled, but paper-clipped together. Submit one original and three photocopies of the article. Please also provide the manuscript on a disk, in any PC or Macintosh word processing program format.

Accepted manuscripts will be edited for clarity, length, and adherence to *Nursing and Health Care Perspectives* editorial style. The author receives an edited copy of the manuscript before publication to check for accuracy of content.

MANUSCRIPT PREPARATION GUIDELINES

Keep in mind that your goal is to engage your reader on a one-to-one basis, so write as clearly as you can. Your audience does not always read when it is fresh, alert, comfortable, and undistracted, so entice the reader. Catch and hold your reader's interest with clear, lively writing. Do not use jargon—it is often an imprecise use of language. Think carefully about what you want to say; then say it as simply and directly as possible. Read *The Elements of Style,* by Strunk and White, for tips on good composition, and examine recent issues of *Nursing and Health Care Perspectives* to get a feel for our style.

Authors should include, on a separate page, their full name, address, and telephone number; professional designations and degrees; current affiliation; and affiliation during preparation of the article. Manuscripts should be in 12-point type, double-spaced on $8\frac{1}{2}$ by 11-inch white paper with $1\frac{1}{2}$-inch margins all around. The average manuscript is 10 to 12 pages in length. Shorter articles are also encouraged.

References should be in APA format. See the APA Style Manual or a recent copy of *Nursing and Health Care Perspectives* for guidance.

Authors are encouraged to provide photographs or other artwork to illustrate their articles. Photographs should be glossy, black and white, and bear the photographer's name and a brief description of what is depicted. Evidence of permission to use or reprint the photograph or other art must be provided by the author.

REFEREED PUBLICATION

All submitted manuscripts undergo evaluation by the editorial staff. Promising manuscripts are reviewed by *Nursing and Health Care Perspectives'* editorial review board. Reviewers judge the manuscript for originality, importance, accuracy, and readability. When we decline a manuscript, we provide a summary of reviewers' comments. The review process is anonymous to ensure fairness and objectivity, so the names and affiliations of authors should not appear in the text but should be provided on a separate page.

COPYRIGHT

Copyright is by the National League for Nursing, Inc., except where otherwise noted.

INDEXED

Nursing and Health Care Perspectives is indexed in *Cumulative Index to Nursing and Allied Health Literature, Information Resources Group, International Nursing Index,* and *MEDLINE.*

SAMPLE JOURNAL ARTICLE TITLES

- "A Student's Experiences in El Salvador"
- "Competency Model 101: The Process of Developing Core Competencies"
- "Critical Thinking Skills of Baccalaureate Nursing Students at Program Entry and Exit"
- "The Development of Online Courses for Undergraduate Nursing Education: A Faculty Perspective"
- "Thinking in Nursing Education: Part I, A Student's Experience Learning to Think"

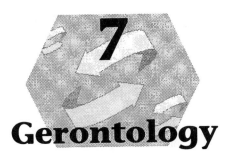

7

Gerontology

Geriatric Nursing

G*eriatric Nursing* is published by Mosby, Inc., and is the official journal of the National Gerontological Nursing Association.

JOURNAL FOCUS/PURPOSE

The primary purpose of *Geriatric Nursing* is to provide timely information on new and innovative programs and practices in clinical care and administration, as well as reporting clinical research findings applicable to practice. *Geriatric Nursing* strives to provide pertinent, pragmatic information, news, continuing education, resources, and guidelines to maximize caregivers' ability to help elders capitalize on their achievements, prevent or modify ill health, and complete the tasks of late life in ways that add to its enjoyment and meaning.

JOURNAL FACTS

Publication schedule: bimonthly
Circulation: 10,400
Submitted papers per year: 80-100

Acceptance rate: not available

Monetary honorarium: None

Average turnaround time: 4-6 weeks

Publishing timetable: approximately 4 months after acceptance

Correspondence:
Mosby, Inc.
11830 Westline Industrial Drive
St. Louis, MO 63146-3318
Telephone: 1-800-453-4351
Fax: (314) 432-1158
E-mail: periodical.service@mosby.com

Internet site: www.mosby.com

MANUSCRIPT SUBMISSION

Communications regarding manuscripts or the editorial management of the journal should be addressed to the editor. Authors are encouraged to write the editor at the address given below. Before submitting a manuscript for review, briefly describe the content of your manuscript and the experience and knowledge that qualify you to discuss the subject. Summarize in about 35 words the main points you plan to make.

Submit manuscripts to:

Priscilla R. Ebersole, PhD, RN, FAAN
Editor, *Geriatric Nursing*
2790 Rollingwood Drive
San Bruno, CA 94066
Telephone: (650) 952-3155
E-mail: ebersole@sfsu.edu

Manuscripts intended for publication in the NGNA section of the journal should be sent directly to:

Ann Schmidt Luggen, PhD, RN, CS, CNAA
751 Locust Corner Road
Cincinnati, OH 45245

Enclose a self-addressed, stamped envelope for return of manuscripts that are not accepted.

All manuscripts are accepted for publication with the understanding that they are contributed solely to *Geriatric Nursing*. On acceptance, manuscripts become the permanent property of the journal and may not be reproduced elsewhere without written permission from the publisher.

In accordance with the Copyright Act of 1976, all manuscripts must be accompanied by the following statement signed by one author:

> The undersigned author transfers all copyright ownership of the manuscript (title of article) to Mosby, Inc., in the event the work is published. The undersigned author warrants that the article is original, is not under consideration by another journal, and has not been previously published.

Statements and opinions expressed in the articles and communications herein are those of the author(s) and not necessarily those of the editor or the publisher. The editor and the publisher disclaim any responsibility or liability for such material and do not guarantee, warrant, or endorse any product or service advertised in this publication, nor do they guarantee any claim made by the manufacturer of such product or service.

Send written permission of the copyright holder and author for any quotation, table, or figure taken from previously published material. Patient or guardian consent must accompany any photograph that shows a recognizable likeness of a person.

MANUSCRIPT PREPARATION GUIDELINES

Submit three copies of the manuscript and supporting materials (abstract, reference list, tables, figures, and figure legends). Type the manuscript on good-quality, white bond paper ($8\frac{1}{2} \times 11$ inches) on one side of the page only, with liberal margins (at least 1 inch on all sides). Use double spacing throughout the paper, including title page, abstract, text, acknowledgments, references, tables, and figure legends. Length of the manuscript depends on nature of the content, but brevity, about 8 to 10 pages, is desirable. All pages should be numbered consecutively (beginning with the title page) in the upper right-hand corner.

Once a manuscript is accepted, the final version of the manuscript should be submitted on diskette along with three copies of the printout. The author accepts responsibility for the submitted diskette's exactly matching the printout of the final version of the manuscript. Files must be saved in a translatable format. Rich text format (RTF) or ASCII is preferred. Guidelines for submission of accepted manuscript on diskette will be sent to the author by the editorial office.

The title page should include the manuscript title (concise but informative); the full names of all authors with their highest earned academic degrees and institutional affiliations; the name of the department and institution to which the work should be attributed; disclaimers if any; the name, address, phone and fax numbers, and e-mail address of the author(s) responsible for correspondence concerning the manuscript, galley proofs, and reprints; and acknowledgment of any financial support (grants, equipment, pharmaceuticals). Each article must be accompanied by an abstract, not to exceed 100 words in length, that summarizes the main points of the article.

References must be cited consecutively in the text as superscript numbers. A reference that is mentioned more than once in the text can be designated by the same superscript number. The reference list must be current and typed double-spaced in numeric order on a separate sheet at the end of the text. The format of the reference list should conform to that set forth in "Uniform Requirements for Manuscripts Submitted to Biomedical Journals" (Vancouver style) (JAMA 1993;269:2282-6).

Examples of journal citations:

> Badaledmant RA, Drago JR. Prostate cancer: promising advances that may alter survival rates. Postgrad Med 1990;87:65-72.
>
> Hanks GE. Radical prostatectomy or radiation therapy for early prostate cancer: two roads to the same end. Cancer 1988;61:2153-60.

For books, include up to the first six author(s) (last name and initials), title of book (lowercase and no quotation marks), edition or column, city of publication, publisher, and year. When particular pages of a book are relevant or when a book is referenced several times, the relevant pages can be listed.

Examples of book citations:

> Strauss AL. Chronic illness and the quality of life. St. Louis: CV Mosby, 1975.
>
> Sulloway FJ. Freud: biologist of the mind. New York: Basic Books, 1979:102-10, 130-1, 194.

Personal communication should not be included in the reference list but may be cited in parentheses in the text.

Illustrations are encouraged. Number figures consecutively in the order of mention; all illustrations must be cited in the text. Mark lightly in pencil on the back of each illustration the figure number and name of first author, and indicate the top. Additionally, the top of the illustration should be indicated with an arrow. Do not mount illustration on cardboard. Original drawings or graphs should be prepared in black India ink or typographic (press-apply) lettering if not done with a laser printer. Typewritten or freehand lettering is unacceptable. All lettering must be done professionally and should be in proportion to the drawing, graph, or photograph. Do not send original artwork or X-ray films. Glossy print photographs, 3×5 inches minimum to 5×7 inches maximum, with good black-and-white contrast color balance, are preferred. Consistency in size within the article is strongly preferred. Any special instructions regarding sizing should be clearly noted. Illustrations will be returned only if the author requests such at the time the manuscript is submitted.

Figure legends should be double-spaced on a separate sheet of paper. Spell out in the legends any abbreviations or acronyms used as labels on the figures. If the figure is taken from previously published material, the legend must give full credit to the original source, and the author must obtain written permission to reproduce previously published material from the original source.

Number tables consecutively in the order of mention; all tables must be mentioned in text. Data appearing in tables should supplement, not duplicate, the text. Provide a brief title for each table. Any abbreviations or acronyms in the table should be spelled out in a footnote or legend to the table. As for figures, if material has been previously published, the table legend must give full credit to the original source, and the author must obtain written permission to reproduce the material from the original source.

REFEREED PUBLICATION

Geriatric Nursing is a refereed journal. Manuscripts are reviewed by at least two editorial advisers and by the editor.

COPYRIGHT

Copyright by Mosby, Inc.

INDEXED

Geriatric Nursing is indexed in the *Cumulative Index to Nursing and Allied Health Literature, Nursing Abstracts, Current Advances in Ecological Sciences, Current Literature on Aging, Hospital Literature Index, Index Medicus, International Nursing Index, International Pharmaceutical Abstracts, Nursing Abstracts, Nutrition Research Newsletter,* and *Psychological Abstracts.*

SAMPLE JOURNAL ARTICLE TITLES

- "Assessing Problem Feeding Behaviors in Mid-Stage Alzheimer's Disease"
- "Medications and the Visually Impaired Elderly"
- "Recognizing and Helping Older Persons With Vision Impairments"
- "Salicylism in the Elderly: 'A Little Aspirin Never Hurt Anybody!'"
- "Sleep Problems and Self-care in Very Old Rural Women: Nursing Implications"

Journal of Gerontological Nursing

The *Journal of Gerontological Nursing* is published by SLACK Incorporated.

JOURNAL FOCUS/PURPOSE

The primary purpose of the *Journal of Gerontological Nursing* is to provide articles dealing with the practice and/or teaching of gerontological nursing.

JOURNAL FACTS

Publication schedule: monthly

Circulation: approximately 10,400

Submitted papers per year: approximately 140

Acceptance rate: 50%

Monetary honorarium: none

Average turnaround time: approximately 4-5 months

Publishing timetable: approximately 4-6 months after acceptance

Correspondence:
SLACK Incorporated
6900 Grove Road
Thorofare, NJ 08086-9447
Telephone: (856) 848-1000
Fax: (856) 853-5991
E-mail: mlong@slackinc.com

Internet site: www.slackinc.com/jgn.htm

MANUSCRIPT SUBMISSION

Manuscripts dealing with the practice and/or teaching of gerontological nursing should be submitted to the editor. Articles are accepted for consideration with the understanding that they are contributed solely to the *Journal of Gerontological Nursing* and have not been published previously.

Manuscripts should include a self-addressed, postage-paid postcard with the title of the manuscript, to be returned to the authors as acknowledgment of receipt. Manuscripts will not be returned to authors after review and will be destroyed in the editorial office. To have manuscripts returned, authors must request it in the submission letter and provide a self-addressed, postage-paid envelope. The Journal is able to offer prompt publication of accepted manuscripts.

Please send materials to:

Kathleen C. Buckwalter, PhD, RN, FAAN
Editor, *Journal of Gerontological Nursing*
6900 Grove Road
Thorofare, NJ 08086
Telephone: (856) 848-1000

If you have manuscript development ideas or questions, contact the managing editor at (856) 848-1000, extension 256, or e-mail: mlong@slackinc.com.

It is not the policy of the Journal to provide monetary compensation for articles. However, complimentary copies of the Journal issue in which a finished article appears will be sent to the author(s).

All manuscripts should be accompanied by a letter of copyright transmittal. This must be signed and dated by all authors. The letter is required before any manuscript can be considered for publication and should contain the following language:

In consideration of SLACK Incorporated's taking action in reviewing and editing my (our) submission, the author(s) undersigned hereby transfers, assigns, or otherwise conveys all copyright ownership to SLACK Incorporated in the event that said work is published by SLACK Incorporated. The copyright so conveyed includes any and all subsidiary forms of publication, such as electronic media. The author(s) declares that the manuscript contains no matter that is, to the best of the author's knowledge, libelous or unlawful, or that infringes upon any U.S. copyright.

MANUSCRIPT PREPARATION GUIDELINES

Five original manuscripts should be submitted, typed, double-spaced with one-inch margins on one side of $8\frac{1}{2} \times 11$-inch paper. Length should be approximately 16 pages. Copies of the manuscripts submitted should be devoid of author identification to facilitate separation for blind peer review. The author's name, address, academic degrees, current position, telephone number, and the complete title of the manuscript should appear at the end of the article on a separate sheet of paper.

Figures, tables, and references should be typed on separate sheets of paper. Number all pages as well as figures and tables. Follow APA style guidelines in preparing references and bibliographic citations. For questions on preferred reference style, please consult the *Publication Manual of the American Psychological Association,* 4th ed. (1994).

Photographs are a positive addition to any manuscript, and a 5×7-inch black-and-white or color format is preferred. Permission to publish pictures must be obtained in writing from all individuals who are photographed. In case studies involving actual persons, their written release is required.

All manuscripts must address the clinical implications of the topic or research being discussed for nurses. These implications should be evident throughout the manuscript.

REFEREED PUBLICATION

The *Journal of Gerontological Nursing* is a juried publication employing the blind peer review system. Following Editorial Board review and review by the editor, the author(s) will be notified of the disposition of the manuscript.

COPYRIGHT

Copyright by SLACK Incorporated.

INDEXED

The *Journal of Gerontological Nursing* is indexed in the *International Nursing Index, Cumulative Index to Nursing and Allied Health Literature, Nursing Abstracts, RNdex Top 100,* and *PsycINFO database.*

SAMPLE JOURNAL ARTICLE TITLES

- "Grief Responses of Senior and Elderly Widows: Practical Implications"
- "Prostate Cancer Elder Alert: Epidemiology, Screening, and Early Detection"
- "Planning an Osteoporosis Education Program for Older Adults in a Residential Setting"
- "Consequences of Not Recognizing Delirium Superimposed or Dementia in Hospitalized Elderly Individuals"
- "Individualized Interventions to Prevent Bed-Related Falls and Reduce Siderail Use"

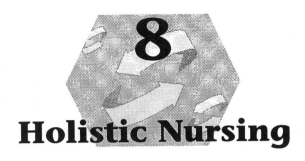

8

Holistic Nursing

Holistic Nursing Practice

Holistic Nursing Practice is published by Aspen Publishers, Inc.

JOURNAL FOCUS/PURPOSE

The primary purposes of *Holistic Nursing Practice* are to explore holistic models of nursing practice and to emphasize the complementarity of traditional and holistic nursing and health care practices.

JOURNAL FACTS

Publication schedule: quarterly

Circulation: approximately 2,000

Submitted papers per year: approximately 116

Acceptance rate: 59%

Monetary honorarium: none

Average turnaround time: 3 to 5 months

Publishing timetable: 6 months after acceptance

Correspondence:
  Customer Services
  200 Orchard Ridge Drive
  Gaithersburg, MD 20878
  Customer service telephone: 1-800-234-1660

Internet site: www.aspenpub.com (enter journal title in search box)

MANUSCRIPT SUBMISSION

Articles are sought that deal with holistic nursing models and theory-based interventions and their outcomes. Articles sought for publication in *HNP* include the following themes: innovations in holistic nursing care practice, exploration of controversies inherent in holistic nursing practice and health care; empirical and historical research related to holistic nursing practice, health care and policy, and values and ethical-legal issues related to holistic care practices. The holistic approach is a worldview that emphasizes the potential for health and healing in human systems rather than the disease process and deficit. Projected topics for future publication are listed on the back of each issue. These topics should not limit submission of articles on other topics by prospective authors.

Research and theory articles: All types of empirical research, including descriptive, quasi-experimental, experimental, basic, and applied. Research articles should include a clear and concise summary of the purpose and problem, a statement of the hypothesis tested, background and significance, theoretical framework, design, methods and procedures, analyses of data, findings, conclusions, and implications for further research and nursing practice. Historical research articles should deal with the history of holistic theory, holistic nursing and health care practices, policy, or related health care issues.

Theory articles: Analyses of holistic concepts and theories germane to nursing intervention and health care. Such articles should include concise classic and modern literature reviews of the concept or theory and implications for nursing practice or research.

Nursing practice articles: Articles on innovative or best practices in nursing/holistic care or related fields.

Creative pieces: Poetry or brief creative essays or thought pieces related to holistic nursing care or human experiences related to health care.

Manuscripts and correspondence regarding publication should be addressed to the journal editor:

Gloria F. Donnelly, PhD, RN, FAAN
Editor, *Holistic Nursing Practice*
312 Penn Road
Wynnewood, PA 19096
E-mail: Gloria.Donnelly@drexel.edu

Submissions must comprise an original and three copies of a manuscript, plus an identical version on disk, to be created on IBM-compatible (PC) equipment using Microsoft Word version 6.0 or 7.0 for Windows 95 or a higher operating system. However, manuscripts created using Microsoft Word 6.0 or 7.0 for a Macintosh System 7 are acceptable. The manuscript must include the following: a completed article submission form, an original, signed copyright transfer form, and an abstract of the manuscript of 100 words or less.

The journal editors will review to determine the article's suitability for publication and will work with the author to ensure that articles meet the journal's needs and adhere to its standards. In addition to the editor's review, all articles are sent to Editorial Board members for review and recommendations. The editors may recommend that an article be revised or rewritten before being accepted for publication. The author may withdraw the article or make revisions according to the editor's recommendations. If the article is revised, the new version will again be subject to review.

Authors must release copyright ownership of their manuscript at the time of its submission to the journal. Articles that are selected for publication are edited by the editorial staff at Aspen and sent to type. Galley proofs will be sent to the author for review and approval.

MANUSCRIPT PREPARATION GUIDELINES

Manuscripts should be created using Aspen's Journals Authoring Template (template is available from your journal editor or from Aspen). Manuscripts should be created on IBM-compatible (PC) equipment using Windows 95 or higher operating system. Our preferred software is Microsoft Word. Hard copy and electronic files should be submitted for all text and all artwork. All disks submitted must be new. Disks should be clearly labeled as to operating system and software application.

Manuscripts should be double-spaced (including quotations, lists, references, footnotes, figure captions, and all parts of tables).

Manuscripts should be ordered as follows: title page, abstracts, text, references, appendixes, tables, and any illustrations.

Each manuscript must include the following:

Title page, including (1) title of the article, (2) author names (with highest academic degrees) and affiliations (including titles, departments, and name and location of institutions of primary employment), and (3) any acknowledgments, credits, or disclaimers

Abstract of no more than 100 words and up to 10 key words that describe the contents of the article like those that appear in the *Cumulative Index to Nursing and Allied Health Literature (CINAHL)* or the *National Library of Medicine's Medical Subject Headings (MeSH)*

Clear indication of the placement of all tables and figures in text

Signed copyright transfer form

Completed article submission form for each contributor

Written permission for any borrowed text, tables, or figures

References must be cited in text and styled in the reference list according to *American Medical Association Manual of Style,* 9th ed. (1998). They must be numbered consecutively in the order they are cited in the text; reference numbers may be used more than once throughout an article. Page numbers should appear with the text citation following a specific quote. References should not be created using Microsoft Word's automatic footnote/endnote feature. References should be included on a separate page at the end of the article and should be double-spaced.

References should also include citations within the text (see examples below).

Citation:

Reliability has been established previously[1,2-8,19]

Citation following a quote should include page numbers:

Jacobsen concluded that "the consequences of muscle strength . . ."[5(pp3,4)]

Reference list style for book:

1. Gregory CF, Chapman MW, Hanse ST Jr. Open fractures. In: Rockwood CA Jr, Green DP, eds. *Fractures.* Philadelphia: JB Lippincott Co; 1984: 169-218.
2. Yando R, Seitz U, Zigler E, et al. *Imitation: A Developmental Perspective.* New York: John Wiley & Sons; 1978.

Reference list style for journal (journal names should be abbreviated as shown):

3. Fielding JW, Hensinger RN, Hawkins RJ. Os Odontoideum. *J Bone Joint Surg Am.* 1980;62:376-383.

Reference list style for unpublished material:

4. Sieger M. The nature and limits of clinical medicine. In: Cassell EJ, Siegler M, eds. *Changing Values in Medicine.* Chicago: University of Chicago Press. In press.

Reference list style for dissertation and thesis:

5. Raymand CA. Uncovering Ideology: Occupational Health in the Mainstream and Advocacy Press, 1970-1982. Ithaca, NY: Cornell University; 1983. Thesis.

Illustrations: Figures should be created using electronic software (i.e., Adobe Illustrator, Corel Draw, and Photoshop). Please save files in both the application in which they were created (i.e., Microsoft Word) and as either EPS or TIFF files. Use computer-generated lettering. Do not use screens, color, shading, or fine lines.

In lieu of original drawings and other material, a sharp, glossy, black-and-white photographic print between 5″ × 7″ and 8″ × 10″ is acceptable.

Each figure should have a label on the back indicating the number of the figure, the names of the authors, and the top of the figure. Do not write on the back of figures, mount them on cardboard, or scratch or mar them using paper clips. Do not bend figures.

Cite each figure in the text in consecutive order. If a figure has been previously published, in part or in total, acknowledge the original source and submit written permission from the copyright holder to reproduce or adapt the material.

Supply a caption for each figure, typed double-spaced on a separate sheet from the artwork. Captions should include the figure title, explanatory statements, notes, or keys as well as source and permission lines.

Provide a camera-ready copy and a separate electronic file for each piece of artwork. Do not embed art in your text file.

Tables should be on a separate page at the end of the manuscript. Number tables consecutively and supply a brief title for each. Include explanatory footnotes for all nonstandard abbreviations. Cite each table in the text in consecutive order. If you use data from another published or unpublished source, obtain permission and acknowledge fully.

Permissions: Authors are responsible for obtaining signed letters from copyright holders granting permission to reprint material being borrowed or adapted from other sources, including previously published material of your own. Authors must obtain written permission for the following material (authors are responsible for any permission fees to reprint borrowed material):

All direct quotes of 300 words or more from any full-length book

All direct quotes of 200 words or more from a periodical article

All excerpts from a newspaper article or other short piece

Any passage from a play or a song

Two or more lines of poetry

Any borrowed table, figure, or illustration being reproduced exactly or adapted to fit the needs of the subject

REFEREED PUBLICATION

Holistic Nursing Practice is a peer-reviewed journal.

COPYRIGHT

Copyright by Aspen Publishers, Inc.

INDEXED

Holistic Nursing Practice is indexed in the *Cumulative Index to Nursing and Allied Health Literature, Family Studies Database, Hospital and Health Administration Index, Health Planning and Administration Database, International Nursing Index, Inventory of Marriage and Family Literature, MEDLINE, Nursing Abstracts, Nursing Scan in Oncology,* and *RNdex Top 100.*

SAMPLE JOURNAL ARTICLE TITLES

- "Attitudes, Concerns, and Fear of Acquired Immunodeficiency Syndrome Among Registered Nurses in the United States"
- "Holism in the Care of the Allogeneic Bone Marrow Transplant Population: Role of the Nurse Practitioner"
- "Interdisciplinary Education in Clinical Ethics: A Work in Progress"
- "Stress, Hope, and Well-Being of Women Caring for Family Members With Alzheimer's Disease"
- "Teaching About the Female Condom"

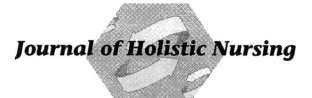

Journal of Holistic Nursing

The *Journal of Holistic Nursing* is published by Sage Publications, Inc., and is the official publication of the American Holistic Nurses' Association.

JOURNAL FOCUS/PURPOSE

The primary purpose of the *Journal of Holistic Nursing* is to publish original articles of merit related to holistic nursing. The emphasis of the journal is on original work, including education, research, and practice.

JOURNAL FACTS

Publication schedule: quarterly

Circulation: 5,000

Submitted papers per year: 70

Acceptance rate: 46%

Monetary honorarium: none

Average turnaround time: 12 weeks

Publishing timetable: 3-6 months after acceptance

Correspondence:
Sage Publications, Inc.
2455 Teller Road
Thousand Oaks, CA 91320
Telephone: (805) 499-0721
Fax: (805) 499-0871

Internet site: www.sagepub.com

MANUSCRIPT SUBMISSION

Manuscripts should be submitted in quadruplicate to:

Dr. Lynn Rew, Editor
Journal of Holistic Nursing
University of Texas—Austin, School of Nursing
1700 Red River
Austin, TX 78701-1412
Telephone: (512) 471-7311
Fax: (512) 471-4910
E-mail: ellerew@mail.utexas.edu

The *Journal of Holistic Nursing* expects that original contributions have not been previously published and are not under simultaneous consideration by another publication.

The *Journal of Holistic Nursing* is a pioneering force in exploring the frontiers of holism. This innovative journal provides an objective forum for researchers, scholars, and practitioners to exchange information, report the results of clinical experiences, and share research pertaining to health care, wellness, healing, and human potential.

MANUSCRIPT PREPARATION GUIDELINES

Manuscripts should be submitted in typewritten, double-spaced form. They should not exceed 18 pages and should not be right-justified. Every element within the manuscript must be double-spaced, including tables and references, and must follow the *Publication Manual of the American Psychological Association* (4th ed.).

The cover page should contain the title of the manuscript, the name(s), highest academic degree(s) earned, institutional affiliation(s), mailing address(es), and telephone/fax numbers of all authors. An abstract of 100 to 150 words should also be included and should contain factual information rather than a general description of the manuscript contents.

Tables should be typed, double-spaced, one to a page and numbered. Their relative placement in the text should be noted. All figures should be in camera-ready form.

Biographical sketches should include name, institutional affiliation, recent publications, and the author's current research interest. Authors are requested to use gender-neutral text unless a direct quote is involved from another author that is not gender neutral or unless the context of the manuscript appropriately calls for a specific gender.

REFEREED PUBLICATION

The *Journal of Holistic Nursing* is a peer-reviewed journal with a blind review process.

COPYRIGHT

Copyright by the American Holistic Nurses' Association.

INDEXED

The *Journal of Holistic Nursing* is indexed in *Bowker Saur, the Cumulative Index to Nursing and Allied Health Literature, International Nursing Index, Family Studies Database, Linguistics and Language Behavior Abstracts, Nursing Abstracts, Nursing Citation Index, Social Planning/Policy and Development Abstracts, Sociological Abstracts,* and *Violence and Abuse Abstracts.*

SAMPLE JOURNAL ARTICLE TITLES

- "Cultural Meanings of Childbirth: Muslim Women Living in Jordan"
- "Faculty's Response to 'The Case of Baby M': Nursing Care in an Ethical Wilderness"
- "Potential Benefits of Pet Ownership in Health Promotion"
- "Spirituality in Terminal Illness: An Alternative View of Theory"
- "Use of Neonatal Boundaries to Improve Outcomes"

Legislative Issues

Journal of Nursing Law

The *Journal of Nursing Law* is published by PESI HealthCare, LLC, and is the official publication of the American Association of Nurse Attorneys.

JOURNAL FOCUS/PURPOSE

The primary purpose of the *Journal of Nursing Law* is to serve the needs of practicing nurses in hospitals, clinics, schools, and elsewhere for solid practical advice on the legal and ethical issues that influence their jobs. In addressing these critical needs, the Journal will also benefit lawyers, risk managers, health care administrators, nursing students, and health care providers who employ nurses.

JOURNAL FACTS

Publication schedule: quarterly

Circulation: 1,000

Submitted papers per year: 24-30

Acceptance rate: 85%

Monetary honorarium: none

Average turnaround time: 3-4 weeks

Publishing timetable: 3-6 months after acceptance

Correspondence:
    PESI HealthCare, LLC
    200 Spring Street
    P.O. Box 1000
    Eau Claire, WI 54702-1000
    Telephone: (715) 833-5288
    Fax: (715) 836-0031
    E-mail: info@pesi.com
Internet site: www.pesihealthcare.com

MANUSCRIPT SUBMISSION

Articles should be 10-20 pages long and cover topics such as: unlicensed assistive personnel (delegation); the nurse's role in informed consent; liability issues concerning documentation; understaffing; analysis of and mechanisms for complying with new federal legislation, such as ADA Patient Self-Determination Act, Medical Devices Safety Act; legal and ethical issues regarding patients and health care workers with infectious diseases; risks of specific areas of nursing practice; issues involving professional liability insurance; legal and ethical trends and events in a state that would be of interest to nurses nationally; and ethical issues affecting nursing.

Articles should address legal or ethical issues affecting nursing practice and include the analysis of cases, laws, and regulations. They should offer possible suggestions for decreasing nursing liability or improving patient care. Inclusion of figures and tables is recommended, where possible. The Journal is interested in identifying legal and procedural trends and discussing their effects on nursing.

Send manuscripts to:

Shelly Kistner, Managing Editor
Journal of Nursing Law
c/o PESI HealthCare, LLC
P.O. Box 1000
Eau Claire, WI 54702-1000
Telephone: (715) 833-5288
Fax: (715) 836-0031
E-mail: skistner@pesihealthcare.com

If your article is published, you will receive three copies of the Journal that includes it.

MANUSCRIPT PREPARATION GUIDELINES

Your manuscript should be 10-20 typed pages long. Please double-space. Along with the manuscript, send a 3½" disk on which the article is saved as a WordPerfect or ASCII file, if available. Include a one-paragraph abstract of the article.

Follow the *Publication Manual of the American Psychological Association,* 4th ed. Send a one-paragraph biography. It will be included with your article in the Journal.

REFEREED PUBLICATION

Each article is subject to a high-quality peer review to ensure accuracy and relevance.

COPYRIGHT

PESI HealthCare, LLC, intends to hold copyright to the articles. Authors will be requested to sign a contributor's agreement that assigns ownership and warrants originality. If the manuscript, any significant portion of it or quotations consisting of 50 or more consecutive words have been published before or if copyright resides other than in the author, reprint permission must be obtained by the author in a form acceptable to PESI HealthCare, LLC. The author accepts responsibility for the accuracy of any cite to statutes, cases, and regulations.

INDEXED

Not indexed.

SAMPLE JOURNAL ARTICLE TITLES

- "Avoiding Malpractice—Beyond the Scope of Employment"
- "Boarder Babies and the Public Trust: A Case Study"
- "Developing a Business Plan for Your Legal Nurse Consulting Practice"
- " 'I Wouldn't Want to Live': The Myth About Attitudes of Terminal Patients"
- "Protecting Patients From Incompetent or Unethical Colleagues: An Important Dimension of the Nurse's Advocacy Role"

The Journal of Legal Nurse Consulting

The *Journal of Legal Nurse Consulting* is published by the American Association of Legal Nurse Consultants and is the official publication of the American Association of Legal Nurse Consultants.

Telephone: (877) 402-2562
Fax: (847) 375-6313
Internet site: www.aalnc.org

JOURNAL FOCUS/PURPOSE

The primary purpose of *The Journal of Legal Nurse Consulting* is to provide current information on medical, legal, and consultant practice issues as well as case law updates and association news. The journal also seeks to promote legal nurse consulting within the medical-legal community, to provide both the novice and the experienced legal nurse consultant with a quality professional publication, and to teach and inform the legal nurse consultant about clinical practice, current national legal issues, and professional development.

JOURNAL FACTS

Publication schedule: quarterly

Circulation: 4,000

Submitted papers per year: 50

Acceptance rate: 80%

Monetary honorarium: none

Average turnaround time: 6-8 weeks

Publishing timetable: 6-8 weeks after acceptance

Correspondence:
   American Association of Legal Nurse
      Consultants
   Jim Gubman, *JLNC*
   Managing Editor
   4700 W. Lake Avenue
   Glenview, IL 60025-1485

MANUSCRIPT SUBMISSION

The journal accepts original articles, case studies, letters, and research. Query letters are welcomed but not required. Material must be original and never published before and should not be submitted to any other journal simultaneously.

Manuscripts should be addressed to:

   JNLC Managing Editor
   4700 W. Lake Avenue
   Glenview, IL 60025-1485

MANUSCRIPT PREPARATION GUIDELINES

Manuscripts must be typed double-spaced on $8\frac{1}{2} \times 11$-inch, plain white paper and should not exceed 12 pages (approximately 3,000 words). The title page should include the title of the manuscript, the authors' names, credentials, work affiliations, and daytime phone and fax numbers. One author should be designated as the corresponding author. The title page, the illustrations, and the reference list should each appear on a separate page. Pages, beginning with the title page, should be numbered consecutively.

It is desirable, but not absolutely necessary, that a manuscript be submitted on a computer disk (either a $3\frac{1}{2}$-in. or $5\frac{1}{4}$-in. disk is acceptable). The file should be saved as ASCII Text Only or Text Only in the dialogue box that appears on the screen when the Save As option is selected. If there is more than one file on the disk, indicate the name of the file that contains your submission.

The Journal of Legal Nurse Consulting follows the manuscript style and reference guidelines of the *Publication Manual of the American Psychological Association* (4th ed.). Legal citations must adhere to the guidelines published in *The Bluebook: A Uniform System of Citation* (15th ed.), Cambridge, MA: The Harvard Law Review Association.

Acquiring permission to reprint previously published material (e.g., illustrations) is the responsibility of the author. Figures include line drawings, diagrams, and graphs. Tables show data in an orderly display of columns and rows, to facilitate comparison. Each illustration should be labeled sequentially (e.g., Figure 1, Figure 2 or Table 1, Table 2) and should correspond to a statement in the text directing the reader to see such a figure or table (e.g., see Figure 1). When using figures from another source, the author must obtain written permission from the original publisher and include that as part of the manuscript submission materials.

All photographs must be black-and-white glossy prints. The author is responsible for obtaining permission for the use of photographs of identifiable persons.

Upon acceptance of the manuscript, the author will yield copyright to *The Journal of Legal Nurse Consulting*. Permission for reprints or reproduction must be obtained from the American Association of Legal Nurse Consultants.

REFEREED PUBLICATION

Manuscript submissions are peer-reviewed by eminent professional legal nurse consultants with diverse professional backgrounds. Manuscript assistance can be provided upon request to the editor. Acceptance will be based on the importance of the material for the audience and the quality of the material.

COPYRIGHT

Copyright by the American Association of Legal Nurse Consultants.

INDEXED

The Journal of Legal Nurse Consulting is indexed in the *Cumulative Index to Nursing and Allied Health Literature.*

SAMPLE JOURNAL ARTICLE TITLES

- "Alternative Dispute Resolution: Mediation and Arbitration"
- "Creating a Resume for the Legal Field, Part I"
- "Imaging of the Lumbar Spine With CT and MRI"
- "Pharmaceutical Products Liability, Part I: Legal Concepts"
- "Selecting Computer Equipment for a Legal Nurse Consulting Practice"

10

Maternal/Child Care

AWHONN Lifelines

AWHONN *Lifelines* is published for the Association of Women's Health, Obstetric and Neonatal Nurses by Lippincott Williams & Wilkins and is an official publication of the Association of Women's Health, Obstetric and Neonatal Nurses.

JOURNAL FOCUS/PURPOSE

The primary purpose of the *AWHONN Lifelines* is to educate, guide, and report on health care trends and current everyday practice issues in women's health, obstetric, and neonatal nursing.

JOURNAL FACTS

Publication schedule: bimonthly
Circulation: 22,500
Submitted papers per year: 288
Acceptance rate: not available
Monetary honorarium: none
Average turnaround time: 4-6 weeks
Publishing timetable: 4 months after acceptance
Correspondence:
    Association of Women's Health, Obstetric and
    Neonatal Nurses

2000 L Street, NW, Suite 740
Washington, DC 20036
Telephone: 1-800-673-8499, ext. 2437
Fax: (202) 728-0575
E-mail: Lifelines@awhonn.org

Or

Lippincott Williams & Wilkins
Business Offices
227 East Washington Square
Philadelphia, PA 19106-3780
Telephone: (215) 238-4200

Or

12107 Insurance Way
Hagerstown, MD 21740
Telephone: (301) 714-2300
Fax: (301) 714-2398
Customer service: 1-800-638-3030

Internet site: www.awhonn.org/lifeline/
    index.html or www.awhonn.org or
    www.nursingcenter.com/journals

MANUSCRIPT SUBMISSION

All documents should be submitted to:
    Carolyn Davis Cockey, Executive Editor
    AWHONN Lifelines
    804 W. Wildwood Avenue
    Ft. Wayne, IN 46807-1643
    Telephone: (877) 744-3899 or (219) 744-3899
    Fax: (219) 744-7443

E-mail: Lifelines@awhonn.org or
carolyndc@awhonn.org

Manuscripts can be submitted in a variety of formats, including features on particular health and nursing issues, case studies, literature review, clinical innovations, opinion pieces, and first-person experiences. We recognize that our writers are nurses, not professional writers. We are willing to help you focus your article's information and coach you in magazine writing style.

AWHONN Lifelines publishes only original works. Manuscripts must not have been previously published and must not be under consideration by another publication. We also retain all rights to works published in print and online. All authors must sign and return the Copyright Transfer and Warranty Agreement with the manuscript.

AWHONN Lifelines welcomes manuscripts on a variety of topics, including innovations and trends within clinical and nursing practice, the management of individual patients and patient populations, the impact of health care systems, the impact of ethical and legal trends on patient care issues and professional practice, the impact of legislative/regulatory actions on health care practice, or any other relevant, newsworthy topic suitable to the mission of *AWHONN Lifelines*. We suggest writers who want to submit articles for consideration to *AWHONN Lifelines* familiarize themselves with the magazine. All features and departments are open for writer submissions based on the following:

- Articles: Should not exceed 2,500 words, or approximately 10 typed pages, including references
- Departments: Should not exceed 1,000 words, or approximately 4 typed pages, including references
- Letters to the Editor: Should not exceed 400 words, or approximately 1.5 typed pages

Authors should also include helpful "sidebar" materials, such as sources for additional reading, WWW sites, and lists of helpful organizations with their WWW addresses and phone numbers to aid readers in gathering additional information.

MANUSCRIPT PREPARATION GUIDELINES

AWHONN Lifelines will accept for consideration articles submitted within the following format:

- Author names should not appear on the manuscript pages; the review process is blinded.
- Manuscripts (articles) must be submitted with signed author application and copyright transfer form.
- Double-spaced with one-inch margins and with type in both upper and lower case.
- Use only one side of the paper, number pages consecutively, beginning with the title page.
- Articles must be submitted on either an IBM-compatible PC diskette with two copies of the file printed out or via e-mail. Articles submitted via e-mail should be sent to Lifelines@awhonn.org.
- If submitting via e-mail, fax one copy of the article to (219) 744-7443, attn: Executive Editor.
- Microsoft Word is preferred for submission of copy on diskette or via e-mail.

Because visual aids enhance reader understanding, writers should include tables, lists, photographs, drawings, illustrations, etc., with their manuscript submission. All authors must provide copies of written permission from copyright holders to reproduce copyrighted materials with their article. All visual and graphics submitted without such permissions will be rejected. Writers must also provide accurate credit information as to the source; this includes names and copyrights where applicable. Every effort will be made to return original art upon request; however, *AWHONN Lifelines* assumes no responsibility for such.

The writing style used in *AWHONN Lifelines* is direct, informative and conversational; *AWHONN Lifelines* reads much the way you speak to your professional colleagues. We encourage writers to include clinical experiences with techniques precisely discussed. Within your article, cite primary references only. Seek out and use the most current and up-to-date references (evidence) in your text; lack of current referencing is the most common reason articles are rejected for publication. Limit your references to no more than 10 sources. Matters of fact that are well established in nursing, such as normal pulse rate ranges, don't need to be referenced. In formatting your cited references, follow the standards set for references in the *Publication Manual of the American Psychological Association.* Use generic names of all drugs and devices; put brand name equivalents (when applicable) in parenthesis on first mention in the text.

AWHONN Lifelines reserves the right to edit all submissions for clarity, accuracy, length, publication style, and standard English use. We don't reject manuscripts just because they might need a little—or a whole lot—of editing. We will work through the editing with you to help you improve your professional writing abilities. But we will ask you to be flexible in matters of publication style and content. Editing effects can range from simple changes in a headline to extensive condensing and redrafting of the article. In all cases, every attempt will be made to have the author review the final edited manuscript, although we reserve the right to recognize that in all cases this will not always be possible.

REFEREED PUBLICATION

All featured articles within *AWHONN Lifelines* are reviewed by up to three reviewers considered familiar with the particular subject matter, including at least one member of the *AWHONN Lifelines* editorial board. When necessary, articles may receive additional review to ensure the accuracy and usefulness. Although *AWHONN Lifelines* works with a panel of selected expert reviewers, we often use professionals outside our organization to further ensure the quality and integrity of the materials published. All articles are sent to our reviewers blinded—that is, with the author's name and credentials deleted—so that the reviewer doesn't know who is authoring the work. We do this because we think we get a more fair and even-handed review of the article based on its merit alone. Questions about reviews should be addressed to the Executive Editor.

COPYRIGHT

Copyright by AWHONN, the Association of Women's Health, Obstetric and Neonatal Nurses.

INDEXED

The *AWHONN Lifelines* is indexed in the *Cumulative Index to Nursing and Allied Health Literature, Index Medicus, International Nursing Index,* and *MEDLINE.*

SAMPLE JOURNAL ARTICLE TITLES

- "Coming to Terms: Electronic Fetal Monitoring Update"

- "Nursing & the 'Net': Exploring World Wide Web Opportunities"
- "Keeping the Faith: Jewish Traditions in Pregnancy & Childbirth"

- "Preventing Osteoporosis"
- "Sexual Health Across the Lifespan: Covering All the Bases: Teaching Women About Their Sexuality"

Issues in Comprehensive Pediatric Nursing

Issues in Comprehensive Pediatric Nursing is published by Taylor & Francis Inc.

Taylor & Francis Inc.
325 Chestnut Street, 8th Floor
Philadelphia, PA 19106
Telephone: (215) 625-8900
Fax: (215) 625-2940

Internet site: www.taylorandfrancis.com or www.taylorandfrancis.com/JNLS/cpn.htm

JOURNAL FOCUS/PURPOSE

The primary purpose of *Issues in Comprehensive Pediatric Nursing* is to contribute to the literature now available to practitioners, researchers, educators, administrators, and students in nursing and other related health disciplines. The journal is devoted to examining the specific needs of children and their families through the framework of state-of-the-art interventions, theory, research, dissemination, and related organizational and management concepts.

JOURNAL FACTS

Publication schedule: quarterly

Circulation: approximately 600

Submitted papers per year: 25-30

Acceptance rate: 85%

Monetary honorarium: none

Average turnaround time: 8-12 weeks

Publishing timetable: 5-6 months after acceptance

Correspondence:

MANUSCRIPT SUBMISSION

Nurse authors as well as coauthors representing health-related disciplines are invited to submit manuscripts. Only unpublished work is invited for submission. If the manuscript is a research report involving human subjects, it must contain a statement indicating that informed consent was obtained. Authors are responsible for obtaining permission to reproduce copyrighted material from other sources and are required to sign an agreement for the transfer of copyright to the publisher. All accepted manuscripts, artwork, and photographs become the property of the publisher. Submission of a manuscript to this journal is understood to imply that it or substantial parts of it have not been published or accepted for publication elsewhere and that it is not under consideration for publication elsewhere. Authors are notified about the decision to publish within 6 to 8 weeks of receipt of a completed manuscript. Please note that e-mail submissions to the editor are welcome.

Send the original manuscript and two copies to the editor:

Jane Bliss-Holtz, DNSc, RN, C
P.O. Box 619
Rocky Hill, NJ 08553
E-mail: janel@idt.net

One set of page proofs is sent to the designated author. Proofs should be checked and returned within 48 hours.

MANUSCRIPT PREPARATION GUIDELINES

Manuscripts must be submitted in the style and format described in the *Publication Manual of the American Psychological Association,* 4th ed. (1994). Copies of the manual can be obtained from the Publication Department of the American Psychological Association, 750 First Street NE, Washington, DC 20002-4242. Telephone: (202) 336-5500.

The manuscript must be typewritten, double-spaced, with 1½″ margins all around. Typically, manuscripts should range in length from 14-16 pages. Manuscripts must be accompanied by a title page and an abstract not to exceed 250 words. Refer to the manual for specifications regarding the title page, running heads, short title, page numbering, abstract, tables/figures, and references.

One set of page proofs is sent to the designated author. Proofs should be checked and returned within 48 hours.

The corresponding author of each article will receive one complete copy of the issue in which the article appears. Reprints of an individual article may be ordered from Taylor & Francis. Use the reprint order form included with page proofs.

REFEREED PUBLICATION

Issues in Comprehensive Pediatric Nursing is a refereed journal.

COPYRIGHT

Copyright by Taylor & Francis Inc.

INDEXED

Issues in Comprehensive Pediatric Nursing is indexed in the *Cumulative Index to Nursing and Allied Health Literature, International Nursing Index, Journal of Abstracts in International Education, Psychology Abstracts, Sage Family Studies Abstracts, SAM Index,* and *Social Abstracts.*

SAMPLE JOURNAL ARTICLE TITLES

- "Influence of Health Locus of Control and Parental Health Perceptions on Follow-Through With School Nurse Referral"
- "Nurses' Assessments and Management of Pain in Children Having Orthopedic Surgery"
- "Preschool Children of Battered Women Identified in a Community Setting"
- "Salivary Cortisol Testing in Children"
- "Spasticity in Children With Cerebral Palsy: A Retrospective Review of the Effects of Intrathecal Baclofen"

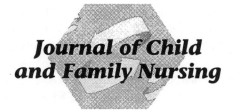

Journal of Child and Family Nursing

The *Journal of Child and Family Nursing* is published by Lippincott Williams & Wilkins.

JOURNAL FOCUS/PURPOSE

The primary purpose of the *Journal of Child and Family Nursing* is to feature a state-of-the-science article on a topic of interest to nurses who work with children.

JOURNAL FACTS

Publication schedule: bimonthly

Circulation: 1,500

Submitted papers per year: 10 review articles

Acceptance rate: 80%

Monetary honorarium: none

Average turnaround time: 4 months

Publishing timetable: 3-4 months after acceptance

Correspondence:
Lippincott Williams & Wilkins
Business Offices
227 East Washington Square
Philadelphia, PA 19106-3780
Telephone: (215) 238-4200

Or
12107 Insurance Way
Hagerstown, MD 21740
Telephone: (301) 714-2300
Fax: (301) 714-2398
Customer services: 1-800-638-3030

Internet site: www.nursingcenter.com/journals

MANUSCRIPT SUBMISSION

Please submit two paper copies and one disk with manuscript on it. If you prefer to send as an attachment to e-mail, that's fine also. Please use text file to save.

For submission of an e-mail attachment send to:
E-mail: mebroome@uwm.edu

For submission of a paper manuscript send to:
Marion E. Broome, RN, PhD, FAAN
P.O. Box 413, Cunningham Hall
University of Wisconsin
Milwaukee, WI 53201
Telephone: (414) 220-4030

Each issue of *Journal of Child and Family Nursing* will feature state-of-the-science articles on a topic of interest to nurses who work with children. Authors who are experts in the field, and accomplished authors, will be invited to submit a manuscript that contains the following:

A. Introduction: This background section should include the significance of the topic to nursing, any relevant historical perspective on the topic and how study of the topic has evolved over time, definitions, and so on.

B. Theoretical perspectives: In this section, the author should outline any theoretical perspectives used to study the topic, along with a critique of the usefulness of each perspective to increasing our understanding of the area.

C. Empirical research: This section presents a synthesis of research in the area and includes a section on limitations of methods used to study the topic.

D. Directions for further research: In this section, the author's recommendations for further research should be described. Please be as specific as possible.

E. Implications for practice: Recommendations, reference to any existing guidelines, and so on should be presented here that would help the practicing nurse guide practice in the area.

The author is encouraged to use charts, figures, algorithms, and the like to help the reader quickly visualize the content. The focus of this review paper is on synthesis, critique, and recommendations, and the author should make it easy for the reader to use the information presented.

MANUSCRIPT PREPARATION GUIDELINES

1. The paper should be 14-16 pages long.
2. APA style of referencing and formatting should be used.

COPYRIGHT

Copyright by Lippincott Williams & Wilkins.

INDEXED

The *Journal of Child and Family Nursing* is indexed in the *Cumulative Index to Nursing and Allied Health Literature* and *MEDLINE.*

SAMPLE JOURNAL ARTICLE TITLES

- "Culturally Competent Nursing Research: Are We There Yet?"
- "Health Promotion for Children"
- "The Child With a Chronic Condition"
- "The Child With an Acute or Critical Illness"
- "Watch Out! The Bogeyman Is in the Hospital Closet: Measurement of Children's Medical Fears"

Journal of Midwifery & Women's Health

The *Journal of Midwifery & Women's Health* (formerly the *Journal of Nurse-Midwifery*) is published by Elsevier Science and is the official journal for the American College of Nurse-Midwives (ACNM).

research and new knowledge within: nurse-midwifery, family-centered childbirth, well-woman gynecology, family planning, women's health, and parent-child health.

JOURNAL FOCUS/PURPOSE

The primary purpose of the *Journal of Midwifery & Women's Health* is to speak with authority on all aspects of nurse-midwifery care today, providing extensive coverage of current

JOURNAL FACTS

Publication schedule: bimonthly

Circulation: 8,000

Submitted papers per year: 70

Acceptance rate: 50%

Monetary honorarium: none

Average turnaround time: 2-3 months

Publishing timetable: 3-6 months after acceptance

Correspondence:
American College of Nurse-Midwives
818 Connecticut Avenue, NW, Suite 900
Washington, DC 20006
Telephone: (202) 728-9860
Fax: (202) 728-9897
E-mail: info@acnm.org

Internet site: www.infor@acnm.org or
www.elsevier.com

MANUSCRIPT SUBMISSION

Authors should submit complete sets of the manuscript and the author checklist that follows to:

Mary Ann Shah, CNM, MS, FACNM
Editor-in-Chief, *Journal of Midwifery &
Women's Health*
67 Tarry Hill Road
Tarrytown, NY 10591-6511
E-mail: jnmmas@aol.com

A 3- to 9-month turnaround time from acceptance to publication should be anticipated.

A submitted manuscript must be accompanied by an agreement signed by each of the authors. A copy of this agreement can be found at the end of the checklist portion of these instructions. By signing the form, each author agrees with the following: (1) that the content of the paper is original and is being contributed solely to *Journal of Midwifery & Women's Health;* (2) that each author has participated meaningfully in the conception, writing, and approval of the manuscript, and to a degree sufficient that he or she can take public responsibility for the work described; (3) that no financial affiliations are held by any author that could represent a potential conflict of interest in terms of the content presented; and (4) that if the paper is ultimately accepted, the copyright will transfer to the ACNM.

MANUSCRIPT PREPARATION GUIDELINES

The Editorial Board of the *Journal of Midwifery & Women's Health* welcomes unsolicited manuscripts that address issues related to women's health, childbearing families, and nurse-midwifery. A manuscript will be accepted for review with the understanding that it has been submitted exclusively to the *Journal of Midwifery & Women's Health,* that the content is not fraudulent, and that the material does not infringe on or violate any copyright agreements or any other personal or proprietary rights. The *Journal of Midwifery & Women's Health* accepts no responsibility for statements made by contributors or claims made by advertisers. In addition, neither the *Journal of Midwifery & Women's Health* nor the ACNM necessarily endorse any viewpoints expressed or implied therein, nor does the inclusion of any product advertisement imply *Journal of Midwifery & Women's Health/*ACNM endorsement.

Manuscripts are subject to modification and revisions to bring them into conformity with the *Uniform Requirements for Manuscripts Submitted to Biomedical Journals* promulgated by the International Committee of Medical Journal Editors. Specific guidelines can be found in *Journal of Nurse-Midwifery,* Volume 37, Number 1, January/February 1992, pp. 71-76.

The *Journal of Midwifery & Women's Health* is not responsible for manuscripts that are lost or destroyed. Manuscripts will be returned only upon request and when accompanied by a self-addressed stamped envelope. Rejected manuscripts will be retained on file for 1 year from date of submission. Thereafter, they will be destroyed.

Authors receive page proofs of their articles to be proofread, corrected, and returned within 48 hours of receipt. Authors will be charged for extensive alterations and revisions made on page proofs. Reprints may be ordered before publication using the price list enclosed with proofs.

REFEREED PUBLICATION

The *Journal of Midwifery & Women's Health* is refereed. Each manuscript submitted to the *Journal of Midwifery & Women's Health* undergoes a blind review by members of the *Journal of Midwifery & Women's Health*'s Peer Review Panel and Editorial Board. Every manuscript that is submitted to the *Journal of Midwifery & Women's Health* for consideration as a full-length article is reviewed by a minimum of five members of the Editorial Board, three peer review panelists, and when appropriate, by one to three research consultants.

COPYRIGHT

Copyright by the American College of Nurse-Midwives.

INDEXED

The *Journal Midwifery & Women's Health* is indexed in the *Cumulative Index to Nursing and Allied Health Literature; Current Contents—Social Sciences Citation Index; Current Contents—Social and Behavioral Sciences; Index Medicus; International Nursing Index; Nursing Abstracts; Nursing Citation Index;* and *RNdex Top 100.*

SAMPLE JOURNAL ARTICLE TITLES

- "Abrupt Onset of Severe Pain at Term: A Case Report"
- "Becoming a Father: First-Time Father's Experience of Labor and Delivery"
- "The Historical Relationship of Nurse-Midwifery With Medicine"
- "The Relationship of Ambulation in Labor to Operative Delivery"
- "Transfer Rates From Freestanding Birth Centers: A Comparison With the National Birth Center Study"

JOGNN, Journal of Obstetric, Gynecologic, and Neonatal Nursing

The *Journal of Obstetric, Gynecologic, and Neonatal Nursing (JOGNN)* is published by Lippincott Williams & Wilkins and is the official journal of the Association of Women's Health, Obstetric and Neonatal Nurses.

JOURNAL FOCUS/PURPOSE

The primary purpose of the *Journal of Obstetric, Gynecologic, and Neonatal Nursing* is to reflect practice, research, opinions, policies, and trends in the nursing care of women, child-bearing families, and newborns.

JOURNAL FACTS

Publication schedule: bimonthly

Circulation: 24,000

Submitted papers per year: 110

Acceptance rate: 65%

Monetary honorarium: none

Average turnaround time: 2-3 months for first review cycle

Publishing timetable: approximately 1 year or less after acceptance

Correspondence:
Association of Women's Health, Obstetric, and Neonatal Nurses
2000 L Street, NW, Suite 740
Washington, DC 20036
Telephone: (202) 261-2438
Fax: (202) 728-0575

Internet site: www.awhonn.org/jognn/jognn.htm or www.awhonn.org or www.nursingcenter.com/journals

MANUSCRIPT SUBMISSION

Mail five copies of the manuscript in a heavy paper envelope. Enclose the manuscript copies, figures, and photographs in cardboard to prevent bending of the materials in the mail. Place photographs and transparencies in a separate heavy paper envelope within the manuscript envelope.

Address manuscripts to:
Lillian Biller, Managing Editor
Journal of Obstetric, Gynecologic, and Neonatal Nursing
2000 L Street, NW, Suite 740
Washington, DC 20036 ·
Telephone: (202) 261-2438

The Current editor is Karen B. Haller, RN, PhD.

MANUSCRIPT PREPARATION GUIDELINES

Type the manuscript on white, 8½ × 11-inch paper. Double-space all the pages, including the title page, abstract, text, acknowledgments, references, tables, and legends. Use 10- or 12-point type, on one side of the paper only. Use uniform margins of 1½ inches (4 cm) at the top, bottom, right, and left. Do not right-justify lines. Do not divide words at the end of a line. Type everything, including titles and headings, in uppercase and lowercase letters.

Number pages consecutively; include a running head (50 characters or fewer) at the top of each page to identify the manuscript. The running head, a shortened version of the title, must not contain any author names or initials. In the left margin, number each line of text. The average length of an article should be 12 to 16 manuscript pages, plus references, tables, illustrations, and callouts.

Refer to the *Publication Manual of the American Psychological Association* (4th ed.) for grammar, punctuation, and style; *Webster's Tenth New Collegiate Dictionary* for spelling of nontechnical words; and *Dorland's Illustrated Medical Dictionary* for spelling of medical terms. Use generic names of all drugs and products. Report physical measures in SI (International System of Units) units. For examples of conversion to SI equivalents, refer to the APA manual.

Limit the title to 10 to 15 words. Be sure that the title summarizes the main idea of the paper, is fully explanatory standing alone, informs readers about the article, avoids words that serve no useful purpose, and avoids the use of the words *method, results, a study,* and *an experimental investigation.*

Abstracts are required for all manuscripts. For Principles & Practice, Thoughts, & Opinions, Case Reports, and Clinical Issues articles, enclose an abstract of no more than 75 words (in paragraph form). The abstract should be factual, not descriptive, giving the main points of the paper. Instead of saying what will be described, describe it. Structured abstracts are required for Clinical Studies (research) articles and In Review articles and should have no more than 200 words. (See JOGNN author guidelines on www.awhonn.org.)

Callouts highlight a major premise or conclusion of an article. The author may use direct quotes from the manuscript or write new sentences. Provide three callouts for each article. Indicate in the manuscript approximately where each callout should appear in the published article. Avoid repeating text found in the abstract or the first page of the article.

Cite primary sources only. Primary references usually should be no more than 5 years old, although classic texts may be referenced if appropriate. Cite references in the text in the style outlined in the *Publication Manual of the American Psychological Association* (4th ed.). All references appearing in the reference list must be called out in the text. The reference list also should be formatted in American Psychological Association style. Use references prudently. Identify sources of quotations and all other borrowed materials. The authors must obtain written permission to reprint long quotations, figures, tables, photographs, and the like from the original authors and publishers. Include the releases with the submitted manuscript.

Written permission must be obtained from the administration of institutions named in the narrative. Letters of permission must be submitted before publication of the manuscript.

Submit camera-ready artwork. Do not include more than six tables. Submit only actual tabular material in table form. Simple lists should be incorporated into the text. Type each table on a separate page with its own title. Number tables consecutively with arabic numerals and cite in numeric order in the text. Number pages with tables following the reference list. The author must obtain written permission to include a previously published table with the article. Each previously published table must carry a credit line stating the original source.

Have all figures, graphs, and illustrations professionally prepared in black ink or produced on a high-quality laser printer and submit unmounted, glossy black-and-white photographs. Each figure, graph, or illustration should be on a separate page with its own title. Number figures consecutively with arabic numerals, and cite each figure in numeric order in the text. Number pages with figures following the reference page(s) and table pages(s). Follow the American Psychological Association style when labeling tables, figures, and photographs. Keep all explanatory material and legends in the captions beneath the figure, graph, or illustration to which they pertain.

The author must obtain subjects' written permission to publish their photographs in the *Journal of Obstetric, Gynecologic, and Neonatal Nursing.* All authors must sign a copyright transfer which is included in the author guidelines available at www.awhonn.org. The authors must disclose any commercial interest they have in the subject of their study as well as the source of any financial or material support.

REFEREED PUBLICATION

The *Journal of Obstetric, Gynecologic, and Neonatal Nursing* is a peer-reviewed journal, and all manuscripts are submitted to referees who decide on publication.

COPYRIGHT

The *Journal of Obstetric, Gynecologic, and Neonatal Nursing* is protected by copyright. Copyright is held by the Association of

Women's Health, Obstetric and Neonatal Nurses.

INDEXED

The *Journal of Obstetric, Gynecologic, and Neonatal Nursing* is indexed in *Index Medicus, International Nursing Index, Cumulative Index of Nursing and Allied Health Literature,* and *RNdex Top 100.*

SAMPLE JOURNAL ARTICLE TITLES

- "Antiphospholipid Antibodies: A Threat Throughout Pregnancy"
- "Breastfeeding Patterns of Low-Birth-Weight Infants After Hospital Discharge"
- "Emergency Contraception: The Nurse's Role in Providing Postcoital Options"
- "Pastoral Care for Perinatal and Neonatal Health Care Providers"
- "Reliability and Validity Testing of Three Breastfeeding Assessment Tools"

Journal of Pediatric Health Care

The *Journal of Pediatric Health Care* is published by Mosby, Inc., and is the official journal of the National Association of Pediatric Nurse Associates & Practitioners.

JOURNAL FOCUS/PURPOSE

The primary purpose of the *Journal of Pediatric Health Care* is to provide pediatric nurses practicing in expanded roles with current didactic and research articles in the following areas: ambulatory care, primary care, home health care, school health, and inpatient care. In addition, articles on health care policy and role issues relevant to the advanced pediatric nurse are provided.

JOURNAL FACTS

Publication schedule: bimonthly

Circulation: approximately 7,800

Submitted papers per year: 185

Acceptance rate: approximately 30%

Monetary honorarium: none

Average turnaround time: 6 weeks

Publishing timetable: 9-12 months after acceptance

Correspondence:
Business Office
Mosby, Inc.
11830 Westline Industrial Drive
St. Louis, MO 63146-3318
Telephone: 1-800-453-4351
Fax: (314) 432-1158
E-mail: periodical.service@mosby.com

Or

National Association of Pediatric Nurse
Associates & Practitioners
NAPNAP National Office
1101 Kings Highway North, Suite 206
Cherry Hill, NJ 08034
Telephone: (856) 667-1773
Fax: (856) 667-7187
E-mail: 74224.51@compuserve.com
Internet site: www.mosby.com

MANUSCRIPT SUBMISSION

All manuscripts should be sent to:

Bobbie Crew Nelms, PhD, RN, CPNP
3133 Barbara Street
San Pedro, CA 90731
E-mail: nelms@csulb.edu

Submit the original and three copies to the editor.

Journal of Pediatric Health Care manuscripts are reviewed by editorial board members and selected experts in appropriate specialties. Authors will be notified on receipt of their manuscripts. Notification of acceptance customarily requires 8 to 12 weeks. Acceptance is based on originality of ideas, significance for pediatric nurses, validity, and adherence to the prescribed submission requirements.

Manuscripts become the permanent property of the *Journal of Pediatric Health Care* and may not be published elsewhere without written permission from the author and journal publisher. All accepted manuscripts are subject to manuscript editing.

Authors should disclose at the time of submission any conflict of interest, especially any financial arrangement with a company whose product is discussed in the manuscript. Such information may be held as confidential during the review process. If the article is accepted for publication, an appropriate disclosure statement will be required.

In accordance with the Copyright Act of 1976, all manuscripts must be accompanied by the following statement signed by one author:

The undersigned author transfers all copyright ownership of the manuscript (title of article) to the National Association of Pediatric Nurse Associates & Practitioners in the event the work is published. The undersigned author also warrants that the article is original, is not under consideration by another journal, and has not been previously published. I sign for and accept responsibility for releasing this material on behalf of any and all coauthors.

MANUSCRIPT PREPARATION GUIDELINES

Manuscripts should not exceed 15 pages. Submit the original and three copies, typed double-spaced, one side only, on $8\frac{1}{2} \times 11$-inch paper, with liberal margins on all four sides. Once a manuscript is accepted, the final version of the manuscript may be submitted on diskette along with three copies of the printout. The author accepts responsibility for the submitted diskette's exactly matching the printout of the final version of the manuscript. Guidelines for submission of accepted manuscripts on diskette will be sent to the author by the editorial office. The text must conform to acceptable English usage. If abbreviations cannot be avoided, use the expanded form when first mentioned and abbreviate thereafter. Use generic drug and equipment names (trade names may be listed in parentheses at the point of first mention). If it is necessary to mention a trade name for equipment, the name must be followed immediately by the manufacturer's name and city/state.

The title page should include the full name(s) of author(s), academic degrees, institutional affiliations, and current status. Give the complete mailing address, business and home telephone numbers, and fax number of the author to whom correspondence and reprint requests should be directed. Do not type the authors' names on the manuscript pages.

Abstracts for nonresearch articles should be limited to 100 words and appear on the first page after the title page. The abstract should be factual, not descriptive, and present the key points in the manuscript. Abstracts for research articles should be limited to 200 words or less, appear after the title page, and use the following headings:

Introduction: State the purpose or objective of the study, including the major hypothesis tested, if any.

Method: Describe the study design, the setting, sample, and measures used to collect data.

Results: Describe the major outcomes and statistical significance, if appropriate.

Discussion: State the significance of the results.

Use the reference style of the *Publication Manual of the American Psychological Association,* 4th ed. (1994). The reference list should appear on a separate page at the end of the text. The list should be double-spaced both between and within references. Only references cited in the text should appear in this list.

Tables should be double-spaced throughout, including column headings, data, and footnotes. Each table should be submitted on a separate sheet of paper. They should be numbered according to their mention in the text. A concise title describing the table's content should be supplied for each table. All footnotes should appear immediately below the table, and all abbreviations not used in the text should be defined in a footnote. If a table or any data therein have been previously published, a footnote must give full credit to the original source.

Illustrations (three sets of glossy prints) should be numbered in the order of their mention in the text and marked lightly on the back with the first author's last name and an arrow to indicate the top edge. Drawings or graphs should be prepared in black India ink or typographic (press-apply) lettering. Typewritten or freehand lettering is unacceptable. All lettering must be done professionally and should be in proportion to the drawing, graph, or photograph. Do not send original artwork, X-ray films, or ECG strips. Glossy print photography, 3 × 4 inches (minimum) to 5 × 7 inches (maximum), with good black-and-white contrast or color balance are preferred. Special arrangements must be made with the editor for color plates or numerous illustrations. Consis-

tency in size of illustrations within the article is strongly preferred. Any special instructions regarding sizing should be clearly noted. Illustrations will not be returned unless specifically requested by the author.

Figures may be submitted in electronic format. All images should be at least 5 inches wide. Images should be provided as EPS or TIFF files on Zip disk, CD, floppy, Jaz, or 3.5 MO. Macintosh or PC is acceptable. Graphics software such as Photoshop and Illustrator, not presentation software such as PowerPoint, CorelDraw, or Harvard Graphics, should be used in the creation of the art. Color images need to be CMYK (cyan-magenta-yellow-black), at least 300 DPI (dots per inch), with a digital color proof, not a color laser print or color photocopy. Note: This proof will be used at press for color reproduction. Gray scale images should be at least 300 DPI with a proof. Gray scale line art should be at least 1,200 DPI with a proof. Please include hardware and software information, in addition to file names and fonts, with the disk.

The legends should be typed double-spaced on a separate sheet of paper and numbered to correspond with the figures. If a figure has been previously published, the legend must give full credit to the original source.

Direct quotations, tables, or illustrations that have appeared in copyrighted material must be accompanied by written permission for their use from the copyright owner and original author along with complete information as to source. Photographs of identifiable persons must be accompanied by signed releases showing informed consent.

REFEREED PUBLICATION

The *Journal of Pediatric Health Care* is a peer-reviewed journal with a blind review process.

COPYRIGHT

INDEXED

The *Journal of Pediatric Health Care* is indexed in the *Cumulative Index to Nursing and Allied Health Literature, International Nursing Index, MEDLINE,* and *Nursing Abstracts.*

SAMPLE JOURNAL ARTICLE TITLES

- "An Asthma Management Program for Urban Minority Children"
- "Attention-Deficit/Hyperactivity Disorder: Focus on Pharmacologic Management"
- "Health Care of the Internationally Adopted Child, Part 1"
- "Neonatal Nurse Practitioner and Physician Use on a Newborn Resuscitation Team in a Community Hospital"
- "Tuberculosis, a Pediatric Concern"

Journal of Pediatric Nursing: Nursing Care of Children and Families

The *Journal of Pediatric Nursing: Nursing Care of Children and Families* is published by W. B. Saunders Company.

JOURNAL FOCUS/PURPOSE

The primary purpose of the *Journal of Pediatric Nursing: Nursing Care of Children and Families* is to disseminate subject matter pertinent to the nursing care needs of healthy and ill infants, children, and adolescents addressing their biopsychosocial needs. Papers are published covering the life span from birth to adolescence.

JOURNAL FACTS

Publication schedule: bimonthly
Circulation: approximately 5,000

Submitted papers per year: more than 120

Acceptance rate: approximately 20-30%

Monetary honorarium: none

Average turnaround time: approximately 2 months

Publishing timetable: approximately 1 year after acceptance

Correspondence:
W. B. Saunders
The Curtis Center
Independence Square West
Philadelphia, PA 19106-3399
Telephone: (215) 238-7800 or 1-800-545-2522

Internet site: www.wbsaunders.com

MANUSCRIPT SUBMISSION

Editorial correspondence and manuscripts should be addressed to:
Cecily Lynn Betz, PhD, RN, FAAN

Editor, *Journal of Pediatric Nursing: Nursing Care of Children and Families*
Department of Nursing, University of Southern California
1540 Alcazar Street, CHP 222
Los Angeles, CA 90033
Voice mail: (323) 342-2001
Fax: (323) 342-2091
E-mail: cbetz@aol.com

One author should be designated as correspondent in the covering letter. Authors should retain a copy of their manuscript; the journal is not responsible in the event that a manuscript is lost.

Authors are encouraged to submit abstracts or outlines of potential articles. Feedback and advice about the topic and its development will be provided.

All manuscripts should be submitted in triplicate without identification of the author's name. A postcard acknowledging receipt of manuscripts can be expected by the primary author. Scoring guides used by the reviewers for clinical and research manuscripts are available from the editors on request.

MANUSCRIPT PREPARATION GUIDELINES

The text and references of the manuscript must conform in style to the *Publication Manual of the American Psychological Association.* The separate title page of the manuscript should be typed double-spaced and include the following information: title of the manuscript, author(s) name(s), institutional affiliation(s), and address and phone number of the author who is to receive correspondence.

An abstract of approximately 50 to 100 words should be included on a separate page. Manuscript length should not exceed 25 pages typed double-spaced. The entire manuscript, including text, figure legends, tables, references, footnotes, appendices, abstracts, excerpts, and the like, must be typed double-spaced. If photographs are used, they must be 5×7 black-and-white glossy prints. Authors are responsible for supplying all photographs.

The manuscript must be original, containing only unpublished material not submitted simultaneously for publication in another journal. Manuscripts that are rejected will not be returned unless a stamped, self-addressed envelope has been provided. However, authors will be sent reviewer comments regarding the rationale for rejection.

Authors are responsible for obtaining permission for reproducing copyrighted material. This applies to text, tables, and photographs. Copies of all permission letters must be forwarded to the editors.

REFEREED PUBLICATION

This is a refereed journal. All manuscripts received by the editor and sent to reviewers are treated as privileged communication. Manuscripts are sent to reviewers for blind review. Generally, manuscripts are sent to two review experts. Manuscripts that have been revised one or more times will be reviewed by the original reviewing team to ensure consistency. The review process takes approximately 2 to 3 months.

COPYRIGHT

INDEXED

The *Journal of Pediatric Nursing: Nursing Care of Children and Families* is indexed in the *Cumulative Index to Nursing and Allied*

Health Literature, Index Medicus, and *Nursing Abstracts.*

SAMPLE JOURNAL ARTICLE TITLES

- "Community-Based Pediatric Experiences: Education for the Future"

- "Family Transition Through the Termination of Private Duty Home Care Nursing"
- "Juvenile Arthritis: A Nursing Perspective"
- "Parenting Attitudes and Behaviors of Low-Income Single Mothers With Young Children"
- "The Multiple Meanings of Long-Term Gastrostomy in Children With Severe Disability"

Journal of Perinatal & Neonatal Nursing

The *Journal of Perinatal & Neonatal Nursing* is published by Aspen Publishers, Inc.

200 Orchard Ridge Drive
Gaithersburg, MD 20878
Customer service telephone: 1-800-234-1660

Internet site: www.aspenpub.com (enter journal title in search box)

JOURNAL FOCUS/PURPOSE

The primary purpose of the *Journal of Perinatal & Neonatal Nursing* is to provide practicing nurses with useful information on perinatal/neonatal nursing. Each issue will feature one topic, to be presented in depth.

JOURNAL FACTS

Publication schedule: quarterly

Circulation: approximately 3,000

Submitted papers per year: approximately 50-60

Acceptance rate: approximately 40-50%

Monetary honorarium: none

Average turnaround time: approximately 2 months

Publishing timetable: 6-12 months or longer after acceptance

Correspondence:
  Customer Services

MANUSCRIPT SUBMISSION

Authors are encouraged to submit to the *Journal of Perinatal & Neonatal Nursing* clinically focused, academically sound articles that (1) add new knowledge to the field of perinatal/neonatal nursing and (2) codify existing knowledge or add to the present and future roles of practitioners in the field.

Manuscripts should encompass both perinatal and neonatal aspects whenever possible. Clinical research articles will also be considered. Acceptance or rejection of articles is based on the judgment of the editors and peer reviewers.

Manuscripts (an original and three copies) and correspondence regarding publication should be addressed to:

Perinatal Section:
Diane J. Angelini, EdD, CNM, CNAA,
FACNM
155 Adirondack Drive
East Greenwich, RI 02818
E-mail: Dangelin@wihri.org
phjrnl@ajj.com

Neonatal Section:
Susan Blackburn, RN, C, PhD, FAAN
Department of Family and Child Nursing
Box 357262, University of Washington
Seattle, WA 98195-7262
E-mail: sblackbn@u.washington.edu

MANUSCRIPT PREPARATION GUIDELINES

Manuscripts should be created using Aspen's Journals Authoring Template (template is available from your journal editor or from Aspen). Manuscripts should be created on IBM-compatible (PC) equipment using Windows 95 or higher operating system. Our preferred software is Microsoft Word. Hard copy and electronic files should be submitted for all text and all artwork. All disks submitted must be new. Disks should be clearly labeled as to operating system and software application.

Manuscripts should be double-spaced (including quotations, lists, references, footnotes, figure captions, and all parts of tables).

Manuscripts should be ordered as follows: title page, abstracts, text, references, appendixes, tables, and any illustrations.

Each manuscript must include the following:

Title page, including (1) title of the article, (2) author names (with highest academic degrees) and affiliations (including titles, departments, and name and location of institutions of primary employment), and (3) any acknowledgments, credits, or disclaimers

Abstract of no more than 100 words and up to 10 key words that describe the contents of the article like those that appear in the *Cumulative Index to Nursing and Allied Health Literature (CINAHL)* or the *National Library of Medicine's Medical Subject Headings (MeSH)*

Clear indication of the placement of all tables and figures in text

Signed copyright transfer form

Completed article submission form for each contributor

Written permission for any borrowed text, tables, or figures

References must be cited in text and styled in the reference list according to the *American Medical Association Manual of Style,* 9th ed. (1998). They must be numbered consecutively in the order they are cited; reference numbers may be used more than once throughout an article. Page numbers should appear with the text citation following a specific quote. References should be double-spaced and placed at the end of the text. References should not be created using Microsoft Word's automatic footnote/endnote feature.

References should be included on a separate page at the end of the article and should be double-spaced. Here are some examples of correctly styled reference list entries:

Journals:

Author, article title, journal, year, volume, inclusive pages.

Doe J. Allied medical education. *JAMA.* 1975;23:170-184.

Books:

Author, book title, place of publication, publisher, year.

Cherry B, Geiger J. *Foundations of Maternal Newborn Nursing*. Philadelphia: W. B. Saunders;1994.

Illustrations: Figures should be created using electronic software (i.e., Adobe Illustrator, Corel Draw, and Photoshop). Please save files in both the application in which they were created (i.e., Microsoft Word) and as either EPS or TIFF files. Use computer-generated lettering. Do not use screens, color, shading, or fine lines.

In lieu of original drawings and other material, a sharp, glossy, black-and-white photographic print between 5″ × 7″ and 8″ × 10″ is acceptable.

Each figure should have a label on the back indicating the number of the figure, the names of the authors, and the top of the figure. Do not write on the back of figures, mount them on cardboard, or scratch or mar them using paper clips. Do not bend figures.

Cite each figure in the text in consecutive order. If a figure has been previously published, in part or in total, acknowledge the original source and submit written permission from the copyright holder to reproduce or adapt the material.

Supply a caption for each figure, typed double-spaced on a separate sheet from the artwork. Captions should include the figure title, explanatory statements, notes, or keys as well as source and permission lines.

Provide a camera-ready copy and a separate electronic file for each piece of artwork. Do not embed art in your text file.

Tables should be on a separate page at the end of the manuscript. Number tables consecutively and supply a brief title for each. Include explanatory footnotes for all nonstandard abbreviations. Cite each table in the text in consecutive order. If you use data from another published or unpublished source, obtain permission and acknowledge fully.

Permissions: Authors are responsible for obtaining signed letters from copyright holders granting permission to reprint material being borrowed or adapted from other sources, including previously published material of your own. Authors must obtain written permission for the following material (authors are responsible for any permission fees to reprint borrowed material):

All direct quotes of 300 words or more from any full-length book

All direct quotes of 200 words or more from a periodical article

All excerpts from a newspaper article or other short piece

Any passage from a play or a song

Two or more lines of poetry

Any borrowed table, figure, or illustration being reproduced exactly or adapted to fit the needs of the subject

REFEREED PUBLICATION

The *Journal of Perinatal & Neonatal Nursing* is a refereed journal. Each issue is peer-reviewed and will feature one topic, to be covered in depth. All manuscripts submitted for publication are reviewed by a minimum of three members of the editorial board. The *Journal of Perinatal & Neonatal Nursing* provides a double-blind, fully masked review in which the reviewers do not know the identities of the authors or the authors' facility or institution.

COPYRIGHT

Copyright by Aspen Publishers, Inc.

INDEXED

The *Journal of Perinatal & Neonatal Nursing* is indexed in the *Cumulative Index to Nursing and Allied Health Literature, Current Contents/Social and Behavioral Sciences, Family Studies Database, Health Promotion and Education Database, International Nursing Index, MEDLINE, Nursing Abstracts, Nursing Scan in Critical Care, Social SciSearch, Research Alert®,* and *RNdex Top 100.*

SAMPLE JOURNAL ARTICLE TITLES

- "Electronic Fetal Monitoring Then and Now"
- "Fetal Oxygen Saturation Monitoring During Labor"
- "Pregnancy-Induced Hypertension, Preeclampsia, and Eclampsia"
- "Preterm Birth in the United States: Current Issues and Future Perspectives"
- "The Human Genome Project and Gene Therapy: A Genetic Counselor's Perspective"

Journal of the Society of Pediatric Nursing

The *Journal of the Society of Pediatric Nursing* is published by Nursecom, Inc., and is the official journal of the Society of Pediatric Nurses.

JOURNAL FOCUS/PURPOSE

The primary purpose of the *Journal of the Society of Pediatric Nursing* is to promote the health of infants, children, and adolescents and their families through the dissemination of evidence to guide clinical decision making within the ethical, financial, and organizational context of care. "Evidence" for decision making includes research- and data-based information, clinical expertise, and the perspectives of children and families.

JOURNAL FACTS

Publication schedule: quarterly
Circulation: 3,000
Submitted papers per year: 125
Acceptance rate: 30%
Monetary honorarium: none
Average turnaround time: 2 months
Publishing timetable: 3-6 months

Correspondence:
Journal of the Society of Pediatric Nursing
Nursecom, Inc.
1211 Locust Street
Philadelphia, PA 19107
Telephone: (215) 545-7222 or 1-800-242-6757
Fax: (215) 545-8107
E-mail: margon@compuserve.com

Internet site: www.nursecominc.com/html/jspn.html or www.nursecominc.com

MANUSCRIPT SUBMISSION

Send manuscripts that describe innovations in clinical practice, education, or administration, case presentations, public policy information, synthesis of research findings, and original research. We are particularly interested in manuscripts, regardless of type, that (a) clearly specify the nursing problems/issues, (b) make a compelling argument for the way in which the author addresses the issues, (c) provide information that will facilitate clinical judgments, (d) describe how clinicians can best use the information presented, and (e) where applicable, include a list of additional resources (including web sites) that provide related information for clinical judgment.

Submit 4 copies of the manuscript to:

Roxie Foster, PhD, RN
Editor, *Journal of the Society of Pediatric Nursing*
School of Nursing, Box C288-10
University of Colorado, Health Sciences Center
4200 E. Ninth Avenue
Denver, CO 80262
E-mail: roxie.foster@UCHSC.edu

Each manuscript must be accompanied by a letter stating the following:

As the author(s) of (title of manuscript), I/we hereby transfer copyright ownership to Nursecom, Inc. if the work is published. I/we warrant that the manuscript is original, has not been submitted to another journal, and has not been previously published.

The letter must be signed by all authors. The manuscript cannot be reviewed until this letter is received by the editor. Please include a copy of any other papers published by the author(s) that are similar to the submitted manuscript or that report data from the same study.

Manuscripts will be sent to reviewers with content/methodological expertise in the area; the decision to publish will be based on their recommendations. All reviewers for manuscripts that report results of research hold doctorates. Reviewers for non-data-based papers hold a master's degree in nursing or higher degree. If accepted, the author(s) must submit the manuscript, including figures and tables, on a disk in WordPerfect or Word or e-mail the manuscript to the editor.

MANUSCRIPT PREPARATION GUIDELINES

All manuscripts must be typed, double-spaced, with 1-inch margins, and no more than 17 pages in length, including abstract, references, tables, and figures. Retain a copy of your manuscript; the *Journal of the Society of Pediatric Nursing* is not responsible in the event that a manuscript is lost. Manuscripts will not be returned after review.

Include a title page with the title of the manuscript and name(s), credentials(s), and institutional affiliation(s) of all authors. Provide full mailing address, phone and fax numbers, and e-mail address for the corresponding author. For blind review, authors' names and other identifying information should appear only on the title page.

Include a structured abstract of 100 to 150 words. Headings for research abstracts are as follows: issue(s) and purpose, design and methods, results, practice implications. For other abstracts, headings are as follows: issue(s), purpose, conclusions, implications for practice. Include key words.

Follow the style of the *Publication Manual of the American Psychological Association,* 4th ed. (1994).

Use generic names for medications. Put all measurements in the metric system. Acknowledge any funding (monetary or in-kind support or provision of equipment) for conduct of the research or preparation of the manuscript. If any author has a financial stake in the funding agency or a product mentioned in the manuscript, state this also.

Authors are responsible for obtaining permission to reproduce any copyrighted material, including text, tables, photographs, and figures. Copies of all permission letters must accompany the manuscript. Pictures can be submitted as a glossy print or an original slide. Be sure to clearly identify the picture with the name of the first author. If photographs of people are used and the person in the picture is identifiable, copies of the person's or parent's permission to use the photograph must accompany the manuscript.

REFEREED PUBLICATION

The *Journal of the Society of Pediatric Nursing* is a peer-reviewed journal.

COPYRIGHT

Copyright by Nursecom, Inc., and the Society of Pediatric Nurses

INDEXED

The *Journal of the Society of Pediatric Nursing* is indexed in the *Cumulative Index to Nursing and Allied Health Literature,* *Excerpta Medica, Index Medicus, Nursing Abstracts,* and *Psychology Abstracts.*

SAMPLE JOURNAL ARTICLE TITLES

- "Broken Past, Fragile Future: Personal Stories of High-Risk Adolescent Mothers"
- "Conflicting Responses: The Experiences of Fathers of Infants Diagnosed With Severe Congenital Heart Disease"
- "Role Play: Clinical Pathways—A Tool to Evaluate Clinical Learning"
- "Using Parents' Concerns to Detect and Address Developmental & Behavioral Problems"

MCN: The American Journal of Maternal/Child Nursing

M*CN: The American Journal of Maternal/ Child Nursing* is published by Lippincott Williams & Wilkins.

JOURNAL FOCUS/PURPOSE

The primary purpose of *MCN: The American Journal of Maternal/Child Nursing* is to provide the most timely, relevant information to nurses practicing in perinatal, neonatal, midwifery, and pediatric specialties.

JOURNAL FACTS

Publication schedule: bimonthly

Circulation: 13,000

Submitted papers per year: 100

Acceptance rate: 30 plus

Monetary honorarium: none

Average turnaround time: 8 weeks

Publishing timetable: 6-12 months after acceptance

Correspondence:
Lippincott Williams & Wilkins
Business Offices
227 East Washington Square
Philadelphia, PA 19106-3780
Telephone: (215) 238-4200

Or

12107 Insurance Way
Hagerstown, MD 21740
Telephone: (301) 714-2300
Fax: (301) 714-2398
Customer service: 1-800-638-3030

Internet site: www.nursingcenter.com/journals

MANUSCRIPT SUBMISSION

Submit four copies of your manuscript to:

Dr. Margaret Comerford Freda
Editor, *MCN*
Albert Einstein College of Medicine,
    Montefiore Medical Center
1695 Eastchester Road, Suite 301
Bronx, NY 10461
Telephone: (718) 405-8161 or (718) 892-9184
Fax: (718) 405-8162
E-mail: freda@aecom.yu.edu

MCN is interested in receiving manuscripts that describe practice issues for perinatal, neonatal, midwifery, and pediatric nursing. In addition, clinically relevant research, literature reviews that clearly describe the state of the science/clinical implications, and descriptions of research utilization projects are especially welcome. Manuscripts describing research utilization projects are desired, as are literature reviews that clearly describe the clinical implications of the state of the science. Letters to the editor that comment on the content of *MCN* are always welcomed.

MANUSCRIPT PREPARATION GUIDELINES

Manuscripts describing research utilization projects are desired, as are literature reviews that clearly describe the clinical implications of the state of the science. Letters to the editor that comment on the content of *MCN* are always welcomed.

Manuscripts should be typed double-spaced, using 12-point type, on one side only, with 1-inch margins. Use a letter-quality printer only. Do not send a disk unless you are requested to do so after the review process.

Follow APA format for cites and references (see the *Publication Manual of the American Psychological Association,* 4th ed., 1994).

Number each line of text in the left margin and each page at the top center. Twenty pages of text are the maximum, including references, tables, and figures.

Provide a running head at the top right of each page that describes the title in four words or less. Put no author identification on any page except the title page. Provide an abstract of 250 words that describes the purpose of the article and the clinical implications. For clinical research, the abstract should be a structured one, with these headings: Purpose, Design, Methods (including data collection, sample, instruments), Results, and Clinical Implications.

The title page should include all the authors with their credentials and primary affiliations. Identify address, home and work phones, fax numbers, and e-mail addresses of the author to be contacted. The second page should include three callouts and four key words. Callouts are single sentences that highlight the main theme, the conclusion, and the clinical implications. Key words are single words that classify the manuscript. Use MeSH® (Index Medicus) key words only. The abstract appears on the third page.

The text begins on the fourth page (labeled as page 1). Twenty pages are the maximum, including references, tables (no more than five), and figures. Manuscripts detailing practice issues should have clearly labeled sections starting with Introduction and ending with Clinical Implications. Clinical research submissions should label sections as Introduction, Study Design and Methods, Results, Clinical Implications. *MCN* is especially interested in research with strong Clinical Implications sections.

References (check each carefully for completeness and accuracy before submitting). Unpublished data, personal communication, submitted manuscripts, and non-peer-reviewed publications may not be listed as references. No more than 30 references should be included. References should not be more than 10 years old.

The combined maximum of tables and figures is five.

REFEREED PUBLICATION

MCN is a peer-reviewed journal that meets its mission by publishing clinically relevant practice and research manuscripts aimed at assisting nurses toward evidence-based practice.

COPYRIGHT

Copyright by Lippincott Williams & Wilkins.

INDEXED

MCN: The American Journal of Maternal/Child Nursing is indexed in the *Cumulative Index to Nursing and Allied Health Literature, Index Medicus, International Nursing Index,* and *RNdex Top 100*.

SAMPLE JOURNAL ARTICLE TITLES

- "Camp Superteens: An Asthma Education Program for Adolescents"
- "Comparisons of a Rocking Bed and Standard Bed for Decreasing Withdrawal Symptoms in Drug-Exposed Infants"
- "Lowering the Rate of Unscheduled Extubations"
- "Oral Rehydration Therapy: A Neglected Treatment for Pediatric Diarrhea"
- "The REST Regimen: An Individualized Nursing Intervention for Infant Irritability"

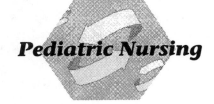

Pediatric Nursing

Pediatric Nursing is published by Jannetti Publications, Inc.

JOURNAL FOCUS/PURPOSE

The primary purpose of *Pediatric Nursing* is to reflect trends, policies, practice, and research in pediatric nursing. Topics should be timely, controversial, and currently unavailable in the literature.

JOURNAL FACTS

Publication schedule: bimonthly

Circulation: 12,000

Submitted papers per year: 50-55

Acceptance rate: 70%

Monetary honorarium: $20 per journal page

Average turnaround time: 9 months

Publishing timetable: 6-12 months after acceptance

Correspondence:
Jannetti Publications, Inc.
East Holly Avenue
Box 56
Pitman, NJ 08071-0056
Telephone: (856) 256-2300
Fax: (856) 589-7463
E-mail: pnjrnl@ajj.com

Internet site: www.ajj.com/jpi or www.ajj.com/jpi/pnj/pnjmain.htm

MANUSCRIPT SUBMISSION

A query letter is requested, including an abstract of the manuscript and the anticipated submission date. Unsolicited manuscripts are welcome, provided that they are for the exclusive use of *Pediatric Nursing* and have not been previously published or accepted for publication or are under consideration elsewhere. Authors are encouraged to use clear, concise, non-discriminatory language.

Authors should send the original and five photocopies of the manuscript to:

Veronica Feeg, PhD, RN, FAAN
Editor, *Pediatric Nursing*
East Holly Avenue
Box 56
Pitman, NJ 08071-0056

A copy of the manuscript should be retained by the authors in the event of damage or loss in transit. Receipt of manuscript is acknowledged by the editor.

MANUSCRIPT PREPARATION GUIDELINES

Manuscripts should be typewritten, double-spaced, on one side of $8\frac{1}{2} \times 11$-inch white paper; maximum length 20 pages (5,000 words). A cover page should include the manuscript title (10-12 words); authors' names, credentials, and primary affiliations; and the address, telephone numbers, and fax number of the primary author. This page should be followed by a substantive abstract of approximately 125-150 words. The manuscript title should be repeated on the first page of the text.

References, photographs, tables, and all other details of style must conform with the *Publication Manual of the American Psychological Association,* 4th ed. (1994). Photographs can be color or black-and-white glossy, 5 × 7 or 8 × 10 inches, and of crisp, clear quality. References in the text should be cited by author and date—for example (Doe & Brown, 1994)—with page numbers cited for direct quotations. The reference list at the end of the manuscript should be double-spaced, include only those references cited in text, and be arranged alphabetically by author. For example:

Journal article:

Doe, J. R., & Brown, M. S. (1994). Coping with hospitalization. Pediatric Nursing, 21(2), 115-120.

Book:

Doe, J. R., & Brown, M. S. (1994). Pediatric nursing care. New York: Academic Press.

Pediatric Nursing reserves the right to edit all manuscripts according to its style and space requirements and to clarify content. Edited copy will be returned for the primary author's approval.

Authors will be notified of a manuscript's acceptance within 12 weeks of receipt, with publication in the next available issue. Manuscripts not accepted for publication will not be returned to the authors.

Disks will be requested for all accepted manuscripts. The Journal will accept both IBM and Macintosh format 3.5″ disks. Most IBM and Macintosh word processor files are acceptable for submission to the Journal.

Each author of a submitted manuscript signs a statement expressly transferring copyright in the event the paper is published. This form will be sent by the editor when receipt of the manuscript is acknowledged.

REFEREED PUBLICATION

Pediatric Nursing is a refereed journal; therefore, each manuscript is reviewed by members of the Manuscript Review Panel as well as the editors. Because manuscripts are reviewed blind (authors anonymous), names of authors should appear only on the cover page. Decisions regarding acceptance for publication are based on the recommendations of the referees.

COPYRIGHT

Copyright on all published articles will be held by *Pediatric Nursing.*

INDEXED

Pediatric Nursing is indexed in *Access to Uncover, Cumulative Index to Nursing and Allied Health Literature, International Nursing Index, Nursing Abstracts, Nursing Citation Index, RNdex Top 100,* and *UMI* (University Microfilms International).

SAMPLE JOURNAL ARTICLE TITLES

- "Accuracy of Tympanic Temperature Readings in Children Under 6 Years of Age"
- "Incidence and Physiologic Characteristics of Hypothermia in the Very Low Birth Weight Infant"
- "Managing Asthma: A Growth and Development Approach"
- "Searching for Normalcy: Mothers' Caregiving for Low Birth Weight Infants"
- "Weight Change of Infants, Age Birth to 12 Months, Born to Abused Women"

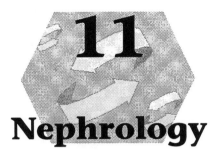

11

Nephrology

Nephrology Nursing Journal

The *Nephrology Nursing Journal* is published by Anthony J. Jannetti, Inc., and is the official journal of the American Nephrology Nurses' Association (ANNA).

JOURNAL FOCUS/PURPOSE

The primary purpose of the *Nephrology Nursing Journal* is to promote excellence and advance nephrology nursing through publication of significant clinical and educational articles, nephrology research, and special features. The *Nephrology Nursing Journal* is a clinical and scientific resource that provides current information to facilitate the practice of professional nephrology nursing. Its purpose is to disseminate the latest information on advances in research, practice, and education to nephrology nurses to positively influence the quality of care they provide.

The *Nephrology Nursing Journal* is designed to meet the education and information needs of nephrology nurses in a variety of roles and at all levels of practice. Its content expands the knowledge base for nephrology nurses, stimulates professional growth, guides research-based practice, presents new technological developments, and provides a forum

for review of critical issues promoting the advancement of nephrology nursing practice.

JOURNAL FACTS

Publication schedule: bimonthly

Circulation: 10,000

Submitted papers per year: 40-45

Acceptance rate: 80%

Monetary honorarium: $100 for continuing education articles only

Average turnaround time: 4-12 months

Publishing timetable: 4-8 months after acceptance

Correspondence:
American Nephrology Nurses' Association
East Holly Avenue
Box 56
Pitman, NJ 08071-0056
Telephone: (856) 256-2320
Fax: (856) 589-7463
E-mail: anna@ajj.com

Internet site: www.annanurse.org

MANUSCRIPT SUBMISSION

Authors should send the original and five photocopies of the manuscript to the Journal office:

Denise Marshall, Editorial Coordinator
Nephrology Nursing Journal

East Holly Avenue
Box 56
Pitman, NJ 08071-0056
Telephone: (856) 256-2320

A copy of the manuscript should be retained by the authors in the event of loss or damage in transit. If you do not receive an acknowledgment within 2 weeks, contact the *Nephrology Nursing Journal,* Editorial Coordinator.

A query letter is requested, including an abstract of the manuscript and the anticipated date of submission. Unsolicited manuscripts are welcome, provided that they are for the exclusive use of the *Nephrology Nursing Journal* and have not been previously published, accepted for publication, or under consideration elsewhere in whole or in part except in abstracted form of 300 words or less.

Authors are encouraged to use clear, concise, nondiscriminatory language and to make readability a priority. Eliminate all discriminatory language by making the preceding referent plural (e.g., nurses . . . they, their)—unless the reference is to a specific person.

Authors of all accepted manuscripts will be asked to submit a disk along with a hard copy of the final edited manuscript following the review process. It is not necessary to submit a disk prior to review. Disk submission guidelines are available through the American Nephrology Nurses' Association National Office or you may download guidelines.

The following are general guidelines to follow when submitting disks to the Journal: The Journal will accept both IBM and Macintosh format disks. All disks should be clearly labeled with your name, manuscript title, disk type (IBM or Macintosh), file name, and word processor name (or file type, if ASCII). Most IBM and Macintosh word processor files are acceptable for submission to the Journal. If possible, all files should be saved as WordPerfect. Please call the Journal office if you have any questions. Please use only common fonts (CG Times, Universe, Helvetica, Courier, etc.) and avoid complex font attributes such as outline. All tables and graphs should be submitted in camera-ready form, if possible. If you will be unable to submit your article on disk, please let us know. If you wish to transfer your article via computer modem, call the Journal office for instructions.

Reprints may be purchased through the National Office.

MANUSCRIPT PREPARATION GUIDELINES

Our manuscript and reference style is based on the *Publication Manual of the American Psychological Association,* 4th ed. (1994). A secondary resource is *The Chicago Manual of Style.*

All material should be typed double-spaced, including abstract, block quotations, reference lists, tables, and figures, on $8\frac{1}{2} \times 11$-inch white paper.

Manuscript titles should be concise, specific, and clear. Generally, they should not be longer that 9-12 words. Avoid unnecessary phrases such as, "the role of . . . ," "use of . . . ," "report of . . . ," "implications of . . . ," and so on. Avoid acronyms. Choose a title that will be accurately indexed (indexers should not have to read the article's abstract to discover what the content is really about). Avoid "cutesy" titles, but make the title interesting enough to attract the reader's attention.

Authors' names should appear only on the title page because manuscripts are reviewed blind (authors remain anonymous to the reviewers). Authors or any other identifying statements such as an acknowledgment should not be identified anywhere within the body of the text.

Biographic information about the author(s) should appear on a separate page. That information should include first name, middle name or initial, and last name; credentials, with highest degree first (e.g., MSN, RN); do not list more than one degree unless there is a compelling reason to do so—for example, PhD, MBA, or MBA, MSN. Give a brief two-sentence autobiographical statement including author's primary affiliation. Do not include additional background information unless it is necessary to explain the author's interest or expertise in the content area.

Sample: Jane Doe, MSN, RN, is Head Nurse for Hemodialysis, Mercy Hospital, Doeville, MA. She is enrolled in the master's program at Doeville University, MA.

The abstract should appear on the first page after the title page. Include a 75-word complete but succinct abstract for all manuscripts. This information should be substantive, accurately reflecting the purpose and content of the manuscript. Include the conclusions.

The introductory information should include a general introduction of the subject and outline what will be covered in the article. No heading labeled "Introduction" is necessary.

The manuscript should be organized in logical subdivisions, according to the outline that was used to develop it. Headings indicate the organization of the manuscript. We use two types of headings: major headings are typed flush with the left margin; paragraph leads are indented at the beginning of a paragraph.

A listing within a paragraph should appear in sentence form and be designated (a) . . . (b) . . . (c) . . . and so on. If major points are made that will be discussed further, each major point should be set off as a paragraph and numbered. For example, "The following action is recommended:"

(1) minor subhead followed by elaboration
(2) minor subhead followed by elaboration

Refer to the *Publication Manual of the American Psychological Association* (1994) for further details.

We strongly encourage the use of graphics to complement and clarify the textual discussion. Your article is also more likely to be read if the text is broken up with tables, figures, or photographs.

Photographs should be black-and-white glossy, 8×10 or 5×7 inches, and of clear, crisp quality. All photos should be accompanied by a caption (on a separate page) that describes the context or names the people in the photo. Authors are responsible for securing photograph permissions and forwarding them to the *ANNA Journal* office before publication.

Figures are those graphics that present nonverbal information—graphs and charts. Each figure should appear on a separate page, should include a number that is referred to in the text (e.g., see Figure 1), should have a title, and should be camera ready. If figures from other sources are used, without changes/adaptations, the author is responsible for securing permission to reproduce the figure. (This permission should be in writing and should accompany the manuscript.)

Tables present either numerical data or verbal information; each table should be typed on a separate page (two short tables may be typed on the same page), should include a title and number (the number should be referred to in text), and should cite the source if it is not original material. The reference source should be placed after the title of the table—for example: Table 1. Etiologies of Acute Renal Failure (Doe & Brown, 1993) (body of the table goes here).

Other graphics may include illustrations that highlight a particular point of the text or summarize and illustrate results of a study.

REFEREED PUBLICATION

Nephrology Nursing Journal is a refereed journal; therefore, the editor assigns each manuscript to reviewers selected from the Editorial Board or the Manuscript Review Panel. The editor completes the final review.

COPYRIGHT

Copyright on all published articles will be held by the *Nephrology Nursing Journal.* Each author of a submitted manuscript must sign a statement expressly transferring copyright in the event the paper is published. This form is sent to the authors by the editorial coordinator when receipt of the manuscript is acknowledged.

INDEXED

The *Nephrology Nursing Journal* is indexed in the *Cumulative Index to Nursing and Allied Health Literature, International Nursing Index,* and *Nursing Abstracts Inc.*

SAMPLE JOURNAL ARTICLE TITLES

- "Discipline and Children With Chronic Illnesses: Strategies to Promote Positive Patient Outcomes"
- "Ethical Conflicts Reported by Certified Nephrology Nurses (CNNs) Practicing in Dialysis Settings"
- "Renal Transplant Recipients' and Their Physicians' Expectations Regarding Return to Work Posttransplant"
- "Research Priorities in Nephrology Nursing: American Nephrology Nurses' Associations Delphi Study"
- "Summer Camps for Children and Adolescents With Kidney Disease"

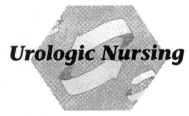

Urologic Nursing

U*rologic Nursing* is published by Anthony J. Jannetti, Inc., and is the official journal of the Society of Urologic Nurses and Associates, Inc., and an official publication of the Urology Nurses of Canada.

JOURNAL FOCUS/PURPOSE

The primary purpose of *Urologic Nursing* is to publish original articles, case studies, letters, descriptions of clinical care, and research.

JOURNAL FACTS

Publication schedule: bimonthly

Circulation: 3,000

Submitted papers per year: 40-50

Acceptance rate: 75%

Monetary honorarium: Articles accepted for continuing education series

Average turnaround time: 4 weeks

Publishing timetable: 9-15 months

Correspondence:
Business Office of Publication Management
Anthony J. Jannetti, Inc.

Urologic Nursing
East Holly Avenue
Box 56
Pitman, NJ 08071-0056
Telephone: (856) 589-2300
Fax: (856) 589-7463
E-mail: uronsg@ajj.com
Internet site: www.ajj.com/jpi

MANUSCRIPT SUBMISSION

Five copies of the manuscript should be submitted to the editorial office; the author retains one copy.

Submit manuscript to:

Editorial Office, *Urologic Nursing*
East Holly Avenue
Box 56
Pitman, NJ 08071-0056
Telephone: (856) 589-2300
Fax: (856) 589-7463

The editor is Catherine-Ann Lawrence, MA, RN, Montefiore Medical Center, Bronx, New York.

E-mail: clawrence@montefiore.org

Manuscripts not accepted for publication will not be returned to the author unless requested within 30 days of notification of rejection.

Upon submission of the manuscript, the author will yield copyright to the journal, contingent on publication of the manuscript. Acquiring permission to reprint previously published material is the responsibility of the author. Manuscripts accepted are subject to copyediting. The author will receive proofs that reflect all editing prior to publication.

In accordance with the Copyright Act of 1976, which became effective on January 1, 1978, all manuscripts must be accompanied by the following written statement signed by the author:

The undersigned author transfers all copyright ownership of the manuscript (title of article) to the Society of Urologic Nurses and Associates, Inc., in the event the work is published. The undersigned author warrants that the article is original, is not under consideration by another journal, and has not been previously published. I sign for and accept responsibility for releasing this material on behalf of any and all coauthors.

Authors will be consulted, when possible, regarding republication of their material.

MANUSCRIPT PREPARATION GUIDELINES

Manuscripts must be typed, double-spaced on 8.5×11-inch white paper. Style should generally follow the *Publication Manual of the American Psychological Association* 4th ed. (1994). Please use the author-date method of citation within the text: (Doe, 1993) or "Doe (1987) states . . ." With multiple authors, the first citation must list all authors; in subsequent citations, list only the name of the first author and et al.

The title page should include the manuscript title, authors' names and credentials, and a biographic statement. Also include a brief abstract of 40 words or less, along with an address for correspondence and day and evening phone numbers.

Double-space all typing, using 1.5- to 2-inch margins. Include the title, or a short descriptor, on top of each page, but do not include authors' names. Include subheadings in the manuscript where possible. Type all subheadings flush with the left margin.

List all references in alphabetical order. Sample references are shown below:

Book:

Doe, J. R. (1993). *Skin and aging processes.* Boca Raton, FL: CRC Press.

Chapter in a book:

Doe, J. R., & Smith, B. (1993). Aging of the human skin. In R. Jones (Ed.), *Handbook on aging* (pp. 123-234). New York: Nostrand-Rheinhold Company.

Periodical

Jones, J.F. (1993). Skin cancer. *American Journal of Nursing, 84*(11), 1234-1456.

Figures include line drawings, photographs, diagrams, and graphs. Each figure must be numbered, and that number must correspond to a statement in the text directing the reader to see that figure. Include a separate legend sheet with double-spaced captions. The author must obtain permission for figures borrowed from another source.

Photographs may be black-and-white, glossy, 5×7 inch or color 5×7 inch or 35 mm slides.

The journal will accept both IBM and Macintosh 3.5" format diskettes sent with manuscripts. All diskettes should be clearly labeled with the author name, manuscript title, disk type (IBM or Macintosh), file name, and word processor name and version (or file type, if ASCII).

Most, but not all, IBM and Macintosh word processor files are acceptable for submission to the journal. When possible, all files should be saved as WordPerfect. Many spreadsheet files may also be acceptable but must be approved prior to sending. To ensure acceptability of your disk, please contact the journal office before sending any material.

Please use only common fonts (CG Times, Universe, Helvetica, Courier, etc.) and avoid complex font attributes such as outline. All graphics (tables, graphs, etc.) must be submitted in camera-ready form.

The editor assumes that articles emanating from a particular institution are submitted with the approval of the requisite authorities, including all matters pertaining to human studies.

REFEREED PUBLICATION

Urologic Nursing is a peer-reviewed journal with a blind review process. The journal is refereed; all manuscripts submitted undergo review by the editor and blind reviews by the manuscript review panel and/or editorial board. Each article is evaluated on its timeliness, importance, accuracy, clarity, and applicability.

COPYRIGHT

Copyright by the Society of Urologic Nurses and Associates, Inc.

INDEXED

Urologic Nursing is indexed in the *International Nursing Index, Cumulative Index to Nursing and Allied Health Literature,* and *Nursing Abstracts.*

SAMPLE JOURNAL ARTICLE TITLES

- "Group Learning Behavior Modification and Exercise for Women With Urinary Incontinence"
- "Key Components of Patient Education for Pelvic Floor Stimulation in the Treatment of Urinary Incontinence"
- "Maintenance Therapy With Bacillus Calmette-Guerin in Patients With Superficial Bladder Cancer"
- "Treatments for Patients With Pelvic Pain"
- "Urinary Outcomes in Older Adults: Research and Clinical Perspectives"

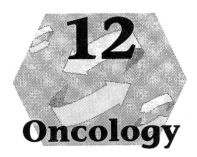

Oncology

Clinical Journal of Oncology Nursing

The *Clinical Journal of Oncology Nursing* is published by Oncology Nursing Press, Inc., and is the official journal of the Oncology Nursing Society.

JOURNAL FOCUS/PURPOSE

The primary purpose of the *Clinical Journal of Oncology Nursing* is to provide clinical information necessary for day-to-day practice.

JOURNAL FACTS

Publication schedule: bimonthly

Circulation: approximately 30,000

Submitted papers per year: approximately 100-120

Acceptance rate: 40%

Monetary honorarium: none

Average turnaround time: 8 weeks

Publishing timetable: 9-12 months

Correspondence:
Oncology Nursing Press, Inc.
501 Holiday Drive
Pittsburgh, PA 15220-2749
Telephone: (412) 921-7373
Fax: (412) 921-6565
E-mail: member@ons.org or
CJONeditor@hotmail.com

Internet site: www.ons.org

MANUSCRIPT SUBMISSION

Articles are to be clear, concise, comprehensive, and well referenced. Manuscripts are accepted for consideration with the understanding that they are contributed solely to this journal, that the material is original, and that the article has not been published previously. If the work has multiple authors, the article is reviewed on the assumption that all authors have granted approval for submission. All submitted articles are subject to blind peer review. Articles will be judged on the quality of the work and the suitability for the audience.

The original and four copies of the entire manuscript should be mailed to:
Oncology Nursing Press, Inc.
501 Holiday Drive
Pittsburgh, PA 15220-2749
Telephone: (412) 921-7373, ext. 554

Receipt of each manuscript will be acknowledged.

Editor: Lisa Schulmeister, RN, MS, CS, OCN
P.O. Box 23868
New Orleans, LA 70183

phone: (504) 739-9462
Fax: (504) 738-2087

We also have an author assistance (mentoring) program for new/novice writers and give an annual award to a new writer.

Accepted manuscripts are subject to editorial revision for clarity, punctuation, grammar, syntax, and conformity to journal style. Substantive revisions, when necessary, will be done by the author based on feedback from the editor and the peer reviewers. The author will have an opportunity to review the final manuscript prior to publication.

Manuscripts must be accompanied by a cover letter designating one author as correspondent with her or his complete mailing address and home and work telephone numbers. Include a photo of the primary author and a short professional biography of each author. The following statement should be typed on a separate piece of paper and signed by all authors. Separately signed statements are acceptable:

I have participated sufficiently in the conception and design of this work ("Name of Work") and the writing of this manuscript to take public responsibility for it. I have reviewed the final version of the submitted manuscript and approve it for publication.

MANUSCRIPT PREPARATION GUIDELINES

Manuscripts should be prepared using IBM-compatible software, typed double-spaced on 8″ × 11″ paper, and printed on a letter-quality printer. Use margins of at least 1 inch on all sides. Number the pages. All elements listed below should begin on separate pages.

Titles should be brief, specific, and descriptive. The full names of all authors, their degrees, titles, and affiliations, and financial disclosures, if applicable, should be included.

An abstract is required for all manuscripts. All abstracts must be double-spaced and must include no more than 100 words summarizing the key points of the article and highlighting the implications for clinical practice.

Prepare articles using standard manuscript form according to the *Publication Manual of the American Psychological Association,* 4th ed. (1994), which can be accessed online at http://webster.commnet.edu/apa. Length should be no more than 10-12 pages (2,000-2,500 words), exclusive of tables, figures, insets, and references.

Use headings and subheadings as appropriate. Cite all tables and figures in the text. Explain abbreviations and acronyms on first mention. If specific drugs or products are included, use the generic name when possible. If you must use the trade name, use the registered (®) or trademark (™) symbol on first reference in the text, and in parentheses include the manufacturer's name and location (city and state).

Visuals should be integrated within the text to create interest and augment learning. Number tables consecutively. Each should be typed on a separate piece of paper at the end of the text.

Figures should be professionally drawn or computer generated. Authors are encouraged to submit photographs that are relevant to their articles for possible use with the article or on the journal cover. Photographs must be of good quality and submitted as black-and-white or color prints. On the back of each photo, indicate the name of the first author, the figure number, and the top of the photo. Any photo showing a patient must include permission from the patient for publication. Type titles and legends for each photograph, double-spaced on separate pages.

The references list (not a bibliography) must be typed double-spaced and must follow

American Psychological Association format (in text and reference list). All references must be cited at least once in the text. Authors are responsible for the accuracy of all reference citations and are expected to have read and verified all of the listed references.

Submitted manuscripts that originated as theses or dissertations prepared by an author on an educational scholarship must cite the name of the scholarship. Authors must disclose any financial interest in products mentioned in the manuscript or in the company who manufactures the product(s), as well as any compensation received for producing the manuscript.

The author is responsible for obtaining written permissions from the author(s) and publisher for the use of any material (text, tables, figures, forms, etc.) previously published or printed elsewhere. Original letters granting this permission must be forwarded with the final manuscript. The author is responsible for obtaining written permission from any patient appearing in a photograph. Both legal and ethical considerations require patient's anonymity; avoid the use of identifying information.

REFEREED PUBLICATION

Clinical Journal of Oncology Nursing is a refereed journal. All submitted papers are subject to blind peer review. The initial review process takes at least 4 months. Reviewers' comments will be shared with the authors.

COPYRIGHT

Copyright by the Oncology Nursing Press, Inc. Authors will be asked to sign a transfer of copyright to the Oncology Nursing Press, Inc., before publication can proceed. Once a manuscript is accepted for publication in the *Clinical Journal of Oncology Nursing* and the copyright transfer is signed, the article becomes the property of the Oncology Nursing Press, Inc.

INDEXED

The *Clinical Journal of Oncology Nursing* is indexed in the *Cumulative Index to Nursing and Allied Health Literature* print index and the *Cumulative Index to Nursing and Allied Health Literature* database, the *International Nursing Index, MEDLINE,* and *RNdex Top 100.*

SAMPLE JOURNAL ARTICLE TITLES

- "A Time to Heal"
- "Harvesting Hope in the Autumn of Life"
- "Method to Determine Age at Which Individual Women Should Begin Mammogram Screening"
- "Nursing Management of Patients Receiving Brachytherapy for Early Stage Prostate Cancer"
- "Sentinel Lymph Node Biopsy in Breast Cancer and the Role of the Oncology Nurse"

Journal of Hospice and Palliative Nursing

The *Journal of Hospice and Palliative Nursing* is published by Nursecom, Inc., and is the official journal of the Hospice and Palliative Nurses Association (HPNA).

JOURNAL FOCUS/PURPOSE

The primary purpose of the *Journal of Hospice and Palliative Nursing* is to explore and report innovations, research, and issues that shape state-of-the-art nursing practice in end-of-life care.

JOURNAL FACTS

Publication schedule: quarterly

Circulation: 3,500

Submitted papers per year: not known, less than 1 year old

Acceptance rate: not yet known, less than 1 year old

Monetary honorarium: none

Average turnaround time: 12 weeks

Publishing timetable: 6-9 months after acceptance

Correspondence:
Journal of Hospice and Palliative Nursing
Nursecom, Inc.
1211 Locust Street
Philadelphia, PA 19107
Telephone: (215) 545-7222 or 1-800-242-6757
Fax: (215) 545-8107
E-mail: margon@compuserve.com

Internet site: www.nursecominc.com or
www.nursecominc.com/html/jhpn.html

MANUSCRIPT SUBMISSION

Papers submitted for consideration are assumed to be original, not previously published, and not under consideration by any other journal.

Send the original and three copies of the entire manuscript to:
Rose Mary Carroll-Johnson, MN, RN
Editor, *Journal of Hospice and Palliative Nursing*
P.O. Box 801360
Santa Clarita, CA 91380-1360
Telephone and fax number: (805) 255-3805
E-mail: rose_mary@earthlink.net

Each manuscript will be acknowledged on receipt. Manuscripts must be accompanied by a cover letter designating one author as correspondent with complete mailing address, home and work telephone and fax numbers, and e-mail address.

When submitting a manuscript for review, include this signed letter of transfer of copyright to *Journal of Hospice and Palliative Nursing:*

I/we hereby transfer copyright ownership to HPNA if the work (insert manuscript title) is published in *JHPN: Journal of Hospice and Palliative Nursing.* I/we warrant that the article is original, has not been submitted to another journal, and has not been previously published.

MANUSCRIPT PREPARATION GUIDELINES

Type manuscripts double-spaced on 8½ × 11″ paper, leaving margins of at least 1″. Number the pages consecutively beginning with the first page of text. Begin each element below on a new page:

1. Title page: Write a brief, specific, and descriptive title. Include the full names of all authors, their degrees, titles, affiliations, and any acknowledgments of financial support.
2. Abstract: Prepare a structured abstract. For research reports (100-120 words): purpose, methods, findings, conclusions, implications for practice. For other articles (75-100 words): purpose, data sources, conclusions, implications for practice. Identify three to five key words for indexing purposes; key words must follow the most recent CINAHL wording.
3. Text: Prepare paper using standard manuscript form according to the *Publication Manual of the American Psychological Association* (APA), 4th ed. (1994). Length should be 12-15 pages inclusive of tables and figures. Use headings and subheadings as appropriate. Identify key sentences or points to help in selecting breakouts for the final manuscript.
4. Tables: Number tables consecutively, cite each one in the text, type each one on a separate page, and place at end of the references.
5. Figures: Follow instructions for tables.
6. Photographs: Send 5″ × 7″ glossy black-and-white photographs. On the back of each one, identify any people (with signature of person photographed, giving permission to publish), include a title, and indicate the name of the first author. Cite each one in the text.
7. References: Use APA format. Cite all references in the text. Authors are responsible for accuracy of all reference citations.

Obtain written permission from the author and publisher for the use of any material (text, tables, figures, photographs, forms) previously published or printed elsewhere. Forward permission letters with the manuscript.

REFEREED PUBLICATION

All submitted papers are subject to blind peer review by a member of the editorial review board and one or more expert reviewers. At time of acceptance, send a copy of the manuscript on a disk in Word or WordPerfect or e-mail the manuscript to the editor.

The initial review process takes 2-3 months. Reviewers' comments will be shared with the authors. Accepted manuscripts are subject to editorial revision for clarity, punctuation, grammar, syntax, and conformity to journal style. Substantive revisions, when necessary, will be done by the author based on feedback from the editor and peer reviewers. The author will have an opportunity to review the final manuscript prior to publication.

COPYRIGHT

Copyright by Nursecom, Inc.

INDEXED

The *Journal of Hospice and Palliative Nursing* is not indexed.

SAMPLE JOURNAL ARTICLE TITLES

- "Case Study: Pain Management in an Elderly Man"

- "Storytelling in Practice: Part One—Mothers' Stories"
- "Storytelling in Practice: Part Two—Professional Storytelling"

- "The Challenge of Pain Management in the Elderly Patient Enrolled in Hospice"
- "What's in the Literature"

Journal of Pediatric Oncology Nursing

The *Journal of Pediatric Oncology Nursing* is published by W. B. Saunders Company and is the official journal of the Association of Pediatric Oncology Nurses.

JOURNAL FOCUS/PURPOSE

The primary purpose of the *Journal of Pediatric Oncology Nursing* is to advance clinical nursing care of children with cancer and their families. Emphasis is on holistic, family-centered care.

JOURNAL FACTS

Publication schedule: quarterly

Circulation: 2,200

Submitted papers per year: 50-65

Acceptance rate: 58-62%

Monetary honorarium: none

Average turnaround time: 1-3 months

Publishing timetable: 4-12 months after acceptance

Correspondence:
W. B. Saunders Company
The Curtis Center
Independence Square West
Philadelphia, PA 19106-3399
Telephone: (215) 238-7800 or 1-800-545-2522

Or

Association of Pediatric Oncology Nurses
National Headquarters Office
4700 W. Lake Avenue
Glenview, IL 60025-1485
Telephone: (847) 375-4724
Fax: (847) 375-4777

Editorial correspondence:
Pamela S. Hinds, PhD, RN, CS, Editor
Journal of Pediatric Oncology Nursing
4677 Normandy Avenue
Memphis, TN 38117

Internet site: www.wbsaunders.com

MANUSCRIPT SUBMISSION

The original and three copies of the manuscript are required.

All manuscripts should be submitted directly to:
Nancy E. Kline, PhD(c), RN, CPNP, CPON, Oncology Nurse Practitioner
Editor, *Journal of Pediatric Oncology Nursing*
Texas Children's Hospital
1102 Bates MC3-3320
Houston, TX 77030

We encourage submission of disks as well as hard copy. Query letters are also welcomed. Manuscripts are accepted for publication on the conditions that they are submitted solely to this journal, that the material is original, and that it has not been previously published.

MANUSCRIPT PREPARATION GUIDELINES

All manuscripts should be submitted on $8\frac{1}{2} \times 11$-inch nonerasable bond paper, typed double-spaced with liberal margins on all sides; each page should be numbered.

The first page of the manuscript should include the following information: (1) title of the paper; (2) author(s') name(s), degree(s), and current position; (3) complete addresses for every author; (4) name and address of the author to whom communications should be addressed. The second page should include a 150- to 200-word abstract.

The use of photographs is encouraged. All figures (photographs and line drawings) should be submitted as clear, glossy, black-and-white prints no larger than $8\frac{1}{2} \times 11$ inches. On the back of each figure, using a soft pencil, identify the figure number and the author.

Figure legends should be typed on a separate sheet and included at the end of the manuscript. A legend must accompany each illustration. Contributors must bear the cost of reproducing color illustrations.

Each table should be typed on a separate sheet. The author should provide table titles on the same sheet as the table. Figures and tables should be cited in order in the text using arabic numerals.

Beginning with the January 1999 issue, references will follow the style used by the American Psychological Association (APA). References should be cited in text with an author-date citation system and are listed alphabetically in the reference section in APA style. They should be typewritten and double-spaced, under the heading REFERENCES.

Journal articles:

Enskar, K., Carlsson, M., Golsater, M., Hamrin, E., & Kreuger, A. (1997). Parental reports of changes and challenges that result from parenting a child with cancer. *Journal of Pediatric Oncology Nursing, 14,* 156-163.

Kennedy, L., & Diamon, J. (1997). Assessment and management of chemotherapy-induced mucositis in children. *Journal of Pediatric Oncology Nursing, 14,* 164-174.

Complete book:

Walker, L. O. (1992). *Parent infant nursing science: Paradigms, phenomena, methods.* Philadelphia: F. A. Davis.

Chapter in a book:

Morris, D.L., & Wykle, M.L. (1994). Minorities in nursing. In J. J. Fitzpatrick & J. S. Stevenson (Eds.), *Annual review of nursing research* (pp. 175-189). New York: Springer Publishing.

Contributors are provided with printed proofs and are asked to proofread them for typesetting errors. Important changes in data are allowed, but authors will be charged for excessive alterations in proof. Proofs should be returned to the publisher within 48 hours.

REFEREED PUBLICATION

The *Journal of Pediatric Oncology Nursing* is a refereed journal with a blind review process. All manuscripts are reviewed by at least three members of the Editorial Board. Accepted manuscripts are subject to editorial revision.

COPYRIGHT

Authors of submitted manuscripts will be asked to sign a transfer of copyright to the Association of Pediatric Oncology Nurses. If the article is not accepted for publication, the copyright consent will be returned.

INDEXED

The *Journal of Pediatric Oncology Nursing* is indexed in the *Cumulative Index to Nursing and Allied Health Literature, Index Medicus, MEDLINE,* and *RNdex Top 100.*

SAMPLE JOURNAL ARTICLE TITLES

- "An International Account: Life Situation and Problems As Reported by Children With Cancer and Their Parents"

- "Behavior Changes Exhibited by Siblings of Pediatric Oncology Patients: A Comparison Between Maternal and Sibling Descriptions"

- "Continuing Education: Conscious Sedation of Pediatric Oncology Patients for Painful Procedures: Development and Implementation of a Clinical Practice Protocol"

- "Hypnosis for Children and Adolescents With Cancer: An Annotated Bibliography, 1985-1995"

- "Research: Challenges of Clinical Research for the Guest Investigator in the Institution"

Oncology Nursing Forum

O*ncology Nursing Forum* is published by Oncology Nursing Press, Inc., and is the official journal of the Oncology Nursing Society.

JOURNAL FOCUS/PURPOSE

The primary purpose of the *Oncology Nursing Forum* is to convey news related to developments in practice, technology, and research to promote a positive image of professional specialized nursing, print timely papers, and stimulate nursing issues in oncology nursing.

JOURNAL FACTS

Publication schedule: 10 times per year

Circulation: approximately 30,000

Submitted papers per year: approximately 110

Acceptance rate: 40%

Monetary honorarium: none

Average turnaround time: 12-16 weeks

Publishing timetable: 3-6 months after acceptance

Correspondence:
Oncology Nursing Society
501 Holiday Drive
Pittsburgh, PA 15220-2749
Telephone: (412) 921-7373
Fax: (412) 921-6565; membership e-mail: member@ons.org; *Oncology Nursing Forum* e-mail: onpress@ons.org

Internet site: www.ons.org

MANUSCRIPT SUBMISSION

The original and three copies of the entire manuscript should be mailed to:

Rose Mary Carroll-Johnson, MN, RN
Editor *Oncology Nursing Forum*
P.O. Box 801360
Santa Clarita, CA 91380-1360
Telephone and fax number: (805) 255-3805
E-mail: rose_mary@earthlink.net

Receipt of each manuscript will be acknowledged. Manuscripts must be accompanied by a cover letter designating one author as correspondent with her or his complete mailing address and home and work telephone numbers. Each listed author must meet authorship requirements. The following statement should be typed on a separate piece of paper and signed by all authors. Separately signed statements are acceptable:

> I have participated sufficiently in the conception and design of this work, the data analysis (when applicable), and the writing of this manuscript to take public responsibility for it. I have reviewed the final version of the submitted manuscript and approve it for publication.

Manuscripts are accepted for consideration with the understanding that they are contributed solely to this journal, that the material is original, and that the article has not been published previously. If the work has multiple authors, the paper is reviewed on the assumption that all authors have granted approval for submission. All submitted papers are subject to blind peer review. Papers will be judged on the quality of the work and suitability for the audience.

The initial review process takes at least 4 months. Reviewers' comments will be shared with the authors. Accepted manuscripts are subject to editorial revision for clarity, punctuation, grammar, syntax, and conformity to journal style. Substantive revisions, when necessary, will be done by the author based on feedback from the editor and the peer reviewers. The author will have an opportunity to review the final manuscript prior to publication.

MANUSCRIPT PREPARATION GUIDELINES

Manuscripts should be prepared using IBM-compatible software, typed double-spaced on $8\frac{1}{2} \times 11$-inch paper, and printed on a letter-quality printer. Use margins of at least 1 inch on all sides. Number the pages. All elements listed below should begin on separate pages.

Titles should be brief, specific, and descriptive. The full names of all authors, their degrees, titles, and affiliations should also be included.

An abstract is required for all manuscripts. All abstracts must be double-spaced and can be written in phrases instead of complete sentences (e.g., "Setting: Rural health clinics in southwestern United States," rather than "Setting: The study was conducted in rural health clinics located in the southwestern United States.").

Research abstracts must be no more than 250 words. The following headings must be included in the abstract: purpose/objectives, design, setting, sample, methods, main research variables, findings, conclusions, and implications for nursing practice. Clearly state the purpose(s) or key objectives of the study and the major hypotheses tested, if any. Describe the basic study design (e.g., descriptive, experimental, survey) or approach (quantitative, qualitative), randomization, blinding, criterion standards, and temporal direction (e.g., prospective, retrospective). Identify the study setting (e.g., primary or tertiary, private or institutional) and other characteristics (e.g., rural, urban, geographic area). Summarize characteristics of the sample (e.g., diagnosis, age range, sex, ethnicity), selection procedures, entry criteria, and number of participants entering and finishing the study. Describe interventions, data-gathering procedures, and instruments (use complete names). Indicate the primary study variables as planned prior to data collection. Describe the hypotheses formulated during or after data collection. Summarize the results of the study, including all significant findings. Describe conclusions supported by the data (avoid speculation and overgeneralization). Give equal emphasis to positive and negative findings. Identify needs for additional research. Describe the specific clinical applications of the research.

Abstracts for clinical, review, or theoretical papers must be no more than 150 words. The following headings must be included in the abstract: purpose/objectives, data sources, data synthesis, conclusions, and implications for nursing practice. State the purpose, key objectives, thesis, organizing construct, and scope (comprehensive or selective) of the review or paper. List all the data sources (e.g., published articles/abstracts, conference proceedings, references from bibliographies of pertinent articles and books, computerized databases) and criteria used for selection of material from reviewed studies or reports. State the main findings and how they relate to the purpose and objectives of the paper. Describe conclusions supported by the evidence reported (avoid speculation and overgeneralization) and the need for additional work/research. State the specific clinical applications of the findings.

Prepare papers using standard manuscript form according to the *Publication Manual of the American Psychological Association,* 4th ed. (1994). Length should be 12-15 pages (4,000 words), exclusive of tables, figures, insets, and references.

Use headings and subheadings as appropriate. Indicate approximate placement of tables and figures in the text. Explain abbreviations on first mention. If specific drugs or products are included, use the generic name when possible. If you must use the trade name, use the registered (®) or trademark (™) symbol on first reference in the text, and in parentheses include the manufacturer's name and location (city and state).

Number tables consecutively. Each should be typed double-spaced on a separate piece of paper at the end of the text. Figures should be professionally drawn or computer generated. Photographs must be of good quality and submitted as black-and-white or color prints. On the back of each photo, indicate the name of the first author, the figure number, and the top of the photo. Type titles and legends for each photograph, double-spaced on separate pages.

The references list (not a bibliography) must be typed double-spaced and must follow American Psychological Association format (in text and reference list). All references must be cited at least once in the text. Authors are responsible for the accuracy of all reference citations.

Submitted manuscripts that are the result of funded research must cite the funding source on the title page. Submitted manuscripts that originated as theses or dissertations prepared by an author on an educational scholarship must cite the name of the scholarship. Authors must disclose any financial interest in products mentioned in the manuscript or in the company who manufactures the product, as well as any compensation received for producing the manuscript.

It is the responsibility of the author to obtain written permissions from the author(s) and publisher for the use of any material (text, tables, figures, forms, etc.) previously published or printed elsewhere. Original letters granting this permission must be forwarded with the final manuscript. Both legal and ethical considerations require patient's anonymity; avoid the use of identifying information. If the manuscript reports the results of an investigational study involving human subjects, the text must include a statement indicating institutional review board approval and informed consent when appropriate. The author is responsible for obtaining permission to include photographs and institution or colleagues' names.

REFEREED PUBLICATION

Oncology Nursing Forum is a refereed journal. All submitted papers are subject to blind peer review.

COPYRIGHT

INDEXED

The *Oncology Nursing Forum* is indexed in the *Cumulative Index to Nursing and Allied Health Literature, Index Medicus, International Nursing Index, MEDLINE, Nursing Citation Index, Nursing Abstracts,* and *SilverPlatter Information, Inc.*

SAMPLE JOURNAL ARTICLE TITLES

- "Extravasation of Liposomal Daunorubicin in Patients With AIDS-Associated Kaposi's Sarcoma: A Report of Four Cases"
- "Gemcitabine: A New Approach to Treating Pancreatic Cancer"
- "Patterns of Fatigue and Activity and Rest During Adjuvant Breast Cancer Chemotherapy"
- "Prostate Cancer Treatment Decisions: A Focus Group Exploration"

13

Operative Nursing

AANA Journal

The *AANA Journal* is published by AANA Publishing, Inc., and is the official scholarly publication of the American Association of Nurse Anesthetists.

JOURNAL FOCUS/PURPOSE

The primary purpose of the *AANA Journal* is to publish manuscripts that foster an understanding of the science of anesthesia delivery and investigate issues, ideas, and innovations that advance the practice of nurse anesthesia.

JOURNAL FACTS

Publication schedule: bimonthly

Circulation: 28,000

Submitted papers per year: 60-70

Acceptance rate: 34%

Monetary honorarium: none

Average turnaround time: 6 weeks

Publishing timetable: 12-18 months after acceptance, depending on the topic

Correspondence:
Editor, *AANA Journal*
222 South Prospect Avenue
Park Ridge, IL 60068-4001

Internet site: www.aana.com

MANUSCRIPT SUBMISSION

The *AANA Journal* welcomes original manuscripts not under consideration by another journal on subjects pertinent to the specialty of anesthesia and those that relate to the broad professional domain of the practicing nurse anesthetist. Manuscripts published in the Journal become the sole property of the American Association of Nurse Anesthetists.

Submitted papers undergo blind review by members of the Editorial Advisory Board. If accepted for publication, editorial revisions may be made to improve presentation without altering meaning. For all papers, edited copy will be submitted to authors for final approval. Authors are responsible for all statements made in their work, including changes made by the copy editor.

Authors are invited to submit inquiry letters or their completed manuscripts to:

Editor
AANA Journal

222 South Prospect Avenue
Park Ridge, IL 60068-4001

MANUSCRIPT PREPARATION GUIDELINES

To avoid delays in the review process, manuscripts should be carefully prepared according to these guidelines and proofread carefully for errors in grammar and spelling. The manuscript should be read for clarity and accuracy by colleagues and/or mentors before submission to the Journal. Write simply and clearly, avoiding jargon and unfamiliar abbreviations. Manuscripts should generally be no more than 12-20 double-spaced pages in length. Authors are invited to submit articles in the following categories in the format described below:

Research articles: A report of an original investigation. Paper should include a title page, abstract page, text (subdivided into Introduction, Materials and Methods, Results, Discussion), acknowledgments page, references, figures and legends, and tables. Manuscripts describing investigations carried out in humans or animals must include a statement indicating that the study was approved by the authors' institutional investigation committee and that written permission was obtained from human subjects.

Case report: A report of a clinical case that is uncommon or of educational value. This category may constitute a brief description of a clinical episode or an in-depth case presentation. The authors must have been personally associated with the case. Paper should include a title page, text that is subdivided into Introduction, Case Summary, Discussion, and References. If applicable, provide figures and legends, and tables.

Survey/review article: Collates, describes, and critically evaluates previously published material to aid in evaluating new concepts. Paper should include a title page, abstract, text (subdivided into Introduction, History/Review of Literature, Discussion of state of the art, Summary), references, figures and legends, and tables.

Letter to the editor. Include brief constructive comments concerning previously published articles or brief notations of general interest.

Professional issue article. The *Journal* will consider publishing professional issues related to the nurse anesthesia practice.

Manuscripts must be typed on a letter-quality printer and submitted in quadruplicate on $8\frac{1}{2} \times 11$-inch white paper with at least $1\frac{1}{2}$-inch margins at top, bottom, and sides. Care should be taken in the preparation of copies to ensure quality reproduction and facilitate readability. The author should retain a copy of the manuscript. Double-space all typing, including references and legends. References should be completed and arranged numerically according to the order in which they appear in the text. Style should conform to the *American Medical Association Manual of Style* for scientific references as follows:

Arrington ME, Gabbert KC, Mazgaj PW, Wolf MT. Multidose vial contamination in anesthesia. *AANA Journal.* 1990;58:462-466.
Moorthy SS. Metabolism and nutrition. In: Stoelting RK, Dierdorf SS. eds. *Anesthesia and Co-existing Disease.* New York, NY: Churchill Livingstone 1983:507-508.

A short biographical sketch of each coauthor with principal author indicated, must accompany each manuscript.

For the title page, include manuscript title, authors' names and credentials, professional position, and affiliations. Furnish a correspondence address, telephone number, and source of grant or financial support.

For indexing purposes, include three to five key words on a separate page or add them to the title page.

The abstract, numbered page 1, will appear as the italicized lead-in portion of the published manuscript. Show manuscript's title, but omit authors' names. Double-space all abstracts. The abstract of original research should include one to three sentences describing the purpose, hypothesis, or theoretical orientation of the paper, followed by two to three sentences describing the method of the study or the nature of the review and how the data was analyzed. Continue with two to three sentences devoted to the major points or results noted in the paper, and conclude with one or two sentences giving the conclusion or take-home message. An abstract of a case report should provide a summary of the case and a discussion. When abstracting a review article, provide a concise summary of the salient points addressed in the review.

The first page of the text should be numbered page 2 with subsequent pages numbered sequentially.

Begin the list of references (only those sources cited in the text) on a new page in the numerical order that they appear in the text. References cited in the paper should be of previously published papers or texts. Cite written personal communications or observations in parentheses in the text. Carefully validate all references to ensure that they are cited accurately, completely, and in the style indicated above. Cite up to six authors. If there are more than six, cite the first three only and add "et al."

A legend should be provided for each illustration or figure and should be double-spaced on a separate page. Photographs, clearly reproducible diagrams, and graphs should be numbered with an arabic numeral and labeled as "Figure 1, Figure 2," and so on and should be cited chronologically in the manuscript. Tables should be typed and double-spaced on a separate page. Tables should be numbered as "Table 1, Table 2," and so on, depending on their sequence in the manuscript, and descriptively titled and cited chronologically in the manuscript.

When employing material previously published, written permission from the original author and publisher is required. Additionally, written permission is required for use of photographs of identifiable individuals.

REFEREED PUBLICATION

AANA Journal is a peer-reviewed journal that undergoes a blind review process.

COPYRIGHT

INDEXED

The *AANA Journal* is indexed in National Library of Medicine's *MEDLINE database, International Nursing Index, Cumulative Index to Nursing and Allied Health Literature, Excerpta Medica,* and *RNdex Top 100.*

SAMPLE JOURNAL ARTICLE TITLES

- "AANA Journal Course: Update for Nurse Anesthetists-Thoracic Trauma"
- "Controlled Drug Misuse by Certified Registered Nurse Anesthetists"
- "Inhaled Nitric Oxide as a Selective Pulmonary Vasodilator in Clinical Anesthesia"
- "Maintaining Intraoperative Normothermia: A Meta-Analysis of Outcomes With Costs"
- "The Expanding Role of the Clinical Coordinator"

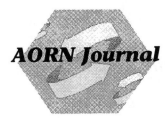

AORN Journal

The *AORN Journal* is published by the AORN (Association of Operating Room Nurses) and is the official publication of the AORN.

JOURNAL FOCUS/PURPOSE

The primary purpose of the *AORN Journal* is to provide its readers with practical and theoretical information that ultimately will result in better patient care and improved standards of perioperative nursing.

JOURNAL FACTS

Publication schedule: monthly

Circulation: 50,000

Submitted papers per year: not available

Acceptance rate: 75%

Monetary honorarium: yes, varies

Average turnaround time: 6-8 weeks

Publishing timetable: 3-6 months after acceptance

Correspondence:
AORN
2170 S. Parker Road, Suite 300
Denver, CO 80231-5711
Telephone: 1-800-755-2676
Fax: 1-800-755-7980
E-mail: bsgd@aol.com

Internet site: www.aorn.org

MANUSCRIPT SUBMISSION

The *AORN Journal* welcomes manuscripts pertaining to perioperative nursing practice. The journal endeavors to publish information on current trends in the health care field and does not adhere to an editorial calendar. Perioperative nurses, educators, researchers, and managers; physicians; other health care professionals; and academicians are invited to submit manuscripts. Short care studies, clinical exemplars, manuscripts about practical innovations, and manuscripts that express professional opinions are welcome.

Manuscripts submitted by RNs will be considered for the journal Home Study Program, which is a continuing education offering. To be selected, manuscripts for the Home Study Program must be comprehensive and written on clinical topics. Authors are not required to write the home study examination questions.

The journal encourages letters to the editor that address articles published within the past 2 months.

Prospective authors are encouraged to write query letters to the editor.

Send manuscripts or queries to:
Editor, *AORN Journal*
2170 S. Parker Road, Suite 300
Denver, CO 80231-5711

The *AORN Journal* accepts manuscripts that are original and have not been published previously. Manuscripts submitted to the journal for review must not be under consideration for publication in other journals. Authors should submit to the editor copies of any published papers or other manuscripts in preparation or submitted elsewhere that are related to the manuscript to be considered by the journal. The journal endeavors to report all sides of controversial issues; however, views and statements are the sole responsibility of the author(s).

If there is a financial association between the author(s) and a commercial company that makes a product featured prominently in the manuscript, the journal requires that the author(s) disclose such an association. Should a conflict of interest exist, the editor reserves the right to reject the manuscript.

All people designated as authors should have contributed significantly to the manuscript to take public responsibility for it. The maximum number of authors is five. Names of those who contributed general support or technical help may be listed in an acknowledgment.

Tear sheets of the article, a copy of the *AORN Journal* containing the article, and an honorarium will be sent to each author after publication.

Submit three copies of the manuscript. After the manuscript has been revised and accepted and if it is prepared with a computer, send a 3½ or 5¼-inch disk with the files saved in word processing format. Indicate the word processing software and version used. Manuscripts should be between 8 and 16 pages long, depending on the topic. Manuscripts submitted for departments should be between 5 and 8 pages.

MANUSCRIPT PREPARATION GUIDELINES

The manuscript must be double-spaced and printed with a quality printer. An outline of the manuscript and a cover letter that includes the home and business addresses and telephone and fax numbers of all authors and a designated senior author for correspondence must be included.

Include manuscript title and authors' names, credentials, and current professional positions. Designate a senior author and give a correspondence address and telephone and fax numbers. The manuscript should have a title.

Include a 100-word informative abstract that follows the manuscript's outline and summarizes the research results (if applicable).

Subheadings should indicate subdivisions in the text. Omit authors' names on text pages. Spell out abbreviations and acronyms on first use, followed by abbreviations in parentheses. Use generic names rather than trade names for medications and devices. Give weights, measurements, and medication dosages in metric units and temperatures in both Fahrenheit and Celsius degrees.

Quotations, statistics, original ideas, or interpretations of works of other authors must be referenced. Number the notes consecutively in the text and provide complete references at the end of the article. Authors also may submit suggested reading of publications pertinent to the article but not cited directly. Notes and suggested reading should follow the style outlined in Kate L. Turabian's *A Manual for Writers of Term Papers, Theses, and Dissertations,* 5th ed. (1987). Books referenced must include the names of all authors, title, volume or edition number, chapter title and author (if applicable), publisher and city, and year of publication. Submit a photocopy of the title page for any books cited. Articles referenced must include names of all authors, title of article, name of publication, volume number, and complete date of publication. References should cite specific page numbers. All references should have been published within the last 5 years unless they are considered classics or they reference historical information. When more than one source is given for a citation, combine the sources into one note. The following are examples of notes.

1. O C Zimmerman, "An article from a journal," *Hospital Topics* 41 (July 1997) 99-102.
2. C E Merriam, M Hodgson, *Book,* third ed (San Antonio: Books Unlimited, 1997) 45.
3. J A Stanton, "A chapter in a book," In *Time Management,* ed P White (New York: Little, Brown & Co, 1997) 146-162; "Positioning the surgical patient," In *AORN Standards, Recommended Practices, and Guide-*

lines (Denver: Association of Operating Room Nurses, Inc., 1997) 211-214.

Photographs and original line drawings are encouraged. Color slides are best, followed by color prints and black-and-white prints. Negatives and Polaroid pictures cannot be used. Illustrations must be labeled on the back with a soft-tip marker or attached to a sheet of paper that is labeled with the figure number and name of author. Do not use paper clips or write heavily on photographs. Photographs in which an individual can be identified must be accompanied by the individual's permission to publish. Send two sets of original illustrations and photographs and one set of photocopies; artwork will not be returned after publication. Captions must be submitted with all photographs and drawings. Tables and figures should be clearly labeled and referred to in the text. They must be referenced if they are not the work of the author.

In consultation with the author(s), the *AORN Journal* reserves the right to edit all manuscripts with regard to length, timeliness, and readability consistent with journal style. Before publication, authors will receive an edited copy of the manuscript for final approval. Upon acceptance of a manuscript, the author transfers all copyright ownership to the Association of Operating Room Nurses, Inc. Published manuscripts become the property of the *AORN Journal* and may not be reproduced without written permission of the managing editor.

Original art ideas are welcomed and republishing previously published work is discouraged. The publisher has a staff of designers and medical illustrators who can develop authors' ideas. If republishing is necessary, the author is responsible for obtaining permission to publish figures and tables from previously published works and for sending copies of permission letters to the *AORN Journal* with the illustrations. The author also is responsible for obtaining permission from photographers and artists to use unpublished photographs and drawings. Permission letters must accompany copyrighted illustrations or the illustrations will not be published.

REFEREED PUBLICATION

The *AORN Journal* is a refereed journal. Manuscripts are evaluated by the editor and by two members of the *AORN Journal* Review Panel. They are judged on accuracy, content, organization, style, contribution to nursing literature, originality, and appearance. Publishing and editorial decisions are based on reviewers' evaluations and the editor's judgment of the quality of the writing, timeliness of the manuscript, and potential interest to readers of the journal. Authors will be notified of the editor's decision approximately 6 to 8 weeks after submitting the manuscript. Manuscripts that are not accepted for publication will be returned.

COPYRIGHT

Copyright by AORN, Inc.

INDEXED

The *AORN Journal* is indexed in the *Cumulative Index to Nursing and Allied Health Literature, Hospital Literature Index, Index Medicus, International Nursing Index, Nursing Abstracts,* and *RNdex Top 100.*

SAMPLE JOURNAL ARTICLE TITLES

- "A Guide to Salivary Gland Disorders"
- "Comparisons of Three Rewarming Methods in a Postanesthesia Care Unit"

- "Preoperative Management of Patients With Major Trauma Injuries"
- "Tongue Reconstruction Procedures for Treatment of Cancer"

- "Treatment of Conductive Hearing Loss With Ossicular Chain Reconstruction Procedures"

CRNA: The Clinical Forum for Nurse Anesthetists

CRNA: The Clinical Forum for Nurse Anesthetists is published by W. B. Saunders Company.

JOURNAL FOCUS/PURPOSE

The primary purpose of *CRNA: The Clinical Forum for Nurse Anesthetists* is to provide nurse anesthetists with in-depth updates of clinical advances. Also included is a section devoted to anesthetic drug interactions.

JOURNAL FACTS

Publication schedule: quarterly

Circulation: approximately 400

Submitted papers per year: approximately 50

Acceptance rate: 80%

Monetary honorarium: none

Average turnaround time: 4-6 weeks

Publishing timetable: dependent on theme

Correspondence:
W. B. Saunders Company
The Curtis Center
Independence Square West
Philadelphia, PA 19106-3399
Telephone: (215) 238-7800 or 1-800-545-2522

Internet site: www.wbsaunders.com

MANUSCRIPT SUBMISSION

The Editorial Board welcomes submissions of manuscripts for review and possible publication in *CRNA: The Clinical Forum for Nurse Anesthetists.*

Please send submissions to:
CDR Frederick C. Hill, Jr., CRNA, MSNA
Editor, *CRNA: The Clinical Forum for Nurse Anesthetists*
401 Tareyton Lane
Portsmouth, VA 23701

Members of the editorial board are available for consultation throughout the development of manuscripts. Guidance should be requested through the editor at the address noted above. Two copies of both manuscript and illustrations, including the original typescript, should be submitted.

MANUSCRIPT PREPARATION GUIDELINES

All parts of the manuscript, including footnotes, abstracts, references, tables, legends, quoted material, and case studies, must be typed double-spaced, with generous margins on both sides and at the top and bottom of every page.

On the title page, please include all of the following information: (1) the names, degrees, and professional affiliations (position, department, institution, location) of all authors; (2) acknowledgment of grant support when appropriate; (3) "Key words," a list of 3 to 10 important words or phrases for indexing; and (4) a complete mailing address for the author to whom galley proofs and reprint requests should be addressed.

A short, concise summary highlighting the main points of the text, including the purpose and conclusions, should be submitted with the manuscript.

Reference numbers in the text follow numerical order and are denoted in text by superscript numbers. References are listed beginning on a separate page at the end of the manuscript text in the order in which they are referred to in the text, not in alphabetical order; they must conform to the style of the following samples. Please note that manuscripts in press may be references; however, manuscripts that have been submitted for publication but not yet accepted should not be referenced. All references must be complete when the manuscript is submitted.

Journal article, one to three authors:

1. Brill JE: Anesthesia for neonatal surgical emergencies. Semin Anesth 7:242-251, 1989

Journal article, more than three authors:

2. Ascah KJ, Stewart WJ, Levine RA, et al: Doppler-echocardiographic assessment of cardiac output. Radiol Clin North Am 23:659-670, 1985

Journal article in press:

3. Whitsett CF: Infections acquired through blood transfusion. Anesth Clin North Am (in press)

Book:

4. Martin JT: Positioning in Anesthesia and Surgery (ed 2), Philadelphia, Saunders, 1988

Chapter of book:

5. Horrow JC: Protamine: A necessary evil, in Ellison N, Jobes DR (eds): Effective Hemostasis in Cardiac Surgery. Philadelphia, Saunders, 1988, pp. 15-39

Abstract:

6. Garson G, Harris B, MacDonald J: Postoperative hemorrhage, Surgery 3:17, 1987 (abstr)

All tables and figures must be cited in the text. The appropriate location of each table or figure should be indicated in the margin of the manuscript in pencil.

Tables are numbered with arabic numerals (Table 1, Table 2) in the order of their text citation. Each table should be typed (double-spaced throughout) on a separate sheet of paper and should have a title. Maximum table width: 144 characters (i.e., letters and spaces). Use spaces, not vertical rules, to separate columns. Each table should have a legend in sufficient detail to allow understanding without reference to the text.

Illustration legends are also numbered with arabic numerals (Fig. 1, Fig. 2). Legends should be typed double-spaced on manuscript paper not attached to the illustrations themselves. Legends should be sufficiently detailed to allow understanding without reference to the text.

Illustrations should be identified (in light pencil on the back) by the author's name as well as by figure number. Top should be marked, and maximum cropping marked. All illustrations must be submitted as glossy black-and-white prints of original artwork of professional quality, ready for printing. The author should retain negatives. Photocopied illustrations or authors' sketches are not suitable for reproduction in the journal (photocopies are acceptable, however, as duplicate copies). Maximum width of illustrations after reduction: 6 inches. The cost of color plates must be borne by the author. Color prints are not acceptable for reproduction as black-and-white prints.

If any illustration has been previously published, a copy of the letter of permission from the copyright holder must accompany the illustration. The source of the illustration should be included among the references to the paper. The figure legend should conclude with "Reprinted with permission" followed by the reference number: e.g., Reprinted with permission. (23)

Contributors are sent galley proofs and asked to proofread them for typographical errors and return them to the publisher within 48 hours. Important changes in data will be accepted, but authors will be charged for excessive alterations in proof.

REFEREED PUBLICATION

All manuscripts are reviewed by at least two members of the Editorial Board.

COPYRIGHT

Copyright by W. B. Saunders Company.

INDEXED

CRNA: The Clinical Forum for Nurse Anesthetists is indexed in the *Cumulative Index to Nursing and Allied Health Literature, Excerpta Medica,* and *RNdex Top 100.*

SAMPLE JOURNAL ARTICLE TITLES

- "Anesthetic Management of Children With Craniofacial Anomalies"
- "Clinical Applications for Pediatric Sedation"
- "Comparison of Ondansetron, Metoclopramide, and Placebo in the Prevention of Postoperative Emesis in Children Undergoing Ophthalmic Surgery"
- "Complications in Anesthesia"
- "Pediatric Trauma"

Journal of PeriAnesthesia Nursing

The *Journal of PeriAnesthesia Nursing* is published by W. B. Saunders Company and is the official journal of the American Society of PeriAnesthesia Nurses.

JOURNAL FOCUS/PURPOSE

The primary purpose of the *Journal of PeriAnesthesia Nursing* is to facilitate communication and promote education specific to the

body of knowledge unique to the practice of perianesthesia nursing.

JOURNAL FACTS

Publication schedule: bimonthly

Circulation: 13,000

Submitted papers per year: approximately 30-40

Acceptance rate: approximately 50%

Monetary honorarium: $25 per published page, $100 maximum per article

Average turnaround time: 6-12 months

Publishing timetable: 4-6 months after acceptance

Correspondence:
W. B. Saunders Company
The Curtis Center
Independence Square West
Philadelphia, PA 19106-3399
Telephone: (215) 238-7800 or 1-800-545-2522

Or
American Society of PeriAnesthesia Nurses
6900 Grove Road
Thorofare, NJ 08086
Telephone: (856) 845-5557
Fax: (856) 848-1881

Internet site: www.wbsaunders.com or www.jopan.org

MANUSCRIPT SUBMISSION

Please address all editorial correspondence and query letters to:

Susan Goodwin, MS, RN, CPAN
Editor, *Journal of PeriAnesthesia Nursing*
1000 Brook Forest Rd
Edmond, OK 73034

Manuscripts should be sent to:

M. Joan Bauer, MS, RN, CPAN
Managing Editor, *Journal of PeriAnesthesia Nursing*
722 Topaz Ln
Madison, WI 53714

The original manuscript plus four copies are required.

The *Journal of PeriAnesthesia Nursing* seeks original articles useful to nurses responsible for all phases of perianesthesia care in surgery facilities, PACUs (postanasthesia care units), and critical care units. Readers are experienced clinicians practicing in diverse areas.

First-time authors as well as those who have published previously are encouraged to submit manuscripts. The editor welcomes manuscripts describing a specific clinical innovation, original research, or case study experiences. Manuscripts may also be submitted for publication in one of the journal's regular sections: Ambulatory Surgery, The Product Page, Practical Points, Pharmacology, Research, Soundwaves, or Management.

The editor invites authors to send a query letter before beginning to write a manuscript. Briefly describe your idea and the primary topics to be covered. The editor will respond with feedback to help you develop the manuscript in accordance with the journal's current needs and policies.

MANUSCRIPT PREPARATION GUIDELINES

All manuscript submissions must include the following:

1. Cover letter specifying the article title and name, home and work addresses, and telephone numbers for the primary author.

2. Copyright release signed by all coauthors.

3. Everything must be typed double-spaced.

4. Title page with article title; full name of each author with credentials, title, and institutional affiliation; and home and business addresses and telephone numbers for each author.

5. A brief abstract (no more than 300 words) summarizing the main focus.

6. Text, references, acknowledgments, tables, and illustrations.

7. All required permissions for tables, illustrations, graphs, photographs, hospital forms and protocols, and so on taken from another source.

A conflict-of-interest statement is required for each manuscript that is submitted for publication. This statement will have no bearing on the editorial decision to publish a manuscript.

The author(s) is (are) asked to provide a statement regarding any relationship existing between a commercial party and material contained in the manuscript that might represent a conflict of interest or to provide a statement declaring that no benefits in any form have been received from a commercial party related directly or indirectly to the subject of the article. The statement will be kept on file in the journal office and published on the title page of the article.

Contributors are provided with page proofs and are asked to proofread them for typesetting errors. Important changes in data are allowed, but authors will be charged for excessive alterations in proof. Proofs must be returned within 48 hours.

Reprints of articles are available to contributors when ordered in advance of publication. An order form showing the cost of reprints is sent with proofs. Readers wishing to obtain reprints of an article can do so by contacting the author at the address given in the journal.

The *Journal of PeriAnesthesia Nursing* subscribes in general to the "Uniform Requirements for Manuscripts Submitted to Biomedical Journals" (N Engl J Med 324:424-428, 1991) and the *Manual for Authors and Editors* of the American Medical Association.

Manuscripts must be neatly typed, double-spaced, on $8\frac{1}{2} \times 11$-inch white bond paper. Use one side of the page only, allowing margins of at least $1\frac{1}{2}$ inches. Do not use eraseable bond.

Use headings and subheadings to separate major sections and ideas within the paper. Describe nursing actions and focus on how to perform. Include the unique contribution of your ideas and experience with the literature review and research presented. Avoid unusual abbreviations.

The text must be accurate. Document content within the text using superscript numbers to designate the references: As the Doe[1] findings indicate . . .

If several consecutive references apply, separate first and last number using a hyphen: As Doe and others[2-8] found . . .

Separate multiple references using commas when they are not consecutive: Several studies [3, 8, 9, 12] show that . . .

If a previously published idea is briefly paraphrased, indicate the source by placing the reference number at the end of the appropriate sentence: One innovative approach to the clinical problem is to institute screening procedures for X, Y and Z.[13]

References should be compiled on a separate page at the end of the article according to the order of citation in the text, not alphabetically. They should be typewritten, double-spaced, under the heading REFERENCES. References should be in the last 5 years. Abbreviations for titles of medical periodicals should conform to those used in the latest edition of Index Medicus. Give inclusive page numbers.

Journal article, one author:

1. O'Connell M: Anxiety reduction in family members of patients in surgery. J. Post Anesth Nurs 4:7-16, 1989

Journal article, two or three authors:

2. Brown MS, Haylor M: Nursing research with preoperational age children. J. Pediatr Nurs 4:19-25, 1989

Journal article, more than three authors:

3. Johnson JM, Hillestad A, Johnson AD, et al: Personalizing the search process. J. Prof Nurs 4:302-307, 1988

Journal article, in press:

4. Shoemaker JK: Nursing diagnosis in graduate curricula. J. Prof Nurs (in press)

Complete book:

5. Bailey BJ, Biller HF: Surgery of the Larynx. Philadelphia, PA, Saunders, 1985, pp 34-113

Chapter of book:

6. Wharam MD: Radiation therapy, in Altman AJ, Schwartz AD (eds): Malignant Diseases. Philadelphia, PA, Saunders, 1983, p. 103

Chapter of book that is part of published meeting:

7. Mitsunaga B: Operationalization of quality dimensions in nursing doctoral programs. Proceedings of the National Forum, Denver, CO, University of Colorado, 1984

Illustrations and tables are encouraged to enhance the text. All illustrations and tables should be numbered consecutively and cited in the text. Mark the position of each table and illustration in the margin of the manuscript. Be sure to include a title for each table and a legend (caption) for each illustration.

Each table should be typed on a separate sheet with its title.

All line drawings must be submitted as clear, glossy, black-and-white, 5″ × 7″ photographs. Black-and-white photographs of clinical procedures, equipment, and the like are also welcomed. On the back of each line drawing, photograph, and table, the figure number, author's name, and running head should be indicated in pencil in the lower left corner. Legends for all illustrations should be typewritten on a separate sheet at the end of the manuscript.

REFEREED PUBLICATION

Manuscripts submitted to the *Journal of PeriAnesthesia Nursing* are subject to review by at least three peers. Reviewers evaluate accuracy and relevance of content, organization, style and clarity, originality, use of verifiable and current references, and the manuscript's contribution to nursing's body of knowledge. The journal staff offers individual feedback based on reviewers' comments to guide revision when necessary. All submissions are subject to editing.

COPYRIGHT

Copyright by the American Society of PeriAnesthesia Nurses.

INDEXED

The *Journal of PeriAnesthesia Nursing* is indexed in the *Cumulative Index to Nursing and Allied Health Literature, International Nursing Index,* and *RNdex Top 100.*

SAMPLE JOURNAL ARTICLE TITLES

- "A Clinical Evaluation of an Operational Postanesthesia Care Unit Source Control System"
- "A Video Approach to Interactive Patient Education"
- "Laryngospasm and Noncardiogenic Pulmonary Edema"
- "Practical Points in the Evaluation of Postoperative Fever"
- "The Physiology and Pharmacology of Pain: A Review of Opioids"

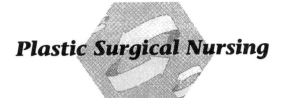

Plastic Surgical Nursing

Plastic Surgical Nursing is published by the American Society of Plastic and Reconstructive Surgical Nurses and is the official journal of the American Society of Plastic and Reconstructive Surgical Nurses.

JOURNAL FOCUS/PURPOSE

The primary purpose of Plastic Surgical Nursing is to inform nurses of the latest advances in plastic and reconstructive surgical nursing practice.

JOURNAL FACTS

Publication schedule: quarterly

Circulation: 2,000

Submitted papers per year: 20-25

Acceptance rate: 90%

Monetary honorarium: none

Average turnaround time: 6 months

Publishing timetable: 1-2 issues after acceptance

Correspondence:
American Society of Plastic and
    Reconstructive Surgical Nurses
East Holly Avenue, Box 56
Pitman, NJ 08071-0056
Telephone: (856) 256-2340
E-mail: psnjrnl@ajj.com

Internet site: www.ajj.com/jpi/psn/psnmain.htm

MANUSCRIPT SUBMISSION

The journal accepts original articles, case studies, letters, and descriptions of clinical care and surgical techniques. Query letters are welcomed, but not required. Material must be original and not previously published. Material is submitted for review with the understanding that it is not being nor will it have been submitted to any other journal prior to final consideration by the journal.

Five copies of the manuscript should be submitted to the editorial office; the author retains one copy. Manuscripts not accepted for publication will not be returned to the author unless requested within 30 days of notification of rejection.

Manuscripts accepted for publication are subject to copyediting. The author will receive an edited copy of the manuscript and galley proofs for review prior to publication.

Manuscripts should be submitted to:
Joyce Black, PhD(c), MSN, RNC, CPSN
Editor, Plastic Surgical Nursing
East Holly Avenue, Box 56
Pitman, NJ 08071-0056
Telephone: (856) 256-2340

The journal will accept both IBM and Macintosh format 3.5″ diskettes sent with manuscripts. All diskettes should be clearly labeled with the author's name, manuscript title, disk type (IBM or Macintosh), file name, and word processor name and version (or file type, if ASCII).

Most, but not all, IBM and Macintosh word processor files are acceptable for submission to the journal. When possible, all files should be saved as WordPerfect. Many spreadsheet files may also be acceptable but must be approved prior to sending. To ensure acceptability of your disk, please contact the journal office before sending any material.

Please use only common fonts (CG Times, Universe, Helvetica, Courier, etc.) and avoid complex font attributes such as outline. All graphics (tables, graphs, etc.) must be submitted in camera-ready form.

MANUSCRIPT PREPARATION GUIDELINES

Manuscripts must be typed, double-spaced on 8.5 × 11-inch white paper. Style should generally follow the *American Psychological Association Publication Manual* (APA). Please use the author-date method of citation within the text—(Doe, 1995) or "Doe (1995) states . . ." With multiple authors, the first citation must list all authors; in subsequent citations list only the name of the first author and et al.

Include the manuscript title, authors' names and credentials, and a biographic statement. Also include a brief abstract of 40 words or less, along with an address for correspondence and day and evening phone numbers.

Double-space all type, using 1.5- to 2-inch margins. Include the title, or a short descriptor, on the top of each page, but do not include authors' names. Include subheadings in the manuscript where possible. Type all subheadings flush with the left margin.

List all references in alphabetical order. Sample references are shown below:

Book:

Doe, J. (1995). *Fundamentals for aesthetic plastic surgery*. Baltimore: Williams & Wilkins.

Chapter in a book:

Doe, J., & Smith, R. (1995). Plastic surgery. In J. Luckmann & K. Sorenson (Eds.), *Medical-surgical nursing* (pp. 1234-1456). Philadelphia: Saunders.

Article in journal:

Doe, J. (1995). Complications following rhytidectomy. *Plastic Surgical Nursing, 7*(3), 67-89.

Figures include line drawings, photographs, diagrams, and graphs. Each figure must be numbered, and that number must correspond to a statement in the text directing the reader to see that figure. Include a separate legend sheet with double-spaced captions. The author must obtain permission for figures borrowed from another source.

Photographs must be black-and-white, glossy, 5 × 7 inch or color 5 × 7 inch or 35 mm slides.

The author is responsible for obtaining permission to use photographs of identifiable persons or those borrowed from other copyright holders.

REFEREED PUBLICATION

Plastic Surgical Nursing is a refereed journal. All manuscripts submitted undergo review by the editor and blind reviews by the manuscript review panel and/or editorial board. Each article is evaluated on its timeliness, importance, accuracy, clarity, and applicability.

COPYRIGHT

Copyright by the American Society of Plastic and Reconstructive Surgical Nurses.

INDEXED

Plastic Surgical Nursing is indexed in *Access to Uncover, Cumulative Index to Nursing and Allied Health Literature, RNdex Top 100,* and *UMI* (University Microfilms International).

SAMPLE JOURNAL ARTICLE TITLES

- "Burn Camp: An Unforgettable Summer Experience for Children and Teenagers"
- "Gaining Commitment to Rehabilitation: Importance of Preoperative Assessment"
- "Laser Resurfacing: A Survey of Pre- and Postprocedural Care"
- "Liposuction: An Overview"
- "Rare Facial Clefts: Craniofacial Anomalies"

14

Orthopedic/ Rehabilitative Nursing

Orthopaedic Nursing

Orthopaedic Nursing is published by the National Association of Orthopaedic Nurses and is the official publication of the National Association of Orthopaedic Nurses.

JOURNAL FOCUS/PURPOSE

The primary purpose of *Orthopaedic Nursing* is to provide continuing education for orthopaedic nurses. It focuses on a wide variety of clinical settings—hospital unit, physician's office, ambulatory care center, emergency room, operating room, rehabilitation facility, community service program, the client's home, and others. It provides departmental sections on current events, organizational activities, research, product and drug information, and literature findings. Articles reflect a commitment to professional development and the nursing profession as well as clinical, administrative, academic, and research areas of the orthopaedic specialty.

JOURNAL FACTS

Publication schedule: bimonthly

Circulation: 12,500

Submitted papers per year: 65

Acceptance rate: 75%

Monetary honorarium: none

Average turnaround time: 4 months

Publishing timetable: 8-12 months after acceptance

Correspondence:
National Association of Orthopaedic Nurses
East Holly Avenue, Box 56
Pitman, NJ 08071-0056
Telephone: (856) 256-2310
Fax: (856) 589-7463
E-mail: naon@mail.ajj.com

Internet site: www.ajj.com/jpi/onj/onjmain.htm

MANUSCRIPT SUBMISSION

Orthopaedic Nursing accepts manuscripts, letters, and case studies. Query letters are welcomed, but not required. Material must be original and never published before. Material is submitted for review with the understanding that it is not submitted to any other journal simultaneously.

Five copies should be sent; author retains the sixth copy.

Manuscripts or query letters should be sent to:

Mary Faut-Rodts, MS, MSA, RN, ONC
Editor, *Orthopaedic Nursing*
East Holly Avenue, Box 56
Pitman, NJ 08071-0056

MANUSCRIPT PREPARATION GUIDELINES

Manuscripts must be typed or word processed on $8\frac{1}{2}'' \times 11''$ paper. Double-space all typing, including references and figure captions.

Style is adapted from the *Publication Manual of the American Psychological Association* (APA), 4th ed. For help in preparation, refer to any article in a recently published issue of *Orthopaedic Nursing*. If you would like to request a recent copy of the journal, call the Editorial Coordinator at the National Office: (856) 256-2310.

On the title page, include manuscript title, authors' names, credentials, and current professional positions. Give a correspondence address and home and work telephone numbers.

On the abstract page, number this as page 1. Double-space. Show manuscript's title, but omit authors' names. Abstracts should be 75-150 words and should summarize essential points of the manuscript.

The first page of the text should be numbered page 2, with subsequent pages numbered sequentially. Omit all authors' names on these text pages. Double-space. Use short paragraph

structure. Refer to any recent *Orthopaedic Nursing* article for style.

Organize information under subheads; do not capitalize subheads. All subheads are flush left, upper- and lowercase. Major subheads are boldfaced. Minor heads are italicized.

Begin the list of references on a separate page. Follow the American Psychological Association style. Where there are six or more authors, list the first three only and add et al. Sample references are shown below.

Book:

Maher, A., Salmond, S., & Pellino, T. (Eds.). (1993). *Orthopaedic nursing*. Philadelphia: Saunders.

Chapter in a book:

Mooney, N. (1994). Assessment and management of pain. In A. Maher, S. Salmond, & T. Pellino (Eds.), *Orthopaedic nursing* (pp. 85-114). Philadelphia: Saunders.

Periodical:

Doheny, P., & Sedlak, C. (1994). So you've been asked to give a presentation. *Orthopaedic Nursing, 14*(2), 21-25.

Figures include photographs, diagrams, line drawings, and graphs. Label each figure: Figure 1. Caption . . . Do not underline. A separate legend sheet must be included, with captions typed double-spaced. When using figures adapted from another source, written permission from the original source is required.

All photographs should be black and white, glossy, preferably $5'' \times 7''$. Mark the back with an adhesive label or with a soft marker, labeling as a figure. Mark top of figure. Written permission is required for use of photographs of identifiable individuals.

Tables include words and/or numbers listed in columns. Do not capitalize or underline the title. Label at the top like this:

Table 2

Title of Table

In consultation with the author, *Orthopaedic Nursing* reserves the right to edit all materials with regard to length, timeliness, and readability consistent with publication style. Copyright on all published materials will be held by *Orthopaedic Nursing*.

When using figures adapted from another source, written permission from the original source is required. Written permission is required for use of photographs of identifiable individuals.

REFEREED PUBLICATION

Orthopaedic Nursing is a refereed journal. All manuscripts submitted undergo review by the editor and blind reviews by three reviewers from the Editorial Board and/or Manuscript Review Panel.

COPYRIGHT

Copyright by the National Association of Orthopaedic Nurses.

INDEXED

Orthopaedic Nursing is indexed in the *Cumulative Index to Nursing and Allied Health Literature, International Nursing Index, MEDLINE, Nursing Abstracts, Nursing Citation Index, RNdex Top 100,* and *UMI* (University Microfilms International).

SAMPLE JOURNAL ARTICLE TITLES

- "Comparing the Effectiveness of Different Educational Programs for Patients With Total Knee Arthroplasty"
- "Meeting the JCAHO Standards for Patient and Family Education"
- "Professional Certification in Orthopaedic Nursing"
- "Proximal Femoral Focal Deficiency"
- "Shoulder Immobilization Devices: Part 2. Shoulder Immobilizers"

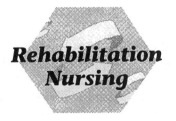

Rehabilitation Nursing is published by the Association of Rehabilitation Nurses and is the official publication of the Association of Rehabilitation Nurses.

JOURNAL FOCUS/PURPOSE

The primary purpose of *Rehabilitation Nursing* is to provide the professional nurse with a quality publication whose focus is rehabilitation nursing, including areas of clinical practice, education, administration, and research; a medium for professional development in the area of rehabilitation; and information of potential interest to rehabilitation nurses.

JOURNAL FACTS

Publication schedule: bimonthly

Circulation: 9,000

Submitted papers per year: 55

Acceptance rate: 70%

Monetary honorarium: none

Average turnaround time: 8-10 weeks

Publishing timetable: 6-12 months after acceptance

Correspondence:
Association of Rehabilitation Nurses
4700 W. Lake Avenue
Glenview, IL 60025-1485
Telephone: 1-800-229-7530 or (847) 375-4710
Fax: (847) 375-4777

Internet site: www.rehabnurse.org

MANUSCRIPT SUBMISSION

Unsolicited manuscripts are welcome. Authors are encouraged to submit abstracts or outlines of potential articles. Feedback and advice about the topic and its development will be provided. Manuscripts that address the relevance to nursing, nursing implications, and contributions to nursing science are valuable to readers.

Submit an original and three copies of the manuscript to:

Susan Dean-Baar, PhD, RN, CRRN, FAAN
Editor, *Rehabilitation Nursing*
4700 W. Lake Avenue
Glenview, IL 60025-1485

One author should be designated as correspondent in the cover letter. The journal is not responsible for lost manuscripts. Authors should retain one copy of their manuscripts.

The manuscript's clarity of purpose, relevance, originality, organization, and interest for *Rehabilitation Nursing* readers are considered during the review process. For research studies, appropriateness of methodology, adequacy of the literature review, and contribution to nursing science are assessed.

MANUSCRIPT PREPARATION GUIDELINES

Manuscripts should be typed double-spaced on $8\frac{1}{2} \times 11$-inch plain white paper, with $1\frac{1}{2}$-inch margins. The title page, abstract, acknowledgments, references, individual tables, and legend each should appear on a separate page. Type the title and page number in the upper right-hand corner of each page. Manuscripts that are 1,000 to 3,000 words (4 to 12 typed pages) will be considered for publication.

The title page should contain the title of the article and the authors' full names, academic degrees, and primary affiliations. Include the corresponding author's name, address, telephone and fax numbers, and e-mail address.

An abstract should state the purpose and principal conclusions presented in the article, and it should not exceed 150 words.

The use of headings within the text makes the manuscript easier to understand. To subdivide the article into main sections, insert subheads in the text. Subheads should be kept short, succinct, and meaningful, and they should be similar in sense and tone.

The author may acknowledge substantive contributions to the article. Grant and contract numbers should be provided.

The style of references is that described in the fourth edition of the *Publication Manual of* the American Psychological Association (APA) (1994). References used in the text should be cited by author's name and date of publication in parentheses (Smith, 1992), with page numbers cited for direct quotations. All references cited in the text must be included in the reference list.

The reference list should be double-spaced and include only references cited in the text in alphabetical order. The references must be verified by the author(s) against the original documents. Examples of correct forms of references follow.

Standard journal article (list all authors):

Ryden, M., Bossenmaier, M., & McLachlan, C. (1991). Aggressive behavior in cognitively impaired nursing home residents. *Research in Nursing and Health, 14*(2), 87-95.

Books and other monographs:

Zejdlik, C. P. (1992). *Management of spinal cord injury* (2nd ed.). Boston: Jones and Bartlett Publishers.

Chapter in edited text:

Fowler, E. (1990). Chronic wounds: An overview. In D. Krasner (Ed.), *Chronic wound care: A clinical source book for healthcare professionals* (pp. 12-18). King of Prussia, PA: Health Management Publications, Inc.

Specific reference by name to commercial entities or products is strongly discouraged in the interest of scientific objectivity. The entity or product should be described in a general fashion. If it is absolutely necessary to use a specific name—such as in a report of a study that compared two very specific products—the appropriate trademark (™) or registered mark (®) should be used with the trade name the first time it is used.

Rehabilitation Nursing welcomes tables, illustrations, and photographs of good quality and encourages authors to submit them with

manuscripts. Note the American Psychological Association format for these.

All manuscripts must be submitted exclusively to *Rehabilitation Nursing* and must not have been published previously. Receipt of manuscripts is acknowledged. Manuscripts are carefully screened for professional content and potential value to the literature. The selection of manuscripts for publication depends primarily on these reviews and recommendations, as well as on long-range editorial plans based on the needs and interests of rehabilitation nurses.

Rehabilitation Nursing reserves the right to edit all manuscripts according to style and space requirements and to clarify content.

Authors will be notified of the disposition of their manuscripts. If a manuscript is accepted for publication, copies of galleys will be sent to the author for review before publication. Manuscripts not accepted for publication will be returned to the author on request.

REFEREED PUBLICATION

Rehabilitation Nursing is a refereed journal with a blind review process.

COPYRIGHT

The Association of Rehabilitation Nurses will hold copyright on all articles published in *Rehabilitation Nursing*. A copyright transfer agreement signed by all authors will be requested on publication of the manuscript.

Manuscripts that are published in the journal become the property of the Association of Rehabilitation Nurses, and reprint or reproduction permission must be obtained from the Association of Rehabilitation Nurses. Reprints can be purchased from the publisher.

INDEXED

Rehabilitation Nursing is indexed in the *Cumulative Index to Nursing and Allied Health Literature, MEDLINE, Nursing Abstracts,* and *RNdex Top 100.*

SAMPLE JOURNAL ARTICLE TITLES

- "Managing Difficult Staff Interactions: Effectiveness of Assertiveness Training for SCI Nursing Staff"

- "Nurses' Assessment of Patients' Cognitive Orientation in a Rehabilitation Setting"
- "Phantom Limb Pain: Elusive, Yet Real"
- "Services That Nursing Facilities Should Provide to Residents With MS: A Survey of Health Professionals"
- "Spinal Cord Injury Rehabilitation in Armenia"

15

Professional Development

Journal of Professional Nursing

The *Journal of Professional Nursing* is published by W. B. Saunders Company and is the official journal of the American Association of Colleges of Nursing.

JOURNAL FOCUS/PURPOSE

The primary purpose of the *Journal of Professional Nursing* is to address the practice, research, and policy roles of nurses with baccalaureate and graduate degrees, the educational and management concerns of the universities in which they are educated, and the settings in which they practice.

JOURNAL FACTS

Publication schedule: bimonthly
Circulation: 2,250
Submitted papers per year: 100
Acceptance rate: 50%
Monetary honorarium: none
Average turnaround time: 2 months
Publishing timetable: 7 months after acceptance
Correspondence:
    W. B. Saunders Company

Editorial Offices
The Curtis Center
Independence Square West
Philadelphia, PA 19106-3399
Telephone: (215) 238-7800 or 1-800-545-2522
Or
American Association of Colleges of Nursing
One Dupont Circle, NW, Suite 530
Washington, DC 20036
Telephone: (202) 463-6930
Fax: (202) 785-8320
E-mail: JPN@aacn.nche.edu
Internet site: www.wbsaunders.com

MANUSCRIPT SUBMISSION

Original contributions that have never been published and are not under simultaneous consideration by another publication should be submitted to:

Eleanor J. Sullivan, Editor
Journal of Professional Nursing
American Association of Colleges of Nursing
One Dupont Circle, NW, Suite 530
Washington, DC 20036

An original manuscript, four manuscript copies, and four sets of illustrations are required for editorial review. Reports of original work, research, reviews, insightful descriptions, and policy papers focusing on professional nursing will be published. Featured columns include Professional Practice, Education, The Nurse Executive, Policy, Research, and Legal and Licensure Issues.

MANUSCRIPT PREPARATION GUIDELINES

Standard manuscript form, double-spaced, is requested. Separate pages should be used for the title, the abstract and key words, the text, acknowledgments, references, tables, and legends. Each page should be numbered consecutively, beginning with the title page. Include each author's name, highest academic degree earned, and institutional affiliation on the title page as well as the mailing address and telephone number of the corresponding author. In the text, avoid the use of abbreviations; spell terms out in full.

Abstracts should contain factual information rather than a general description of the manuscript's contents. Abstracts should contain 150 to 200 words stating the topic investigated, methods, results, and conclusions. Up to five index words should be listed at the end of the abstract.

Illustrations are preferred in the form of 5 × 7-inch glossy unmounted photographs. Code letters, symbols, arrows, and labeling should be done professionally in black (or white on dark areas). Spelling and abbreviations should correspond to the text. Consistency in style and size of labels is desirable for uniformity. Labels on large illustrations must be large enough to be legible when reduced to journal size. Number each illustration on the back. The first author's name should be marked on the back of each illustration, and an arrow should be drawn to indicate the "top." A reference to each illustration should appear in the text in consecutive numeric order. Color illustrations cannot be reproduced as such unless the cost is subsidized by the author. Such photographs often contain illustrative value even printed in black and white. Legends for the illustrations should be typed, double-spaced, on a separate sheet of paper attached to the manuscript.

Tables should be contained on separate sheets and numbered. Please indicate their placement in the text in consecutive numeric order.

References should be styled according to the guidelines in the *Publication Manual of the American Psychological Association.*

Journal article:

> Massey, J., & Loomis, M. (1988). When should nurses use research findings? *Applied Nursing Research, 1,* 32-40.

Journal article in a journal paginated by issue:

> Mooney, N. E. (1982). Coping with chronic pain in rheumatoid arthritis. Patients' behaviors and nursing interventions. *Orthopedic Nursing, 1*(3), 21-25.

Complete book:

> Pollack, M. L., Wilmore, J. H., & Fox, S. M., III (1984). *Exercise in health and disease.* Philadelphia: W. B. Saunders.

Chapter in a book:

> Dracup, K. (1987). Critical care nursing. In J. J. Fitzpatrick & R. L. Tauton (Eds.), *Annual review of nursing research* (pp. 107-133). New York: Springer.

Letters to the editor are published at the editor's discretion. They will be subject to editing. The use of several references is permissible. A transmittal letter containing copyright assignment should accompany the letter to the editor. The letter to the editor itself should be typed, double-spaced, like a regular manuscript.

Transmittal letters should designate the author to whom correspondence should be sent and give that author's current address and telephone number. In compliance with the Copyright Revision Act of 1976, transmittal letters should contain the following statement:

> In consideration of the Journal of Professional Nursing's reviewing and editing my submission, the author(s) undersigned transfers, assigns and otherwise conveys all copyright ownership to W. B. Saunders Company in the event that such work is published in the Journal of Professional Nursing.

Please indicate whether the manuscript was prepared while the author(s) was an employee of the U.S. government.

Letters of consent for publication must accompany patient photographs in which identification is possible. Parental consent or consent of legal guardian must be obtained to permit publication of a photograph of a minor.

Borrowed material: Illustrations, tables, or quotations must be fully identified as to author and source. If text material totaling 200 words or more is borrowed verbatim, or if illustrations or tables are borrowed, written permission must be obtained from both the publisher and the author. Letters granting this permission should be forwarded with the manuscript.

REFEREED PUBLICATION

Submissions will be peer-reviewed by eminent professional nurses of diverse backgrounds. Acceptance will be based on the importance of the material for the audience and the quality of the material. Final decisions about publication will be made by the editor.

COPYRIGHT

Copyright by W. B. Saunders Company.

INDEXED

The *Journal of Professional Nursing* is indexed in the *Cumulative Index to Nursing and Allied Health Literature, Index Medicus,* and *RNdex Top 100.*

SAMPLE JOURNAL ARTICLE TITLES

- "Curriculum Revision Isn't Just Change: It's Transition"
- "Ethics and Research Priorities in Academic Administration"
- "Retooling Faculty Orientation"
- "Professional Nurses in Unions: Working Together Pays Off"
- "Utilizing Narrative Inquiry to Evaluate a Nursing Doctorate Program Professional Residency"

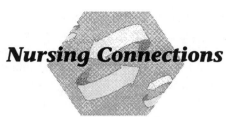

Nursing Connections

Nursing Connections is published by Springer Publishing Company, Inc.

JOURNAL FOCUS/PURPOSE

The primary purpose of *Nursing Connections* is to promote dialogue on the issues confronting us and the commonalities uniting us and to demonstrate the resultant power of collaboration. Manuscripts that reflect this interdependence among the professional specialties in and out of nursing or companion pieces on contrasting viewpoints are actively solicited. Singly or jointly authored papers are welcome.

JOURNAL FACTS

Publication schedule: quarterly

Circulation: 1,000

Submitted papers per year: 30-35

Acceptance rate: 65%

Monetary honorarium: none

Average turnaround time: 4 months

Publishing timetable: 2-3 months after acceptance

Correspondence:
Nursing Connections
Room 1B-41, The Washington Hospital Center
110 Irving Street, NW
Washington, DC 20010
Telephone: (202) 877-3048
Fax: (202) 877-8082
E-mail: mcb3@mhg.edu

Internet site: not available

MANUSCRIPT SUBMISSION

Send manuscripts and all correspondence to:
Molly Billingsley, RN, EdD
Editor-in-Chief, *Nursing Connections*
Room 1B-41, The Washington Hospital Center
110 Irving Street, NW
Washington, DC 20010
E-mail: mcb3@mhg.edu

Query letters or telephone calls to the editor are appropriate in some instances but are not mandatory. Authors are encouraged to submit abstracts or detailed outlines of potential articles. The editor will provide direction on the subsequent development. It is possible that substantive assistance may be provided to authors having problems developing a concept considered to be vitally important and timely. Please note that neither of these processes ensures final referee approval.

MANUSCRIPT PREPARATION GUIDELINES

Nursing Connections welcomes original articles that detail collaborative efforts and ideas of interest to advanced level nurses in each of the four roles. *Nursing Connections* is a periodical from the Washington Hospital Center for nurses who recognize the interdependence of administration, education, clinical practice, and research.

The editors strongly believe that the successful future of nursing in this age of superspecialization and fragmentation depends on increasing our communication and thus better understanding, valuing, and utilizing the diverse skills and expertise within the profession. There is further belief that nurses can benefit from studying related disciplines outside the profession and integrating useful concepts into nursing systems. Computer science, ethics, and business administration are but a few examples that have been learned and applied by nurses in solving professional problems and proposing alternatives to traditional practices.

The title page should include the article title and the name, academic degrees, and institutional affiliation of each author. The title page is the only page of the manuscript that should contain identifying information about the authors. Attach an abstract of not over 100 words.

The style of *Nursing Connections* is scholarly yet not arcane. A major editorial thrust is that the ideas and experiences offered, while soundly and explicitly based on theory, are directly usable to the interested reader. Grammatically, the editors request only that contrivances such as "He/She" be avoided. Authors are referred to the *Publication Manual of the American Psychological Association,* 4th ed. (1994), for reference, footnotes, or citation guidelines. Abbreviations should be spelled out the first time they are used. Addenda are not to be included. Tables should be typed, one per page, and placement should be noted in the text.

Manuscripts should be prepared via typewriter or word processor and should not exceed 14 double-spaced pages, including tables, figures, and references list. Articles should be submitted in triplicate. No manuscripts are returned to the authors. *Nursing Connections* is not responsible for lost manuscripts; authors are urged to retain a personal copy. Designate the person (including address and telephone and fax numbers) to whom all correspondence relating to the manuscript should be directed. Curriculum vitae, including work addresses and telephone numbers, for each author are also requested.

Decisions are rendered within a 3- to 5-month time frame. Articles accepted for publication will by copyedited as well as edited for house style by the staff. A complimentary issue will be mailed to each author on publication.

Manuscripts submitted to *Nursing Connections* must not be under consideration by any other journal. Should your manuscript be selected, it immediately becomes the property of *Nursing Connections* and may not be published elsewhere without permission. Articles are accepted on a nonremunerative basis.

REFEREED PUBLICATION

Nursing Connections is a refereed journal. Manuscripts are peer-reviewed by two or more referees from the Editorial Board.

COPYRIGHT

Copyright by Washington Hospital Center.

INDEXED

Nursing Connections is indexed in the *Cumulative Index to Nursing and Allied Health Literature, International Nursing Index, Nursing Abstracts,* and *Nursing Citation Index.*

SAMPLE JOURNAL ARTICLE TITLES

- "A Study of Preceptor Roles in Clinical Teaching"
- "Health Promotion and Social Support for Community-Based Clients With Chronic Mental Illness"
- "Optimizing Nursing Through Reorganization: Mandates for the New Millennium"

- "Problem-Based Learning in a Home Health Course"

- "The Use of Complementary Therapies by Cancer Patients"

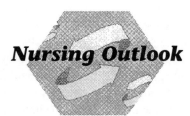

Nursing Outlook

Nursing Outlook is published by Mosby, Inc., and is the official journal of the American Academy of Nursing.

JOURNAL FOCUS/PURPOSE

The primary purpose of *Nursing Outlook* is to provide critical and timely analyses of emerging professional and health care issues of importance to all nurses. The primary editorial goals of the journal are these:

1. To publish innovative, original articles that stimulate thoughtful discussion and scholarly debate among nurses and other health care professionals
2. To inform readers about the diversity of opinion on controversial professional and health care matters facing nursing
3. To provide a multidisciplinary forum for discussion of current and future practice and health policy alternatives
4. To disseminate information about creative, alternative, and forward-looking models of education and practice as they relate to changing systems of health care
5. To promote the use of scientific knowledge in a timely fashion by nurses to enhance the quality and efficiency of health care
6. To provide information about leadership and leadership development opportunities for nurses, including professional meetings, hearings, forums, fellowships, and internships
7. To increase critical awareness of technologies, products, and services that have the potential for increasing the effectiveness of nurses in all settings

JOURNAL FACTS

Publication schedule: bimonthly

Circulation: 6,650

Submitted papers per year: 112 (average)

Acceptance rate: 26 (average)

Monetary honorarium: none

Average turnaround time: 2 months

Publishing timetable: not available

Correspondence:
  Business Office
  Mosby, Inc.
  11830 Westline Industrial Drive
  St. Louis, MO 63146-3318
  Telephone: 1-800-453-4351
  Fax: (314) 432-1158
  E-mail: periodical.service@mosby.com
Internet site: www.mosby.com

MANUSCRIPT SUBMISSION

Nursing Outlook welcomes unsolicited manuscripts related to nursing education, practice, or research or to health care policy and delivery. All manuscripts are accepted for publication with the understanding that they are contributed solely to *Nursing Outlook*. On acceptance, manuscripts become the permanent property of the Journal and may not be reproduced elsewhere without written permission from the publisher. Those not accepted will be returned only if a self-addressed stamped envelope is enclosed.

Submit manuscripts to:

Carole A. Anderson, PhD, RN, FAAN
Editor, *Nursing Outlook*
The Ohio State University, College of Nursing
1585 Neil Avenue
Columbus, OH 43210-1289
Fax: (614) 292-4535
E-mail: Anderson.32@osu.edu

Submit three copies of the manuscript and supporting materials (reference list, tables, figures, and figure legends) to the editor at the above address.

MANUSCRIPT PREPARATION GUIDELINES

Manuscripts should be prepared in accordance with the "Uniform Requirements for Manuscripts Submitted to Biomedical Journals." For detailed instructions, refer to the requirements as published (*Ann Intern Med* 1997;126:36-47).

General Requirements. Type all manuscripts on $8\frac{1}{2} \times 11$-inch paper on one side of the page, with liberal margins. Double-space all typewritten material, including the reference list, tables, and figure legends.

Number all pages of the manuscript (including reference list, tables, and figure legends) in the upper right-hand corner of the page, beginning with the title page. The body of the manuscript and supporting materials should not contain any reference to identify the author(s).

Once a manuscript has been accepted, the final version of the manuscript must be submitted on diskette along with three copies of the printout. The author accepts responsibility for the submitted diskette's exactly matching the printout of the final version of the manuscript. Guidelines for submission of the accepted manuscript on diskette will be sent to the author by the editorial office.

The text must conform to acceptable English usage. If unusual abbreviations cannot be avoided, use the expanded form with the abbreviation in parentheses when first mentioned and abbreviate thereafter. Use generic drug and equipment names; trademarks may be listed in parentheses at the point of first mention. If it is necessary to use a trademark for equipment, supply the manufacturer's name, city, and state.

The title page should include the manuscript title and the full names of the authors, their highest earned academic degrees, and their institutional affiliations and status. Give the complete mailing address, business and home telephone numbers, and fax number of the author to whom correspondence and galley proofs should be directed. If applicable, include a brief acknowledgment of grants or other financial assistance. Provide a one- or two-sentence miniabstract.

References must be cited consecutively in the text as superscript numbers. A reference that is mentioned more than once in the text can be designated by the same superscript number. The reference list must be typed double-spaced in numeric order on a separate sheet at the end of the text. The format of the reference list should conform to that set forth in "Uniform Requirements for Manuscripts Submitted to Biomedical Journals" (*Ann Intern Med* 1997;126:36-47).

Number figures consecutively in the order of text mention; all illustrations must be mentioned in text. Mark lightly in pencil on the back of each illustration the figure number and name of first author, and indicate the top. Do not mount illustrations on cardboard. Do not send original artwork or X-ray films. Illustrations will be returned only if the author requests such at the time the manuscript is submitted. Special arrangements must be made with the publisher for color illustrations. Type legends double-spaced on a separate sheet of paper. Spell out in the legends any abbreviations used as labels on figures. If the figure is taken from previously published material, the legend must give full credit to the original source.

Figures may be submitted in the electronic format. All images should be at least 5 inches wide. Images should be provided as EPS or TIFF files on Zip disk, CD, floppy, Jaz, or 3.5 MO. Macintosh or PC is acceptable. Graphics software such as Photoshop and Illustrator, not presentation software such as PowerPoint, CorelDraw, or Harvard Graphics, should be used in the creation of the art. Gray scale images should be at least 300 DPI with a proof. Combinations of gray scale and line art should be at least 1,200 DPI with a proof. Line art (black and white or color) should be at least 1,200 DPI with a proof. Please include hardware and software information, in addition to the file names, with the disk.

Number tables consecutively in the order of text mention; all tables must be mentioned in the text. Data appearing in tables should supplement, not duplicate, the text. Provide a brief title for each table, and provide a footnote to the table spelling out any abbreviations used therein. If the table is taken from previously published material, a footnote must give full credit to the original source.

In accordance with the Copyright Act of 1976, all manuscripts must be accompanied by the following statement signed by all authors:

> The undersigned authors transfer all copyright ownership of the manuscript (title of article) to Mosby, Inc., in the event the work is published. The undersigned authors warrant that the article is original, is not under consideration by another journal, and has not been previously published.

Send written permission of the copyright holder and author for any quotation, table, or figure taken from previously published material. Patient or guardian consent must accompany any photograph that shows a recognizable likeness of a person.

REFEREED PUBLICATION

Nursing Outlook is a peer-reviewed journal with a blind review process.

COPYRIGHT

Copyright by Mosby, Inc.

INDEXED

Nursing Outlook is indexed in *Abstracts of Hospital Management Studies, Cumulative Index to Nursing and Allied Health Literature, Exceptional Child Education Abstracts, Hospital Literature Index, Index Medicus, International Nursing Index, International Pharmaceutical Abstracts, Nursing Abstracts, Nursing Studies Index, Psychological Abstracts, Social Services Index,* and *Social Work Research and Abstracts.*

SAMPLE JOURNAL ARTICLE TITLES

- "Cancer Fatalism Among African-Americans: A Review of the Literature"
- "Federal Support of Graduate Nursing Education: Rationale and Policy Options"
- "Men Researching Women Working"
- "Nursing in the Political and Economic Marketplace: Challenges for the 21st Century"
- "Students' Perceptions of Ideal and Nursing Career Choices"

16

Psychiatric Nursing

Archives of Psychiatric Nursing

Archives of Psychiatric Nursing is published by W. B. Saunders Company and is the official journal of the Society for Education and Research in Psychiatric-Mental Health Nursing.

JOURNAL FOCUS/PURPOSE

The primary purpose of *Archives of Psychiatric Nursing* is to disseminate knowledge to guide practitioners of psychiatric and mental health nursing. The *Archives of Psychiatric Nursing* considers psychiatric and mental health nursing in its broadest perspective, including theory, practice, education, research, and policy applications related to all ages, special populations, settings, mental health disciplines, and both the public and private sectors. The *Archives of Psychiatric Nursing* is a medium for clinician-scholars to provide theoretical linkages among diverse areas of practice. Manuscripts are sought and published that will inform current practice and shape public policy for the delivery of psychiatric and mental health nursing services.

JOURNAL FACTS

Publication schedule: bimonthly
Circulation: approximately 3,500
Submitted papers per year: approximately 100-120
Acceptance rate: 30% (60% for resubmissions)
Monetary honorarium: none
Average turnaround time: 2-3 months
Publishing timetable: 3-4 months after acceptance
Correspondence:
    W. B. Saunders Company
    Editorial Offices
    The Curtis Center
    Independence Square West
    Philadelphia, PA 19106-3399
    Telephone: (215) 238-7800 or 1-800-545-2522
Internet site: www.wbsaunders.com

MANUSCRIPT SUBMISSION

Four copies of the manuscript and four camera-ready copies of each illustration should be sent to:

Judith B. Krauss, Editor
Archives of Psychiatric Nursing
Yale University School of Nursing
100 Church St. South
P.O. Box 9740
New Haven, CT 06536-0740

Refer style questions to the production editor at W. B. Saunders Company: (215) 238-5028.

The *Archives of Psychiatric Nursing* reserves the right to edit all manuscripts for its style and space requirements and for the purpose of clarity. The editor of the *Archives of Psychiatric Nursing* will determine in which volume and issue accepted manuscripts will appear. Authors will receive proofs and are responsible for proofreading and checking the accuracy of material as it appears in edited copy.

MANUSCRIPT PREPARATION GUIDELINES

Manuscripts should be printed on a high-quality printer, double-spaced, with one and one-half inch margins. Two face sheets should be included. One face sheet should carry the title of the manuscript, the name and address of the author(s), institution affiliations, and reprint address. The other face sheet should carry only the title, with no identifying author information, for use as the only face sheet during review. Manuscripts should not exceed 16 pages (4,000 words), exclusive of references. Line drawings or other illustrations must be camera-ready copy; photocopies are not acceptable. Photographs, if used, must be 5″ × 7″ glossy black-and-white prints.

The fourth edition of the *Publication Manual of the American Psychological Association* (1994) provides the format for text and references. Titles should be short. Abbreviations should be spelled out for the first time they are used. Symbols, other than standard statistical symbols, should be identified the first time they are used. An abstract, not to exceed 100 words, should be included as a separate page. Tables and figures should be typed or drawn on one page, and relative placement should be noted in the text.

Authors are responsible for obtaining permission for reproducing copyrighted materials and for sending a copy of that permission to the publisher before publication.

REFEREED PUBLICATION

Manuscripts are reviewed by an editor and at least two individuals from the editorial review board: Decisions for publication are made on the basis of these reviews. No manuscripts will be returned to the author(s). Correspondence regarding permission to reprint all or part of any article published in this journal should be addressed to Journal Permissions Dept., W. B. Saunders Company, Orlando, FL 32887. Telephone: (407) 345-2500.

COPYRIGHT

Copyright is by W. B. Saunders Company.

INDEXED

Archives of Psychiatric Nursing is indexed in the *Cumulative Index to Nursing and Allied Health Literature; Current Contents: Social and Behavioral Sciences; Nursing Abstracts; PsycINFO;* and *RNdex Top 100.*

SAMPLE JOURNAL ARTICLE TITLES

- "Deconstructing Progress Notes in Psychiatric Settings"
- "Evolution of Community Mental Health Case Management: Consideration for Clinical Practice"

- "Psychobiology and Psychopharmaco-therapy of Unipolar Major Depression: A Review"
- "The Lifeworld of the Chronic Mentally Ill: Analysis of 40 Written Personal Accounts"

- "Voices From Practice: Mental Health Nurses Identify Research Priorities"

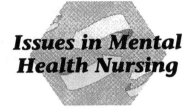

Issues in Mental Health Nursing

I*ssues in Mental Health Nursing* is published by Taylor & Francis, Inc.

JOURNAL FOCUS/PURPOSE

The primary purpose of *Issues in Mental Health Nursing* is to expand the literature on the psychosocial and mental health aspects of nursing care currently available to students, educators, and practitioners. It deals with new, innovative approaches to client care, analysis of current issues, and nursing research findings.

JOURNAL FACTS

Publication schedule: bimonthly

Circulation: approximately 900

Submitted papers per year: approximately 60

Acceptance rate: approximately 70%

Monetary honorarium: none

Average turnaround time: 3 months

Publishing timetable: 6-9 months after acceptance

Correspondence:
Taylor & Francis, Inc.
325 Chestnut Street, 8th Floor
Philadelphia, PA 19106
Telephone: (215) 625-8900
Fax: (215) 625-2940

Internet site: www.taylorandfrancis.com

MANUSCRIPT SUBMISSION

Because clinical research is the primary vehicle for the development of nursing science, *Issues in Mental Health Nursing* presents articles that report research findings and lists studies conducted by nurses that focus on the caretaking process. The journal also presents articles that address the application of the nursing process to clients and families for the purpose of mental health promotion, prevention of psychosocial dysfunction, and the resolution or amelioration of existing problems.

A holistic approach to mental health care emphasizes the need to acknowledge the mutual interaction and influence between the client and the environment. Families, caretakers, the proximate milieu, and society are significant influential dimensions of this environment that nurses need to understand. Articles covering current social issues that either directly or indirectly influence the practice of mental health nursing are welcome.

Address manuscripts to
Sandra P. Thomas, PhD, RN, FAAN
Editor, *Issues in Mental Health Nursing*
College of Nursing, University of Tennessee—Knoxville
1200 Volunteer Blvd.
Knoxville, TN 37996-4180
Telephone: (423) 974-7581

Fax: (423) 974-3569
E-mail: sthomas@utk.edu

Submission of a manuscript to this journal is understood to imply that it or substantial parts of it have not been published or accepted for publication elsewhere.

MANUSCRIPT PREPARATION GUIDELINES

Manuscripts should be typewritten double-spaced throughout, including references, tables, footnotes, and figure legends, on $8\frac{1}{2} \times 11$ regular bond paper (not erasable bond). Submit all manuscripts in triplicate (the original and two copies), including illustrations and tables. All accepted manuscripts, artwork, and photographs become the property of the publisher.

The title page should contain the names, degrees, and institutional affiliations of all authors and the complete mailing address and telephone of the author to whom all correspondence should be sent.

The abstract should be typed on a separate page and should not exceed 150 words. This is an essential part of the paper; lack of an abstract may delay publication.

Tables should be typed on a separate sheet of paper and numbered consecutively with respect to text citation. They should be self-explanatory and should supplement, not duplicate, the text. Illustrations or tables from other publications must be accompanied by letters of permission from the copyright holder, and the permission should be acknowledged in the figure legends or table titles. Figures should also be numbered consecutively. All tables and figures must be referred to in the text.

Line illustrations should be professionally made, with maximum contrast and sharp, even lettering. Photocopies are unacceptable. Number consecutively with single arabic numerals and note in text where each should be placed. Type captions on a separate sheet of paper and place figures and captions following tables. All photographs must be glossy and have good contrast. Four-color illustrations will be considered for publication; however, the author will be required to bear the full cost involved in their printing and publication. The charge for the first figure is $1,200. Subsequent figures, totaling no more than four text pages, are $500.00 each. Good-quality color prints should be provided, in their final size. Figures needing reduction or enlargement will be charged an additional 25%. The publisher has the right to refuse publication of color prints deemed unacceptable.

Cite references in the text by author and date (Smith, 1983). Prepare reference list in accordance with the *Publication Manual of the American Psychological Association* (APA), 4th ed.

Journal:

> Tsai, M., & Wagner, N. N. (1978). Therapy groups for women sexually molested as children. *Archives of Sexual Behavior, 7,* 417-427.

Book:

> Miliman, M. (1980). *Such a pretty face.* New York: W. W. Norton.

Contribution to a book:

> Hartley, J. T., & Walsh, D. A. (1980). Contemporary issues in adult development of learning. In L. W. Poon (Ed.), *Aging in the 1980s* (pp. 239-252). Washington, DC: American Psychological Association.

For spelling, follow *Merriam Webster's Collegiate Dictionary, Tenth Edition,* and *Dorland's Illustrated Medical Dictionary* for medical terms. Page proofs are sent to the designated author. They must be carefully checked and returned within 48 hours of receipt.

The corresponding author of each article will receive one complete copy of the issue in which the article appears. Reprints of an individual article may be ordered from Taylor & Francis, Inc. Use the reprint order form included with page proofs.

REFEREED PUBLICATION

Issues in Mental Health Nursing is a refereed journal with a blind review process.

COPYRIGHT

Copyright by Taylor & Francis, Inc. All papers accepted for publication must be accompanied by a copyright release form signed by the author. A signed copyright form also acknowledges that the author recognizes full responsibility for obtaining permission to reproduce copyrighted material from other sources.

This form is available from the editor or online (requires Adobe Acrobat Reader©).

INDEXED

Issues in Mental Health Nursing is indexed in *Human Resources Abstract, International Nursing Index, MEDLINE, Nursing Abstracts, PsycINFO, Sociological Abstracts,* and *RNdex Top 100.*

SAMPLE JOURNAL ARTICLE TITLES

- "Comparison of Registered Nurses' and Nursing Assistants' Choices of Intervention for Aggressive Behaviors"
- "Severely and Persistently Mentally Ill in Hawaii: Profile and Implications"
- "The Caregiving Story: How the Narrative Approach Informs Caregiving Burden"
- "The Lived Experience of Aloneness for Older Women Currently Being Treated for Depression"
- "Therapy With Male Survivors of Sexual Abuse: The Client Perspective"

Journal of Child and Adolescent Psychiatric Nursing

The *Journal of Child and Adolescent Psychiatric Nursing* is published by Nursecom, Inc., and is the official journal of the Association of Child and Adolescent Psychiatric Nurses, a division of the International Society of Psychiatric-Mental Health Nurses.

JOURNAL FOCUS/PURPOSE

The primary purpose of the *Journal of Child and Adolescent Psychiatric Nursing* is to reflect the broad spectrum of issues relevant to the practice, education, and research of child and adolescent psychiatric and mental health nurses.

JOURNAL FACTS

Publication schedule: quarterly

Circulation: 1,500

Submitted papers per year: 40

Acceptance rate: 25%

Monetary honorarium: none

Average turnaround time: 3 months

Publishing timetable: 4-6 months after acceptance

Correspondence:
  Journal of Child and Adolescent Psychiatric Nursing
  Nursecom, Inc.
  1211 Locust Street
  Philadelphia, PA 19107
  Telephone: (215) 545-7222 or 1-800-242-6757
  Fax: (215) 545-8107
  E-mail: margon@compuserve.com

Internet site: www.nursecominc.com

MANUSCRIPT SUBMISSION

Send four copies of the manuscript to:

  Dr. E. Poster
  University of Texas at Arlington
  Box 19407
  Arlington, TX 76019
  E-mail: poster@uta.edu

All submissions must be accompanied by the following statement signed by the author(s):

As the author(s) of (title of article), I/we hereby transfer copyright ownership to Nursecom, Inc. if the work is published. I/we warrant that the article is original, has not been submitted to another journal, and has not been previously published.

MANUSCRIPT PREPARATION GUIDELINES

Typed double-spaced with 1-inch margins; maximum 15 pages + references, tables, figures. Include a title page with title of article, author(s) full name(s), academic degrees, affiliation, title(s). List references on a separate page; use American Psychological Association style.

Type each figure, chart, table on a separate page. Reference each one in the text. Write a short legend for each one. Include permissions for all artwork, as necessary, and for use of copyrighted material.

Include a structured abstract of 75-100 words. For nonresearch articles, include topic, purpose, sources used, and conclusions. For research articles, include problem, methods, findings, and conclusions. Add 3-5 key words.

Identify corresponding author, including home address, telephone number, and e-mail address.

At time of acceptance, send a disk with your manuscript in Word or WordPerfect or e-mail manuscript to margon@compuserve.com. Check all disks for a virus before sending.

All manuscripts will be edited to conform to the style of this journal. The author is responsible for the content of the original and edited manuscript, once it is approved, and for the accuracy of references, quoted material, and for any violation of copyright.

Illustrations, charts, tables: Photographs, line drawings, graphs, tables, and charts are encouraged if they enhance or amplify the text and are of publishable quality. All need to be referenced in the text. Photographs of people must be accompanied by a signed statement by the individual(s) photographed or the person with the legal right to sign such a statement.

REFEREED PUBLICATION

All manuscripts will be reviewed by the editor and at least two members of the review panel before a decision to publish is made. Accepted manuscripts may be revised in order to conform to the standards and style of this journal.

COPYRIGHT

Copyright by Nursecom, Inc.

INDEXED

The *Journal of Child and Adolescent Psychiatric Nursing* is indexed in *Cumulative Index to Nursing and Allied Health Literature (CINAHL), Index Medicus,* and *International Nursing Index.*

SAMPLE JOURNAL ARTICLE TITLES

- "Adolescent Suicide as a Public Health Threat"
- "Childhood Memories About Food: The Successful Dieter's Project"
- "Homeless Parents Perceptions of Parenting Stress"
- "Psychopharmacology Notes: Pharmacotherapy in Children and Adolescents With Pervasive Developmental Disorders"
- "Reframing the Future—Optimistic Thinking"

Journal of Psychosocial Nursing and Mental Health Services

The *Journal of Psychosocial Nursing and Mental Health Services* is published by SLACK Incorporated.

JOURNAL FOCUS/PURPOSE

The primary purpose of the *Journal of Psychosocial Nursing and Mental Health Services* is to provide the most up-to-date practical information available for today's psychosocial nurse.

JOURNAL FACTS

Publication schedule: monthly

Circulation: 9,000

Submitted papers per year: not available

Acceptance rate: not available

Monetary honorarium: none

Average turnaround time: 4-5 months

Publishing timetable: 2-3 months after acceptance

Correspondence:
Business Office, SLACK Incorporated
6900 Grove Road
Thorofare, NJ 08086-9447

Telephone: (856) 848-1000 or 1-800-257-8290
Fax: (856) 853-5991
E-mail: jpn@slackinc.com

Internet site: www.slackinc.com/jpn.htm

MANUSCRIPT SUBMISSION

The *Journal of Psychosocial Nursing and Mental Health Services* accepts original articles as well as letters to the editor.

All materials should be submitted to:

Dr. Shirley Smoyak
Journal of Psychosocial Nursing and Mental Health Services
6900 Grove Road
Thorofare, NJ 08086

Readers are also encouraged to submit ideas that may be developed into articles, suggestions for news stories, and topics for the "Your Turn" and "Professionally Speaking" columns.

All manuscripts should be accompanied by a letter of copyright transmittal. This must be signed and dated by all authors. The letter is required before any manuscript can be considered for publication and should contain the following language:

In consideration of SLACK Incorporated taking action in reviewing and editing my (our) submission, the author(s) undersigned hereby transfers, assigns, or otherwise conveys all copyright ownership to SLACK Incorporated. The copyright so conveyed includes any and all subsidiary forms of publication, such as electronic media. The author(s) declares that the manuscript contains no matter that is, to the best of the author's knowledge, libelous or unlawful, or that infringes upon any US copyright.

MANUSCRIPT PREPARATION GUIDELINES

Manuscripts are accepted for review with the understanding that they are submitted solely to the Journal and have not been published previously. Receipt of manuscripts will be acknowledged within 30 days.

Four copies of the manuscript should be submitted, typewritten on one side of $8\frac{1}{2} \times 11$-inch paper, double-spaced with 1-inch margins. Contributors should retain a complete copy of the manuscript. Manuscripts between 8 and 12 pages are acceptable. The title page should be separate and should include the following: title; author(s) identification, including degrees and titles; institution of origin, including city and state; reprint address; telephone number; and acknowledgment of grant support.

Manuscript style should follow the *Publication Manual of the American Psychological Association*. References should be held to a maximum of 15. Consult the APA manual for additional questions regarding the style or format for statistics, text citations, or references. The Journal reserves the right to edit manuscripts, delete extraneous or excess material, and change titles and headings.

Manuscripts should include a self-addressed postage-paid postcard with the title of the manuscript, to be returned to the author as acknowledgment of receipt. Manuscripts will not be returned to authors after review and will be destroyed in the editorial office. To have manuscripts returned, authors must request it in their submission letter and provide a postage-paid self-addressed envelope.

Contributors are encouraged to submit appropriate tables, figures, photographs, or illustrations to accompany their articles. It is the responsibility of the author(s) to obtain permission to publish from each individual pictured in photographs. Proper photo credit should be cited.

An order form for reprints will accompany the five complimentary copies of the Journal sent to the primary author.

If academic, hospital, or institutional affiliations are given or are referred to in the manuscript, it is the responsibility of the author to obtain permission from the proper authorities to use the names of such.

REFEREED PUBLICATION

Manuscripts are peer-reviewed. All manuscripts submitted to the Journal go through the classic peer-review procedure common to the most respected professional journals. Your anonymous peers approve or disapprove your manuscripts based on merit and clarity of presentation. This process, we believe, reinforces the integrity not only of the *Journal of Psychosocial Nursing and Mental Health Services* but also our profession through the dissemination of professional knowledge. The Journal does not provide critique of articles not accepted for publication.

COPYRIGHT

Copyright by SLACK Incorporated.

INDEXED

The *Journal of Psychosocial Nursing and Mental Health Services* is indexed in *Adolescent Mental Health Abstracts, Cumulative Index to Nursing and Allied Health Literature, Index Medicus, International Nursing Index, Nursing Abstracts, Nurse Search, Psychiatric Journal Review,* and *Psychological Abstracts.*

SAMPLE JOURNAL ARTICLE TITLES

- "Attitudes Toward Medication Among Persons With Severe Mental Illness"
- "New Hope for a Disabling Condition: Cognitive-Behavioral Approaches to Panic Disorder"
- "Music Therapy as a Nursing Intervention"
- "Use of Physical Restraints on Hospitalized Psychogeriatric Patients"
- "The Impact of the Number of Young Adults on an Inpatient Psychiatric Unit"

Journal of the American Psychiatric Nurses Association

The *Journal of the American Psychiatric Nurses Association* is published by Mosby, Inc. and is the official journal of the American Psychiatric Nurses Association.

JOURNAL FOCUS/PURPOSE

The primary purpose of the *Journal of the American Psychiatric Nurses Association* is to inform psychiatric nurses about important clinical and useful psychiatric care developments.

JOURNAL FACTS

Publication schedule: bimonthly

Circulation: 4,800

Submitted papers per year: not available

Acceptance rate: not available

Monetary honorarium: none

Average turnaround time: 3 months

Publishing timetable: 6-12 months after acceptance

Correspondence:
Business Office
Mosby, Inc.
11830 Westline Industrial Drive
St. Louis, MO 63146-3318
Telephone: 1-800-453-4351
Fax: (314) 432-1158
E-mail: periodical.service@mosby.com

Internet site: www.mosby.com or www.apna.org

MANUSCRIPT SUBMISSION

Manuscripts and correspondence should be sent to either of the following editors:

Nikki S. Polis, RN, PhD
University MacDonald Women's Hospital
Frances Payne Bolton School of Nursing
Mail Stop: MAC 5033
11100 Euclid Avenue
Cleveland, OH 44106
Telephone: (216) 844-1939
Fax: (216) 844-1284
E-mail: Nikki.Polis@uhhs.com

Grayce M. Sills, RN, PhD, FAAN
366 Carilla Lane
Columbus, OH 43228-1315
Telephone: (614) 878-4467
Fax: (614) 878-9233
E-mail: sills.1@osu.edu

Submit the original and three high-quality copies.

MANUSCRIPT PREPARATION GUIDELINES

Prepare manuscripts using the style and standards outlines in the *Publication Manual of the American Psychological Association,* 4th edition. Type the manuscript on $8\frac{1}{2} \times 11$-inch paper, one sided, 1-inch margins on all sides, and double-spaced, including references and tables. Number pages consecutively beginning with the title page. Limit manuscript length to 15 pages, excluding supporting material such as tables, figures, and illustrations. With acceptance of the manuscript, the final version of the manuscript may be submitted on disk with a copy of the printout.

For the title page, on the original, include the title of the manuscript, author(s) name(s) with full credentials, job title(s), and institutional affiliations with city and state. Provide the complete mailing address, business and home telephone numbers, and fax number of the corresponding author. Acknowledgments of support can be included. On the copies, include only the title of the manuscript.

Use a summary abstract format, limited to 100 words, for clinical and issues articles. A structured abstract, limited to 150 words, is to be used with research articles. The abstract is to include five sections with the following headings: Background, Objective(s), Study Design, Results, and Conclusions.

The editors assume that articles from a particular institution are submitted with the approval of the requisite authorities, including all matters pertaining to human subjects.

REFEREED PUBLICATION

The *Journal of the American Psychiatric Nurses Association* is a professional, peer-reviewed journal that welcomes original articles in English.

The corresponding author will receive written notice that the manuscript has been received. All manuscripts are subject to blind review by three experts in fields related to the topic or methods of the manuscript. The corresponding author will receive written notice regarding the outcome of the review process. Revised and resubmitted manuscripts will be reviewed by the same reviewers who evaluated the original submission. All manuscripts will be edited to conform to the standards and style of the *Journal of the American Psychiatric Nurses Association.*

COPYRIGHT

INDEXED

The *Journal of the American Psychiatric Nurses Association* is indexed in the *Cumulative Index to Nursing and Allied Health Literature* and *Nursing Abstracts.*

SAMPLE JOURNAL ARTICLE TITLES

- "An Individualized Music Intervention for Agitation"
- "Leadership in Nursing: Psychiatric Nurses Make a Difference"
- "Mental Health Parity: Victory on the Horizon"
- "Multiphasic Short-term Therapy for Dissociative Identity Disorder"
- "The Ins and Outs of Psychiatric-Mental Health Nursing and the American Nurses Association"

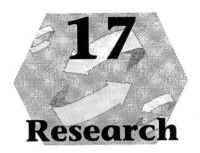

Research

Advances in Nursing Science

Advances in Nursing Science is published by Aspen Publishers, Inc.

JOURNAL FOCUS/PURPOSE

The primary purposes of *Advances in Nursing Science* are to contribute to the development of nursing science and to promote the application of emerging theories and research findings to practice.

JOURNAL FACTS

Publication schedule: quarterly

Circulation: 4,000

Submitted papers per year: 120

Acceptance rate: 15-20%

Monetary honorarium: none

Average turnaround time: 8-10 weeks

Publishing timetable: 2 months after acceptance

Correspondence:
  Customer Services
  200 Orchard Ridge Drive
  Gaithersburg, MD 20878
  Customer service telephone: 1-800-234-1660

Internet site: www.aspenpub.com (enter journal title in search box) or www.nursing.uconn.edu/ans.html

MANUSCRIPT SUBMISSION

Articles sought deal with any of the processes of science, including research, theory development, concept analysis, practical application of research and theory, and investigation of the values and ethics that influence the practice and research endeavors of nursing sciences. Acceptance or rejection of an article is based on the judgment of peer reviewers. A general description of the focus and suggested content for both types of articles follows:

Research articles: *Empirical research* (descriptive, quasi-experimental, experimental, basic) should include a clear and concise summary of the purpose and problem, a statement of the hypothesis tested, background and significance, theoretical framework, design, methods and procedures, analyses of data, findings, conclusions, and implications for further research and nursing practice. *Historical research* articles dealing with the history of nursing practice or nursing science, or related phenomena that have influenced the development of nursing practice and nursing science.

Theory articles: *Concept analyses* are identified as important for nursing and should include a thorough review of existing literature—

both theory and research—related to the concept under examination. Implications for nursing research and for development of nursing theory should also be included. *Theory analyses and development* is an in-depth analysis of existing theory and development of extensions or alternative theory based on the existing theory; comparative analyses of different related theories. A summary of implications for nursing research or nursing practice should be included.

Manuscripts and correspondence regarding publication should be addressed to:

Peggy L. Chinn, Editor
University of Connecticut, School of Nursing
231 Glenbrook Rd.
Storrs, CT 06269-2026

Submissions must comprise an original copy of a manuscript, plus an identical version on a PC-formatted diskette in the Windows 95 version of Microsoft Word 7.0, or send a Microsoft Word (version 7.0 for Windows 95) file via e-mail to PLChinn@uconnvm.uconn.edu.

MANUSCRIPT PREPARATION GUIDELINES

Manuscripts for *ANS* must accompany the following components: Abstract and key words—include an abstract of 100 words or less. The abstract should briefly summarize the major issue, problem, or topic being addressed, and the findings and/or conclusions of the article. Also include up to ten key words that describe the contents of the article like those that appear in *Cumulative Index to Nursing & Allied Health Literature* (CINAHL) or the *National Library of Medicine's Medical Subject Headings* (MeSH).

Title page—include title of the article, author name(s) with highest academic degrees and affiliation (e.g., professional title, name of department or division, name and location of business or institution in which the work should be attributed), and any acknowledgments, credits, or disclaimers.

References: Manuscripts should also include a reference list that is styled according to the *American Medical Association Manual of Style,* 9th ed. (1998). References should also include citations within the text (see examples below):

Citation:

Reliability has been established previously,[1,2-8,19]

Citation following a quote should include page numbers:

Jacobsen concluded that "the consequences of muscle strength . . ."[5(pp3,4)]

Reference list style for book:

1. Gregory CF, Chapman MW, Hanse ST Jr. Open fractures. In: Rockwood CA Jr, Green DP, eds. *Fractures.* Philadelphia: JB Lippincott Co; 1984: 169-218.
2. Yando R, Seitz U, Zigler E, et al. *Imitation: A Developmental Perspective.* New York: John Wiley & Sons; 1978.

Reference list style for journal (journal names should be abbreviated as shown):

3. Fielding JW, Hensinger RN, Hawkins RJ. Os Odontoideum. *J Bone Joint Surg Am.* 1980;62:376-383.

Reference list style for unpublished material:

4. Sieger M. The nature and limits of clinical medicine. In: Cassell EJ, Siegler M, eds.

Changing Values in Medicine. Chicago: University of Chicago Press. In press.

Reference list style for dissertation and thesis:

5. Raymand CA. Uncovering Ideology: Occupational Health in the Mainstream and Advocacy Press, 1970-1982. Ithaca, NY: Cornell University; 1983. Thesis.

Manuscripts should be created using Aspen's Journals Authoring Template (template is available from your journal editor or from Aspen). Manuscripts should be created on IBM-compatible (PC) equipment using Windows 95 or higher operating system. Our preferred software is Microsoft Word. Hard copy and electronic files should be submitted for all text and all artwork. All disks submitted must be new. Disks should be clearly labeled as to operating system and software application.

Manuscripts should be double-spaced (including quotations, lists, references, footnotes, figure captions, and all parts of tables).

Manuscripts should be ordered as follows: title page, abstracts, text, references, appendixes, tables, and any illustrations.

Each manuscript must include the following:

Title page, including (1) title of the article, (2) author names (with highest academic degrees) and affiliations (including titles, departments, and name and location of institutions of primary employment), and (3) any acknowledgments, credits, or disclaimers

Abstract of no more than 100 words and up to 10 key words that describe the contents of the article like those that appear in the *Cumulative Index to Nursing and Allied Health Literature (CINAHL)* or the *National Library of Medicine's Medical Subject Headings (MeSH)*

Clear indication of the placement of all tables and figures in text

Completed article submission form for each contributor

Written permission for any borrowed text, tables, or figures

References must be cited in text and styled in the reference list according to the *American Medical Association Manual of Style,* 9th ed. (1998), with the following exceptions: They must be numbered consecutively in the order they are cited; reference numbers may be used more than once throughout an article. Page numbers should appear with the text citation following a specific quote.

References should not be created using Microsoft Word's automatic footnote/endnote feature. References should be included on a separate page at the end of the article and should be double-spaced.

Illustrations: Figures should be created using electronic software (i.e., Adobe Illustrator, Corel Draw, and Photoshop). Please save files in both the application in which they were created (i.e., Microsoft Word) and as either EPS or TIFF files. Use computer-generated lettering. Do not use screens, color, shading, or fine lines.

In lieu of original drawings and other material, a sharp, glossy, black-and-white photographic print between 5″ × 7″ and 8″ × 10″ is acceptable.

Each figure should have a label on the back indicating the number of the figure, the names of the authors, and the top of the figure. Do not write on the back of figures, mount them on cardboard, or scratch or mar them using paper clips. Do not bend figures.

Cite each figure in the text in consecutive order. If a figure has been previously published, in part or in total, acknowledge the original source and submit written permission from the copyright holder to reproduce or adapt the material.

Supply a caption for each figure, typed double-spaced on a separate sheet from the artwork. Captions should include the figure title, explanatory statements, notes, or keys as well as source and permission lines.

Provide a camera-ready copy and a separate electronic file for each piece of artwork. Do not embed art in your text file.

Tables should be on a separate page at the end of the manuscript. Number tables consecutively and supply a brief title for each. Include explanatory footnotes for all nonstandard abbreviations. Cite each table in the text in consecutive order. If you use data from another published or unpublished source, obtain permission and acknowledge fully.

Permissions: Authors are responsible for obtaining signed letters from copyright holders granting permission to reprint material being borrowed or adapted from other sources, including previously published material of your own. Authors must obtain written permission for the following material (authors are responsible for any permission fees to reprint borrowed material):

All direct quotes of 300 words or more from any full-length book

All direct quotes of 200 words or more from a periodical article

All excerpts from a newspaper article or other short piece

Any passage from a play or a song

Two or more lines of poetry

Any borrowed table, figure, or illustration being reproduced exactly or adapted to fit the needs of the subject

REFEREED PUBLICATION

It is understood that articles are submitted solely to *ANS* and have not been published previously. Manuscripts should not contain identifying information, since the editorial review is anonymous. Authors should provide their name(s) and affiliation(s) on a cover sheet only. There are three stages of manuscript review prior to final publication of the article. They are as follows:

1. Editorial Board review to determine the scholarly merit of the article. All manuscripts are reviewed by three members of the editorial board. Members of the board evaluate manuscripts based on the following criteria: concise, logical ordering of ideas; sound argument and defense of original ideas; accuracy of content; adequacy of documentation; use of sound methods of research or other forms of scholarly investigation; and consistency with the purposes of the journal and the projected issue topic for which the article is intended.

Manuscripts are sent to the reviewers anonymously, with a form for recording their evaluation according to the criteria. The comments of each reviewer are returned to the editor.

2. Every effort is made to complete this stage of the review within 6 to 8 weeks after initiating the review. In this review, the editor makes a decision regarding the eligibility of the article for selection based on the comments and recommendations of the Editorial Board reviewers. The anonymous reviewers' comments and the editor's summary are returned to the first author. At least two reviewers must recommend the article for publication if the article is to be eligible for selection. Based on the editorial review, the editor makes one of the following decisions:

   a. Article is eligible for selection as submitted.

   b. Article is eligible for selection after completion of minor revisions as suggested by the reviewers and the editor.

   c. Article must be revised and resubmitted for review by the deadline date provided by the editor.

   d. Article rejected based on the reviewers' evaluation.

3. Selection of articles for publication. Because *Advances in Nursing Science* is a topical journal, final selection of articles for each issue is made approximately 4 months prior to publication of each issue. Selection of articles is made from those articles that have been determined to be eligible for publication based on the results of the first two stages of the review process. This review is made by the editor and the editorial staff at Aspen. The selection is based on the following criteria: (a) strength of the reviewers' comments and recommendations for publication; (b) congruence of the content of the article with the projected issue topics; (c) overall balance in the type of articles selected for inclusion; that is, an attempt is made to include a balance of theory-related and research articles; and (d) space available for inclusion in the projected issue.

The first author of each article that is eligible for selection is notified by the editor of the status of the article for publication approximately 4 months prior to the projected publication date. If an article has been determined to be eligible for selection but is not selected, the rights of the article revert to the author(s). Unless the article is considered to be of exceptional merit by the reviewers and the editor, it cannot be held for future publication in *Advances in Nursing Science.*

Articles that are selected for publication are edited by the associate editor at Aspen and sent to type. Galley proofs will be sent to the author for review and approval.

COPYRIGHT

Copyright by Aspen Publishers, Inc.

INDEXED

Advances in Nursing Science is indexed in *Behavioral Medicine Abstracts, Cumulative Index to Nursing and Allied Health Literature, Current Contents, Index Medicus, International Nursing Index, Inventory of Marriage and Family Literature, Nursing Abstracts, Psychiatric Journal Review, PsycINFO, Psychological Abstracts,* and *Social Sciences Citation Index.*

SAMPLE JOURNAL ARTICLE TITLES

- "A Concept Analysis on the Process of Empowerment"
- "A Model for Describing Low-Income African American Women's Participation in Breast and Cervical Cancer Early Detection and Screening"
- "Conformity With Nature: A Theory of Chinese American Elders' Health Promotion and Illness Prevention Processes"
- "Culturally Competent Scholarship: Substance and Rigor"
- "Sources of Stigma Associated With Women With HIV"

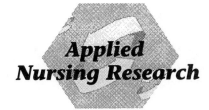

Applied Nursing Research

Applied *Nursing Research* is published by W. B. Saunders Company.

JOURNAL FOCUS/PURPOSE

The primary purpose of *Applied Nursing Research* is to unite the efforts of all professional nurses to advance nursing as a research-based profession. *Applied Nursing Research* will present nursing research in a clear, straightforward style to emphasize results and encourage readers to apply findings in their own practice. Our efforts are focused on bridging the gap between research and practice.

JOURNAL FACTS

Publication schedule: quarterly

Circulation: not available

Submitted papers per year: not available

Acceptance rate: approximately 20%

Monetary honorarium: none

Average turnaround time: 3 months

Publishing timetable: approximately 1 year after acceptance

Correspondence:
W. B. Saunders
The Curtis Center
Independence Square West
Philadelphia, PA 19106-3399
Telephone: (215) 238-7800 or 1-800-545-2522

Internet site: www.wbsaunders.com

MANUSCRIPT SUBMISSION

A query letter or fax before manuscript submission is welcome but not mandatory. Please send query to the journal editor.

Send five copies of the submitted manuscript to:

Joyce J. Fitzpatrick, PhD, FAAN
Editor, *Applied Nursing Research*
New York University, Division of Nursing
429 Shimkin Hall
50 West 4th Street
New York, NY 10012-1165
Telephone: (212) 998-5798
Fax: (212) 995-4679

Authors should submit a cover letter explicitly stating the section of the journal for which the manuscript is being submitted. Also, please include, with the submitted manuscript, any publication where the same content or data set has been used, and summarize in your cover letter how this submitted manuscript is different. If there are no other publications, please state this in your letter. Manuscripts that do not comply with the format and submission guidelines will be returned to the authors without being reviewed. Direct editorial questions to Joyce J. Fitzpatrick at the above address. The review decision is sent to the first author or the designated corresponding author. Edited manuscripts are submitted to the first author for approval.

Manuscripts are accepted for publication on the conditions that they are submitted solely to this journal, that the material is original, and that it has not been previously published.

Galley proofs are sent to the first author. They are to be checked for errors and returned to the publisher within 48 hours. Important changes in data will be accepted, but authors will be charged for excessive alterations in proofs.

MANUSCRIPT PREPARATION GUIDELINES

Authors are asked to focus on research findings and how those findings can be applied to practice. The manuscript should convey the author's enthusiasm for the specific advances in clinical practice indicated by the research. In the manuscript, clearly articulate the research purpose(s) and/or questions. Include a brief description of the study background, including rationale for the research. Provide a summary of the study methods (e.g., design, sample, instrumentation, and procedures). Authors are asked to present material in a framework and style that highlight and explain results and emphasize applications for nursing practice. Key references are to be included—limited to 15, please. Figures, photographs, and illustrations are welcome.

Manuscripts representing all clinical nursing specialties are invited. Studies related to nursing management, nursing roles, and professional development are also welcome.

Original article submissions are reviewed by two pairs of research-clinician referees. Publication decisions are based on the referees' evaluation. Authors of original and feature articles receive complimentary copies of the journal issue in which their articles appear. All complimentary copies are sent to the first-named author for distribution to coauthors.

In Clinical Methods, issues related to and effective techniques for conducting studies within clinical settings are presented. Papers selected for publication address methodological issues or techniques that are of concern to nurses conducting clinical research. Clinical Methods articles are reviewed by two researcher-clinician teams. Figures/illustrations and photographs are encouraged.

Abstracts of research in progress or completed pilot research are invited. The emphasis should be on preliminary results and directions for continuing research.

Special features have been designed to promote a communication loop and foster interchange among nurses. Papers on timely issues or topics related to the "state of nursing research" are desired. Special features are peer-reviewed.

The feature, Ask an Expert, provides practicing nurses with an opportunity to ask questions or seek advice from expert nurse researchers. Please submit questions regarding clinical research issues to the journal editor. Responses to selected questions will be published.

All manuscripts must be submitted in typed, double-spaced form with pages numbered. On the cover sheet of the original, include the title of the manuscript and names, complete addresses, and telephone numbers (i.e., work, home, and fax) of all authors. Also, provide the complete credentials and clinical and/or academic affiliation of all authors, and any acknowledgments on the cover page of the original. On the additional four copies, provide only the title of the manuscript on the cover sheet. Author(s) identification should not appear elsewhere.

With the original typed manuscripts, submit a matching electronic file, preferably in Word or WordPerfect, on a $3\frac{1}{2}$-inch disk formatted for the PC. A matching electronic file should also accompany any revised manuscripts. Manuscripts for Original Articles or Special Features should be no less than 10 and no more than 15 double-spaced typewritten pages, excluding tables, illustrations/figures, and references (generally limited to 15). A brief abstract, no more than 100 words, should emphasize the findings and clinical implications. Authors may wish to suggest appropriate callouts, that is, phrases or brief sentences extracted from the manuscript that highlight key points. Callouts should be listed on a separate sheet.

Papers submitted for publication in the Clinical Methods section should be 8 to 12 double-spaced, typewritten pages, including tables, illustrations/figures, and key references. Research Briefs should be 5 to 7 double-spaced, typewritten pages with key references included.

For submissions to all sections, guidelines in the *Publication Manual of the American Psychological Association* (4th ed.) should be used for manuscript format (e.g., short title on each page, style and inclusion of tables, statistics reporting, and references). Drawings or illustrations must be submitted as camera-ready art; photographs must be black and white and of a quality that can be clearly reproduced.

Journal article in a journal with continuous pagination:

Troy, N.W. (1993). Early contact and maternal attachment among women using public health care facilities. *Applied Nursing Research, 6,* 161-166.

Journal article in a journal paginated by issue:

Wimpsett, J. (1994). Nursing case management: Outcomes in a rural environment. *Nursing Management, 25*(11), 41-43.

Complete book:

Burns, N., & Grove, S. (1994). *The practice of nursing research: Conduct, critique, & utilization* (2nd ed.). Philadelphia: Saunders.

Chapter in a book:

Morris, D. L., & Wykle, M.L. (1994). Minorities in nursing. In J.J. Fitzpatrick & J.S. Stevenson (Eds.), *Annual review of nursing research* (pp. 175-189). New York: Springer Publishing.

Illustrations, black-and-white photographs, diagrams, and graphs are highly recommended to illustrate findings and emphasize clinical applications. Photographs are to be 5 × 8-inch glossies. Photographs of recognizable individuals must be accompanied by releases signed by each person appearing in the photograph. Guardians must sign for minors. Photographs of clinical actions are preferred.

Diagrams, graphs, and line drawings must be professionally rendered and submitted as camera-ready art. Laser-printed graphics that have been computer-generated are acceptable. Please call the production editor at (215) 238-5633 if you have questions regarding illustrations.

If any table, photograph, or illustration has been published previously, a copy of the letter or permission from the copyright holder must accompany the manuscript. The source should be included among the references to the paper. The table or illustration legend should conclude with the "Reprinted with permission" information. See the *Publication Manual of the American Psychological Association* (4th ed.) for the specific format.

A sidebar is a brief, boxed segment of text that appears within an original article. It can be used to present a case study, report the author's experience related to the topic of the study, or discuss similar experiences in other settings. Recommendations for further research, policy implications, or "consumer highlights" (e.g., what would be of interest regarding your research to health care consumers?) can be submitted as a sidebar. Sidebars should be typed, double-spaced, on a separate sheet of paper with the heading "Sidebar" and the article title appearing at the top of each page. Generally, a sidebar is no more than two pages, and only one sidebar should be submitted with each article.

REFEREED PUBLICATION

Applied Nursing Research is a refereed research journal.

COPYRIGHT

Copyright by W. B. Saunders Company.

INDEXED

Applied Nursing Research is indexed in the *Cumulative Index to Nursing and Allied Health Literature, Index Medicus, MEDLARS,* and *RNdex Top 100.*

SAMPLE JOURNAL ARTICLE TITLES

- "Home Care Nurses' Inferences and Decisions"
- "Impact of Liver Transplantation on Quality of Life: A Longitudinal Perspective"
- "Postural Control and Strength and Mood Among Older Adults"
- "Research Utilization: Development of a Central Venous Catheter Procedure"
- "Suicidal Adolescent Perceptions After an Art Future Image Intervention"

Journal of Nursing Scholarship

The *Journal of Nursing Scholarship* is published by Center Press and is the official journal of Sigma Theta Tau International, Honor Society of Nursing, Inc.

JOURNAL FOCUS/PURPOSE

The *Journal of Nursing Scholarship* is intended to provide a forum for the publication of superior nursing thought in the general areas of clinical scholarship and policy. Research reports, reviews of literature, and discursive pieces are desired.

JOURNAL FACTS

Publication schedule: quarterly

Circulation: 120,000

Submitted papers per year: 300

Acceptance rate: 15-20%

Monetary honorarium: none

Average turnaround time: 2-3 months

Publishing timetable: 6-12 months after acceptance

Correspondence:
Business Office
Sigma Theta Tau International Honor Society
550 W. North Street
Indianapolis, IN 46202

For general information:
Toll free (U.S. and Canada): 1-888-634-7575
Toll free (outside U.S. and Canada): 1-800-634-7575-1
Fax: (317) 634-8188
E-mail: melody@stti.iupui.edu or
tjns@u.washington.edu

Internet site: www.nursingsociety.org

MANUSCRIPT SUBMISSION

Manuscripts are voluntary contributions submitted for the exclusive attention of the *Journal of Nursing Scholarship.* Authors submitting manuscripts agree to use e-mail and the Internet whenever possible for all communications about manuscripts.

A diskette and four copies of the manuscript should be sent to:

Journal of Nursing Scholarship
c/o Sigma Theta Tau International
550 W. North Street
Indianapolis, IN 46202
E-mail: melody@stti.iupui.edu

Manuscripts containing original material are accepted for consideration if neither the article nor any part of its essential substance, tables, or figures has been or will be published or submitted elsewhere before appearing in the journal. This restriction does not apply to abstracts or press reports published in connection with scientific meetings.

MANUSCRIPT PREPARATION GUIDELINES

A structured abstract with headings should accompany all full articles. Abstract headings for research articles are purpose (include background and significance), design (include population, sample, setting, years), methods (include intervention, measures), findings (or results), and conclusions (include implications). Abstract headings for review or theoretical articles are purpose (include background and significance), organizing construct (include scope), sources, methods (include source, data extraction, and validation), findings, and conclusions (include implications).

Manuscripts (including abstract) on diskette should be submitted as a text file only—for example, ASCII text or DOS text. Hard copies of manuscript (including abstracts) should be in 12-point type, printed on a letter-quality printer, double-spaced, with reasonably wide margins. Fancy typefaces, italics, and underlines are not in order. Manuscripts should not exceed 20 pages, including references, tables, and figures. Line drawings and illustrations should be camera-ready. The author is responsible for compliance with APA format and for the accuracy of all information, including citations and verification of all references with citations in the text. Spelling may be either American or British English.

A face sheet for the manuscript (electronic and print) should state the title of the manuscript, disk file name, keywords, author(s) name(s), mailing address(es), and e-mail address(es) in APA format. Indicate which author should receive correspondence. Also include a running head of fewer than 40 letter spaces. Authors' names should not appear in headers. Identification will be removed before manuscripts are assigned for peer review.

Material taken from other sources must be accompanied by a written statement from both first author and publisher giving permission to the journal for reproduction.

The *Publication Manual of the American Psychological Association* (4th ed.) provides the format for references, headings, and all other matters. Titles should be short and should not require a colon or any punctuation. Addendums and appendices are not accepted. Tables should be typed one to a page and relative placement of tables noted in text. All tables and figures should follow the reference list.

Abstracts of about 400-500 words require APA format without headings. Abstracts of an empirical research study should describe the problem and significance; design and methods; sample, procedure, and years of data collection; validity and findings; conclusions and implications. Abstracts for a review or theoretical study should describe the topic; purpose and significance; organizing construct and scope; sources, methods for data extractions, validity; conclusions and implications.

Documentation of all references is required—for example, by photocopy of the first page of the work with citation or photocopy of electronic citation. The journal reserves the right to edit all manuscript to its style and space requirements. Authors will receive proofs for approval. Authors are responsible for checking the accuracy of material as it appears in the edited copy. References must be verified by the author(s) against the original source document.

REFEREED PUBLICATION

Letters of inquiry to the editor are welcomed but not required. Manuscripts are ex-amined by the editorial staff and are sent for double-blind peer review. Decisions for publication are made on the basis of reviews usually within 3 months. Manuscripts are not returned to the authors.

COPYRIGHT

Upon acceptance for publication, authors will be asked to provide a biographical sketch and grant permission to publish, assigning copyright to Sigma Theta Tau International.

INDEXED

Journal of Nursing Scholarship is indexed in the *Cumulative Index to Nursing and Allied Health Literature, Nursing Abstracts, Psychological Abstracts, International Nursing Index,* and *RNdex Top 100.*

SAMPLE JOURNAL ARTICLE TITLES

- "Classifying Nursing-Sensitive Patient Outcomes"
- "Collaborative Research by Graduate Students"
- "Life-Span Perspective of Personality in Dementia"
- "Nursing Practice Theory of Exercise as Self-Care"
- "Toward a Model for Nursing Informatics"

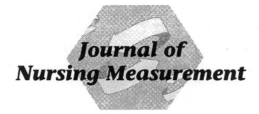

Journal of Nursing Measurement

Journal of Nursing Measurement is published by Springer Publishing Company.

JOURNAL FOCUS/PURPOSE

The primary purpose of the *Journal of Nursing Measurement* is to serve as a forum for the dissemination of information regarding instruments, tools, approaches, or procedures developed or utilized for the measurement of variables for nursing practice, education, and research.

JOURNAL FACTS

Publication schedule: twice a year

Circulation: not sure

Submitted papers per year: 60

Acceptance rate: 12%

Monetary honorarium: none

Average turnaround time: 6 months

Publishing timetable: 3 to 4 months after acceptance

Correspondence:
Springer Publishing Company
536 Broadway
New York, NY 10012-9904
Telephone: (212) 431-4370
Fax: (212) 941-7842
E-mail: contactus@springerjournals.com or editorial@springerpub.com

Internet site: www.springerpub.com

MANUSCRIPT SUBMISSION

The *Journal of Nursing Measurement* invites manuscripts directed to the interest of nurse clinicians, educators, and researchers. Particularly welcome are manuscripts of studies on the development and testing of nursing measures, and evidence for the reliability and validity or sensitivity and testing of nursing measures, and evidence for the reliability and validity or sensitivity and specificity of such instruments. Innovative discussions of theories, principles, practices, and issues relevant to nursing measurement are invited as well. Letters and comments on published articles are welcome.

Manuscripts will be acknowledged on receipt. Following preliminary review by the editors, they will be sent to members of the Editorial Board.

Submit manuscripts to:
Ora L. Strickland, PhD, RN, FAAN
Editor, *Journal of Nursing Measurement*
Nell Hodgson Woodruff School of Nursing,
   Emory University
Atlanta, GA 30322
Telephone: (404) 727-7941
Fax: (404) 727-0536

Authors should submit the original and three copies of manuscripts professionally prepared in accordance with the *Publication Manual of the American Psychological Association,* 4th ed. (1994). A copy of the instrument(s) may be included in an appendix. Instruments will be published at the discretion of the editors.

MANUSCRIPT PREPARATION GUIDELINES

The following are guidelines for developing and submitting a manuscript. Manuscripts that do not conform to these guidelines will be returned to the author without review.

Include an abstract of approximately 125 words. Letters to the editors should be under 300 words. Those accepted for publication may be edited or abridged.

The original manuscript should be typed on 8.5 × 11-inch nontranslucent white paper. Do not use onionskin or erasable bond. Double-space everything, including references, quotations, tables, and figures. Leave generous margins (at least 1 inch all around) on each page. Type cannot exceed 18 characters per inch.

Avoid footnotes whenever possible. Place authors' names, positions, titles, place of employment, and mailing addresses on the cover pages so that the manuscripts may be reviewed anonymously. Upon acceptance, computer disks should be mailed to the editor.

Authors bear full responsibility for the accuracy of references, quotations, tables, and figures. Quotations of 300 words or more from one source require written permission from the copyright holder for reproduction. Adaptation of tables and figures also requires reproduction approval from the copyrighted source. It is the author's responsibility to secure such permission, and a copy of the publishers' written permission must be provided to the journal editors immediately upon acceptance of the manuscript for publication.

REFEREED PUBLICATION

The *Journal of Nursing Measurement* is a refereed journal. Articles will be reviewed by members of the Editorial Review Board, comprised of measurement experts with backgrounds in a variety of clinical and functional areas. Each manuscript will be reviewed by at least two experts on the topic. On publication, each author will receive a copy of the journal in which his or her manuscript appears.

COPYRIGHT

INDEXED

The *Journal of Nursing Measurement* is indexed/abstracted in *AgeLine, CINAHL, Index Medicus, MEDLINE, International Nursing Index, Psychological Abstracts, PsycINFO & PsycLIT, RNdex Top 100, Social Planning/Policy & Development Abstracts,* and *Sociological Abstracts.*

SAMPLE JOURNAL ARTICLE TITLES

- "Adequacy of Two Organizing Principles for the Classification of Lay Caregiving Decisions"
- "Development and Psychometric Evaluation of an Instrument to Measure Staff Nurses' Perception of Uncertainty in the Hospital Environment"
- "Measuring Expectations for Participative Decision Making Among Graduating Nurses"
- "Nursing Students' Evaluation of Classroom Teaching: Developing and Testing an Instrument"
- "The Index of Self-Regulation: Development and Psychometric Analysis"

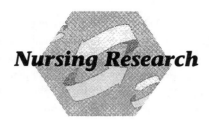

Nursing Research

Nursing Research is published by Lippincott Williams & Wilkins.

Telephone: (301) 714-2300
Fax: (301) 714-2398
Customer service: 1-800-638-3030
Internet site: www.nursingcenter.com/journals

JOURNAL FOCUS/PURPOSE

The primary purposes of *Nursing Research* are to (a) report research, both completed and that which is in progress, that contributes to the knowledge base of the discipline of nursing and that provides a better understanding of human responses to illness and the promotion of health; (b) serve an educational function through presenting reports and critiques of methodology and research design; and (c) serve as a medium for the stimulation for ideas and exchange of information about nursing research and practice.

JOURNAL FACTS

Publication schedule: bimonthly

Circulation: 12,400

Submitted papers per year: approximately 200-250

Acceptance rate: approximately 40%

Monetary honorarium: none

Average turnaround time: 4-6 weeks

Publishing timetable: approximately 6-12 months after acceptance

Correspondence:
Lippincott Williams & Wilkins
Business Offices
227 East Washington Square
Philadelphia, PA 19106-3780
Telephone: (215) 238-4200

Or
12107 Insurance Way
Hagerstown, MD 21740

MANUSCRIPT SUBMISSION

The editor of *Nursing Research* welcomes manuscripts of relevance and interest to those concerned with the conduct of results of research in nursing.

Manuscripts should be sent to:
Molly C. Dougherty, PhD, RN, FAAN
Editor, *Nursing Research*
School of Nursing, CB# 7460 Carrington Hall
University of North Carolina
Chapel Hill, NC 27599-7460
Telephone: (919) 966-9415
Fax: (919) 966-9736
E-mail: m_dougherty@unc.edu

Submit four paper copies and a disk copy of the manuscript. It should not be possible for reviewers to identify authors from the manuscript. It is advisable to precede submission with a letter of inquiry to the editor, describing the article. It is understood that submitted manuscripts are prepared specifically and solely for *Nursing Research.* Accepted manuscripts become the property of *Nursing Research* and may be reproduced in other publications in whole or in part only with the permission of *Nursing Research. Nursing Research* has exclusive rights to the article and to its reproduction and sale in all countries.

Nursing Research reserves the right to edit all manuscripts to its style and space requirements, and to clarify the presentation. Declined manuscripts are not returned; therefore, authors should retain at least one copy. *Nursing Research* reserves the right to edit all manuscripts to its style and space requirements and to clarify the presentation. Before publication, proofs of edited copy are submitted to the corresponding author who is responsible for checking the accuracy of the material. Authors will receive tear sheets of the article and may order reprints with order forms sent with proofs.

MANUSCRIPT PREPARATION GUIDELINES

Full-length manuscripts are limited to 14-16 typewritten pages; Brief Reports and Methodology are limited to 8 pages. These limits do not include the abstract, references, tables, or figures. Prepare manuscripts according to the *Publication Manual of the American Psychological Association* (4th ed.) unless otherwise indicated in the section below on organization of the manuscript. Do not attempt to prepare manuscripts as they appear in the journal.

Double-space manuscripts—including abstract, text, references, and tables—with 1-inch margins on all sides. Use a 12-point font. Do not justify the text.

Nursing Research is concerned with the protection of the rights and dignity of all subjects involved in research. An explicit statement should be made in the manuscript or cover letter affirming the status of human or animal subjects institutional review.

If aspects of the research are reported elsewhere, include a copy of the publication(s).

Include all material in one computer file (do not separate the abstract, tables, figures). Save your file as MS Word or WordPerfect for Windows (any version up to 1998) or in rich text format. Put your disk in a cardboard disk mailer, or it will be destroyed by the mail system.

If you would like to include your e-mail address for communication with readers or URLs of relevant Websites with your printed article, please indicate those on your cover page.

Organize the manuscript in the following order: title page, acknowledgments, abstract, text, references, tables, figure legends, and figures. Do not use addenda or appendices.

- Title page: Include job titles, professional letters, and institutions for each author. Indicate an e-mail address for the corresponding author.
- Acknowledgments: Limit acknowledgments to key contributors.
- Abstract: Prepare a structured abstract with the following sections (include these headings). The abstract should be less than one double-spaced page, with no citations.
  Background: Summarize the literature review in one sentence, demonstrating the need for this study.
  Objectives: Clearly state the main question or hypothesis of this study in one sentence.
  Method: Describe the study design, participants, and measurements used in 3-4 sentences.
  Results: Describe the main results in a concise paragraph. This section should be the most descriptive. Note levels of statistical significance and confidence intervals where appropriate.
  Conclusion(s): Make conclusions based only on the reported results. Describe any further study needed.
  Key words: The indexers use MeSH® guidelines to index articles. Provide 2-3 key words; be very specific in your word choice. Use MeSH® key words when possible.
- Text: No more than 4 citations should be used to support a single idea. Avoid citation of personal communications or unpublished material.
- References: Verify all information included in references carefully; it is essential that readers be able to look up the cited material.
- Tables/figures: Tables and figures are printed only when they express more than can be done by words in the same amount of space. Do not indicate placement of tables or figures in the text—the copy editor will automatically place your tables and figures.

- Figure legends: These should be on one separate page before the figures (not on the same page as the figures).

REFEREED PUBLICATION

Manuscripts are reviewed anonymously by members of an expert panel. The decision with regard to publication is based on the reviews. Authors should not identify themselves or their institutions in the manuscript other than on the title page, which is removed before review.

COPYRIGHT

Copyright by Lippincott Williams & Wilkins. You are free to quote up to 500 words, with credit to *Nursing Research,* except articles bearing the copyright of others, without further permission form *Nursing Research.* We ask that when you quote, you send us a copy of your publication.

INDEXED

Nursing Research is indexed in *Cumulative Index to Nursing and Allied Health Literature, MEDLINE, HealthStar,* and *PsycINFO.*

SAMPLE JOURNAL ARTICLE TITLES

- "Avoiding Common Mistakes in APA Style: The Briefest of Guidelines"
- "Cooling Effects and Comfort of Four Cooling Blanket Temperatures in Humans With Fever"
- "Physiological Responses of Preterm Infants to Breast-Feeding and Bottle-Feeding With the Orthodontic Nipple"
- "Using the SAS System to Perform Discriminant Analysis of Type A/B Behavior"
- "Verification Bias: A Pitfall in Evaluating Screening Tests"

Nursing Science Quarterly

Nursing Science Quarterly is published by Sage Publications, Inc.

tive research related to existing nursing frameworks.

JOURNAL FOCUS/PURPOSE

The primary purpose of *Nursing Science Quarterly* is the enhancement of nursing knowledge. The major purpose of the journal is to publish original manuscripts focusing on nursing theory development, nursing theory-guided practice, and quantitative and qualita-

JOURNAL FACTS

Publication schedule: quarterly

Circulation: 3,000-4,000

Submitted papers per year: 50 plus

Acceptance rate: 30%

Monetary honorarium: none

Average turnaround time: 2 months

Publishing timetable: 6-12 months after acceptance

Correspondence:

    Sage Publications, Inc.
    2455 Teller Road
    Thousand Oaks, CA 91320
    Telephone: (805) 499-0721
    Fax: (805) 499-0871

Internet site: www.sagepub.com

MANUSCRIPT SUBMISSION

Manuscripts are accepted for exclusive publication in *Nursing Science Quarterly*. The editor reserves the right to accept or reject all submitted manuscripts. Accepted manuscripts become the property of Sage Publications and may be reproduced in other publications in whole or in part only with permission from the editor and publisher. Upon acceptance of a manuscript, it will be necessary for the editorial office to receive in writing the assignment of copyright from all authors of the manuscript. Manuscripts that are rejected will not be returned.

The manuscript must be written clearly, presented logically, and must not have been published previously or concurrently in another journal, nor be under simultaneous consideration. *Nursing Science Quarterly* reserves the right to edit all manuscripts for clarity and conformation to its style and space requirements. Edited copy will be submitted to authors for approval. Authors are responsible for checking the accuracy of the copy as it appears in the edited version. Authors may be billed for extensive alterations in the page proofs. Accepted manuscripts must be submitted on a 3½″ disk in IBM Microsoft Word or in ASCII/Text Only format. Make sure hard copy is printed before the document is converted to ASCII. Identify format and software on the disk label.

Submit to:

Rosemarie Rizzo Parse, RN, PhD, FAAN
Editor, *Nursing Science Quarterly*
320 Fort Duquesne Boulevard, Suite 25J
Pittsburgh, PA 15222
Telephone: (412) 391-8471
Fax: (412) 391-8458
E-mail: rparse@orion.it.luc.edu

MANUSCRIPT PREPARATION GUIDELINES

Authors should submit four double-spaced copies of the original manuscript on 8½ × 11-inch paper, with 1-inch margins. Right margins should not be justified. Use 12-point Times Roman font exclusively. Include separate double-spaced pages for title page, tables, and legends for figures. Type page numbers consecutively in the top right-hand corner of each page, beginning with the abstract and text. We do not accept for review manuscripts that exceed 25 pages. On a separate page, the author should sign a statement as follows:

> The author guarantees that neither all nor part of this manuscript has been published elsewhere in its present form, in another publication or under a different title by either this author(s) or another author(s). It is also acknowledged that this manuscript is not currently under review by any other publication.

Do not send a computer disk. Further instructions will be sent at the time of tentative acceptance.

All manuscripts should contain the following sections in the order listed.

Identification Page. List for all authors: name, address, office and home phone, fax number, and e-mail address. Identify corresponding author and preferred mailing address.

Title Page. Include a brief informative title of no more than two lines and running title of three or four words. Include the first name, middle initial, and last name of each author with highest academic degree and FAAN (if application), position/title, and institutional affiliation. List three or four keywords for indexing purposes. Acknowledgments should be limited to institutions supplying grants.

Abstract. Include an abstract of no more than 100 words that includes the central theme of the paper. An abstract for a research paper should include the general purpose, methodology, results, and conclusions of the study. The abstract should not contain abbreviations, acronyms, or references.

Text. Articles about nursing theory and theory development should include a brief introduction followed by the body of the article. Subheadings should be used to divide areas of the article. Articles on practice should include assumptions, propositions, or concepts from a nursing perspective, with detailed examples of how theory is used in practice. Subheadings should be used to divide areas of the article. Articles reporting findings of quantitative and qualitative nursing research should include a brief introduction, the research question, frame of reference, brief review of literature, methodology, findings, and conclusions of the study as related to theory development, further research, and practice.

Use of Tables and Figures. Tables and figures are used only when they express more clearly and briefly than can be done by words in the same amount of space. All tables and figures should be referred to in the text but should be largely self-explanatory and should not duplicate the text.

Tables. Type each table, double-spaced, on a separate sheet of $8\frac{1}{2} \times 11$-inch paper. Number tables consecutively, supply a brief descrip-

tive title for each, and indicate the source of the data. Any inconsistencies in marginal totals or other figures should be explained in a table footnote. Charts and tables should be complete.

Figures. Figures should be professionally drawn and photographed; free-hand or typewritten lettering is unacceptable. Send sharp, glossy black-and-white prints (unmounted) no larger than 8×10 inches. High-quality, computer-generated, laser-printed figures are also acceptable. The name(s) of the author(s) and figure number should be written lightly on a label on the back of each figure to avoid impressions onto the front that cannot be eliminated by the printer. Indicate "top" with an arrow on the back of each figure. On a separate page, type the legend for each figure.

Permission to Reprint. If the manuscript contains direct use of previously published material, signed permission of the author and publisher of such works must be submitted with the manuscript.

Style and Format. Authors should follow the *Publication Manual of the American Psychological Association* (4th ed.).

Acronyms and Special Symbols. A term should be spelled out the first time it is used, followed by the acronym in parentheses. Greek letters or other special symbols should be identified the first time they are used. (This does not apply to the standard symbols used in statistical tests.) Addenda and appendixes are not used.

Footnotes and References. Incidental comments and qualifications should be worked into the text and not included as footnotes. Personal communications should not be included in the references: list in parentheses in the text with the date and communicator's name. References should be limited to those directly pertinent to the paper and be listed at the end of the paper according to APA format. For example:

Journal article, two authors:

> Spetch, M. L., & Wilkie, D. M. (1983). Subjective shortening: A model of pigeons' memory for event duration. *Journal of Experimental Psychology: Animal Behavior Processes, 9,* 14-30.

Chapter in a book:

> Hartley, J. T., Harker, J. O., & Walsh, D. A. (1980). Contemporary issues and new directions in adult development of learning and memory. In L. W. Poon (Ed.), *Aging in the 1980s: Psychological issues* (pp. 239-252). Washington, DC: American Psychological Association.

Complete book:

> Strunk, W., & White, E. B. (1972). *The elements of style.* New York: Macmillan.

Edited book:

> Bernstein, T. M. (Ed.). (1965). *The careful writer: A modern guide to English usage.* New York: Atheneum.

REFEREED PUBLICATION

Nursing Science Quarterly is a peer-reviewed journal. All submitted manuscripts are subject to review by the editor and are then forwarded to a minimum of two anonymous reviewers for blind review.

COPYRIGHT

Copyright by Sage Publications, Inc.

INDEXED

Nursing Science Quarterly is indexed in the *Cumulative Index to Nursing and Allied Health Literature, International Nursing Index,* and *Nursing Abstracts.*

SAMPLE JOURNAL ARTICLE TITLES

- "Clarifying Contributions of Qualitative Research Findings"
- "Feeling Uncomfortable: Children in Families With No Place for Their Own"
- "Mexican American Family Processes: Nurturing, Support, and Socialization"
- "The Philosophical Core of King's Conceptual System"
- "The Meaning of Alcohol to Traditional Muscogee Creek Indians"

Research in Nursing and Health

Research in Nursing and Health is published by John Wiley & Sons, Inc.

JOURNAL FOCUS/PURPOSE

The primary purpose of *Research in Nursing and Health* is to publish a wide range of research and theory that will inform the practice of nursing and other health disciplines.

JOURNAL FACTS

Publication schedule: bimonthly

Circulation: unavailable

Submitted papers per year: approximately 180-200

Acceptance rate: approximately 25%

Monetary honorarium: none

Average turnaround time: 3 months

Publishing timetable: 6-9 months after acceptance

Correspondence:
John Wiley & Sons, Inc.
605 Third Avenue
New York, NY, 10158-0012

Internet site: www.interscience.wiley.com/jpages/0160-6891/info.html

MANUSCRIPT SUBMISSION

The editors invite research reports on nursing practice, education, administration, and history, on health issues relevant to nursing, and on the testing of research findings in practice. Papers on research methods and techniques are appropriate if they go beyond what is already generally available in the literature. Theory papers are accepted if knowledge is advanced; preference is given to papers in which theory is developed rather than simply reviewed. Integrative reviews of the literature are accepted if gaps in knowledge are identified and directions for future research provided. Critical reviews of new books and other publications on research and theory may be included. Letters to the editor commenting on published articles or research and theory issues are welcome.

Authors are urged to seek colleague peer review prior to submission of manuscripts.

Submit an original and three additional copies of the complete manuscript (including title page, abstract, and all tables and figures) to:

Madeline Schmitt, RN, PhD, FAAN
Editor, *Research in Nursing and Health*
School of Nursing, University of Rochester
601 Elmwood Avenue, Box SON
Rochester, NY 14642
Telephone: (716) 275-6946
E-mail: mads@son.rochester.edu

Submission should be accompanied by a cover letter (see APA *Publication Manual* for guidelines); a signed publication agreement; and, if appropriate, permissions to use copyrighted material. Related previous publications also should be included. Authors will receive notification of the receipt of the manuscript within a few weeks of submission.

MANUSCRIPT PREPARATION GUIDELINES

Papers must adhere to the style and format described in the *Publication Manual of the American Psychological Association,* 4th ed. (1994), in all respects except the title page. The title page should contain the following information: article title; name, degrees, title, and institutional affiliation of all authors; telephone number for corresponding author; acknowledgment of financial and other support; key words; running head; and address for reprint requests.

The general text format for empirical studies, review articles, and theory articles is outlined in the APA *Publication Manual.* This format must be adapted for reports of historical research and those employing qualitative methods. Guidelines for reporting qualitative research may be found in Knafl and Howard (1984) (*Research in Nursing and Health, 7,* 17-24). Authors also should review back issues of the journal for samples of the style used in various types of articles.

Manuscript length will vary with the type of article. In general, the text (exclusive of title page, abstract, references, tables, and figures) should be no more than 15-18 pages.

Manuscripts should be printed in letter-quality type, double-spaced, on $8\frac{1}{2} \times 11$-inch paper, using a 12-point typeface. Figures (graphs, charts, illustrations, and halftones) should be professionally prepared or computer generated with a good-quality laser printer (glossy photographs also are acceptable). All figures should be submitted in camera-ready form. Color illustrations may be submitted to the journal. Authors are asked to bear the cost of printing the color illustrations. Charges for reproducing the art will be approved by the contributor before processing. Color proofs will be sent to the contributor for approval prior to printing.

A final version of your accepted manuscript should be submitted on diskette as well as hard copy, using the guidelines for Diskette Submission Instructions form usually included in most issues of the journal.

The journal strongly encourages authors to deliver the final, revised version of their accepted manuscripts (text, tables, and, if possible, illustrations) on disk. Given the near-universal use of computer word processing for manuscript preparation, we anticipate that providing a disk will be convenient for you, and it carries the added advantages of maintaining the integrity of your keystrokes and expediting typesetting. Please return the disk submission slip below with your manuscript and labeled disk(s).

- File names: Submit the text and tables of each manuscript as a single file. Name each file with your last name (up to eight letters). Text files should be given the three-letter extension that identifies the file format. Macintosh users should maintain the MS-DOS "eight dot three" file-naming convention.

- Labels: Label all disks with your name, the file name, and the word processing program and version used.

- Illustrations: All print reproduction requires file for full color images to be in a CMYK color space. If possible, ICC or ColorSyne profiles of your output device should accompany all digital image submissions.

- Storage medium: Submit as separate files from text files, on separate disks or cartridges. If feasible, full color file should be submitted on separate disks from other images files, $3\frac{1}{2}''$ high-density disks, CD, Iomega Zip, and $5\frac{1}{4}''$ 44- or 88-MB SyQuest cartridges can be submitted. At authors' request, cartridges and disks will be returned after publication.

- Software and format: All illustration files should be in TIFF or EPS (with preview) formats. Do not submit native application formats.

- Resolution: Journal quality reproduction will require gray scale and color files at resolutions yielding approximately 300 DPI. Bitmapped line art should be submitted at resolutions yielding 600-1,200 DPI. These resolutions refer to the output size of the file; if you anticipate that your images will be enlarged or reduced, resolutions should be adjusted accordingly.

- File names: Illustration files should be given the 2- or 3-letter extension that identifies the file format used (i.e., .tif, .eps).

- Labels: Label all disks and cartridges with your name, the file names, formats, and compression schemes (if any) used. Hard copy output must accompany all files.

REFEREED PUBLICATION

Research in Nursing and Health is a general, peer-reviewed research journal. All manuscripts are sent simultaneously to three referees for blind peer review. Authors will receive notification of the publication decision, along with copies of the reviews and instructions for revision, if appropriate, approximately 3 months after receipt of the submission.

COPYRIGHT

Copyright by John Wiley & Sons, Inc.

INDEXED

Research in Nursing and Health is indexed in *Current Contents/Social and Behavioral Sciences, Cumulative Index to Nursing and Allied Health Literature, Hospital Literature Index, Index Medicus, International Nursing Index, Nursing Abstracts, Psychological Abstracts, Research Alert, Social Sciences Citation Index,* and *Sociological Abstracts.*

SAMPLE JOURNAL ARTICLE TITLES

- "Collaboration Between Local Public Health and Community Mental Health Agencies"
- "Effects of Family Structure Information on Nurses' Impression Formation and Verbal Responses"
- "Further Validation of the AIDS Attitude Scale"
- "Relationships Between Patient Attitudes, Subjective Norms, Perceived Control, and Analgesic Use Following Elective Orthopedic Surgery"
- "Pathways to Depressed Mood for Midlife Women: Observations From the Seattle Midlife Health Study"

Western Journal of Nursing Research

The *Western Journal of Nursing Research* is published by Sage Publications, Inc.

JOURNAL FOCUS/PURPOSE

The primary purpose of the *Western Journal of Nursing Research* is to disseminate research studies, book reviews, discussion and debate, and meeting calendars to a general nursing audience.

JOURNAL FACTS

Publication schedule: bimonthly
Circulation: 1,297
Submitted papers per year: approximately 90

Acceptance rate: approximately 50%

Monetary honorarium: none

Average turnaround time: approximately 3.5 months

Publishing timetable: 6 to 18 months after acceptance

Correspondence:
Sage Publications, Inc.
2455 Teller Road
Thousand Oaks, CA 91320
Telephone: (805) 499-0721
Fax: (805) 499-0871
Internet site: www.ua-nursing.ualberta.ca

MANUSCRIPT SUBMISSION

Submit four copies of your manuscript directly to:

Pamela J. Brink, RN, PhD, FAAN
Editor, *Western Journal of Nursing Research*
Faculty of Nursing, University of Alberta
3rd Floor, Clinical Sciences Building
Edmonton, Alberta T6G 2G3
Canada
Telephone: (780) 492-1037
Fax: (780) 492-2551
E-mail: peggy.pilgrim@ualberta.ca

A copy of the final revised manuscript saved on an IBM-compatible disk should accompany the final revised hard copy.

MANUSCRIPT PREPARATION GUIDELINES

Limit the title to eight words. Do not include a subtitle or a colon.

The *Western Journal of Nursing Research* now publishes abstracts. Please include a half-page, double-spaced abstract to precede the text.

Use the fourth edition of the *Publication Manual of the American Psychological Association* for your reference style and endnotes. Pay particular attention to the section on sexist language and English usage.

On the cover page, with the title: list all information, including all authors' titles, credentials, initials, current complete mailing addresses (including zip or postal codes), phone numbers, fax numbers, and e-mail addresses, as well as authors' affiliations as you wish to see them in print. On the first page after the abstract, place the title, followed by the content. Do not place authors' names on this page (or any other page, except the cover page) of the manuscript.

Manuscripts must be paginated. Number all pages, including abstract, references, and pages of table and figures. Acknowledgments are treated as endnotes and are placed at the end of the manuscript on a separate page, titled "Notes."

You will need to submit camera-ready figures. Submit original line (or laser printer) drawings, ready for photographing. One figure per page, please. Place pages containing tables and figures at the end of the manuscript. Do not embed tables within the manuscript text. Tables must be double-spaced and are limited to one manuscript page. If a table exceeds one page, it will be counted as more than one table. Limit the total number of tables and figures to three (one table per page).

The maximum allowable pages, including tables and figures, is 20 double-spaced pages (excluding references and indented quotations), with a minimum of 1″ (one inch) margins all around. Please use a typesize of no more than 12 characters per inch.

Include with your manuscript a typed covering letter, stating that you and your named coauthors (if any) are submitting this manuscript (give title) exclusively to the *Western Journal of Nursing Research*. Manuscripts without covering letters will not be sent out for peer review until said letter is received.

Manuscripts must be in dark print (typewriter, laser or dark ink-jet—no line printers or dot-matrix, please) and left-justified. Do not right-justify (fully justify) your manuscript.

The format for organization of a research reports for the *Western Journal of Nursing Research* is as follows:

Introduction. This is not more than one paragraph of what the study is about. The introduction does not have a heading; it follows the title of the manuscript on the first page.

Problem. This section includes the rationale for the study, the theoretical or conceptual framework, and the literature review—all rolled into one, brief section. Give this section a descriptive title that reflects its content. Please do not call it "Problem," "Literature Review," "Rationale," or "Conceptual Framework."

Purpose of Study. Label this brief paragraph as either "Purpose," "Research Questions," or "Hypothesis," whichever is the most descriptive of the content. Do not write "null" hypotheses; they are not appropriate. Write positive research hypotheses (in paragraph—not point—form), if you have any at all. Operational definitions of major terms used in the hypothesis, questions, or research statement follow the purpose of the study.

Design. Please specify the type of design in no more than two sentences.

Sample. Specify how many subjects were obtained, how they were obtained, and what their characteristics were. Ethics review of your study and informed consent of the subjects must also be dealt with in this section. If yours is an experimental design, the exact method of random assignment should be described. Identify the type of probability or nonprobability sample used.

Methods. Be clear about procedures, as well as the actual methods. Do not submit the instrument. If you want to share an instrument, provide an address from which it can be obtained, in the "Notes" section of your manuscript. Describe reliability and validity tests used in full.

Analysis of Data. Provide a complete description.

Findings. Write these our descriptively. Limit yourself to the major, relevant findings. Please do not write "The first hypothesis was upheld," or "The second hypothesis was rejected." Simply state the findings (in paragraph form, with references to tables, if appropriate).

Discussion. This section is the "meat" of the article. Describe what you think is important about your study, what it contributes to the research in the field, and its limitations. Do not include "Implications for Nursing" or "Suggestions for Further Research" in your discussion.

Notes. The "Notes" section appears on a separate page, at the end of the manuscript and contains all content notes, acknowledgments, and instrument access information.

A word about "It . . . that" type clauses: "It . . . that" clauses are the most common, and most annoying, style errors in manuscripts submitted to the *Western Journal of Nursing Research.* They create a passive voice: By simply eliminating them, you make your sentences active. Before you send your manuscript to us, be sure to eliminate all "it . . . that" clauses. (You should not have any sentences that begin with "However," either.)

REFEREED PUBLICATION

The *Western Journal of Nursing Research* is a peer-reviewed journal. The peer review process takes at least 8 weeks to complete (due to editorial office scheduling, the vagaries of Canada Post, and the workloads of reviewers), and the journal production schedule at Sage Publications requires 6 months from hard copy to published issues. For these reasons, time between receipt of a manuscript and publication is at least 1 year.

As a result, the review process takes longer and the time from acceptance to publication depends on available space. Manuscripts submitted during the summer months generally take longer for review.

COPYRIGHT

Copyright by Sage Publications, Inc.

INDEXED

The *Western Journal of Nursing Research* is indexed in *ASSIA: Applied Social Sciences Index and Abstracts; Behavioral Medicine Abstracts; Cumulative Index to Nursing and Allied Health Literature; Current Contents: Social & Behavioral Sciences; Health Instrument File; Human Resources Abstracts; Index Medicus; International Nursing Index; Nursing Abstracts; Nursing Citation Index; Psychological Abstracts; PsycINFO;* and *RNdex Top 100.*

SAMPLE JOURNAL ARTICLE TITLES

- "First-Year Swedish Nursing Students' Experiences With Elderly Patients"
- "Manager Leadership and Retention of Hospital Staff Nurses"
- "Professional Classifications of American Nurses, 1910 to 1935"
- "Studies of Ethical Conflicts by Nursing Practice Settings or Roles"
- "The Meanings of Home in the Stories of Older Women"

18

Skin and Wound Care

Dermatology Nursing

Dermatology Nursing is published by Jannetti Publications, Inc., and is the official journal of the Dermatology Nurses' Association (DNA).

JOURNAL FOCUS/PURPOSE

The primary purpose of *Dermatology Nursing* is to inform nurses of advances in all areas of dermatology nursing care.

JOURNAL FACTS

Publication schedule: bimonthly

Circulation: 6,000

Submitted papers per year: variable

Acceptance rate: 50%-90%

Monetary honorarium: $15/published page, $200 CE series honorarium

Average turnaround time: 6-8 weeks

Publishing timetable: 2-6 months after acceptance

Correspondence:
Jannetti Publications, Inc.
East Holly Avenue
Box 56
Pitman, NJ 08071-0056
Telephone: (856) 256-2300

Internet site: www.ajj.com/jpi or www.inurse.com/jpi

MANUSCRIPT SUBMISSION

The journal accepts original articles, case studies, letters, descriptions of clinical care, and research. Query letters are welcomed, but not required. Material must be original and never published before. Material is submitted for review with the understanding that it is not being submitted to any other journal prior to final consideration by the journal.

Five copies of the manuscript should be submitted to the editorial office; the author retains one copy. Manuscripts not accepted for publication will not be returned to the author unless requested within 30 days of notification of rejection.

Manuscripts should be submitted to:
Marcia Hill, MS, RN
Editor, *Dermatology Nursing*
East Holly Avenue
Box 56
Pitman, NJ 08071-0056

Dermatology Nursing provides its readers with the multifaceted information they need to provide clinically excellent patient care and to enhance their patient care practice. *Dermatology Nursing* publishes clinical and theoretical information relevant to specialists in dermatology and nurses in other specialties who deliver comprehensive, quality care. *Dermatology Nursing* supports DNA's mission to develop and foster the highest standards of dermatology nursing skin and wound care through education and research. The journal provides its readers with the best clinical information available so that they may better care for and educate their patients.

MANUSCRIPT PREPARATION GUIDELINES

Manuscripts must be typed, double-spaced on 8.5 × 11-inch white paper. Style should generally follow the *Publication Manual of the American Psychological Association* (APA). Please use the author-date method of citation within the text—(Doe, 1993) or "Doe (1987) states . . ." With multiple authors, the first citation must list all authors; in subsequent citations, list only the last name of the first author and et al.

Include the manuscript title, authors' names and credentials, and a biographic statement. Also include a brief abstract of 40 words or less, along with an address for correspondence and day and evening phone numbers.

Double-space all typing, using 1.5- to 2-inch margins. Include the title, or short descriptor, on top of each page, but do not include authors' names.

Include subheadings in the manuscript where possible. Type all subheadings flush with the left margin.

List all references in alphabetical order. Sample references are shown below:

Book:

Doe, J.R. (1993). *Skin and aging processes.* Boca Raton, FL: CRC Press.

Chapter in a book:

Doe, J.R., & Smith, B. (1993). Aging of the human skin. In R. Jones (Ed.), *Handbook on aging* (pp. 123-234). New York: Nostrand-Rheinhold Company.

Periodical

Jones, J.F. (1993). Skin cancer. *American Journal of Nursing, 843*(11), 1234-1456.

Figures include line drawings, photographs, diagrams, and graphs. Each figure must be numbered, and that number must correspond to a statement in the text directing the reader to see that figure. Include a separate legend sheet with double-spaced captions. The author must obtain permission for figures borrowed from another source. Photographs may be black-and-white, glossy, 5 × 7 inch, or color 5 × 7 inch or 35 mm slides.

The journal will accept both IBM and Macintosh format diskettes sent with manuscripts. All diskettes should be clearly labeled with the author name, manuscript title, disk type (IBM or Macintosh), file name, and word processor name and version (or file type, if ASCII). IBM diskette densities should be 1.2 MB or lower for 5.25" and 1.44 MB or lower for 3.5"; Macintosh diskette density should be 1.44 MB or lower.

Most, but not all, IBM and Macintosh word processor files are acceptable for submission to the journal. When possible, all files should be saved as WordPerfect. Many spreadsheet files may also be acceptable but must be approved prior to sending. To ensure acceptability of your disk, please contact the journal office before sending any material.

Please use only common fonts (CG Times, Univers, Helvetica, Courier, etc.) and avoid complex font attributes such as outline. All graphics (tables, graphs, etc.) must be submitted in camera-ready form.

REFEREED PUBLICATION

Dermatology Nursing is a refereed journal. All manuscripts submitted undergo review by the editor and blind reviews by the manuscript review panel and/or editorial board. Each article is evaluated on its timeliness, importance, accuracy, clarity, and applicability. Manuscripts accepted are subject to copyediting. The author will receive proofs for review prior to publication.

COPYRIGHT

Copyright by Jannetti Publications, Inc.

INDEXED

Dermatology Nursing is indexed in *Access to Uncover, Cumulative Index to Nursing and Allied Health Literature, Nursing Abstracts, RNdex Top 100,* and *UMI* (University Microfilms International).

SAMPLE JOURNAL ARTICLE TITLES

- "Cutaneous Laser Resurfacing: A Nursing Guide"
- "Heparin-Induced Skin Necrosis: Nurses Beware"
- "Management of Hemangiomas"
- "Pressure Ulcers: A Public Health Problem, An Integrated Hospital's Solution"
- "Smoking Cessation: Information for Specialists"

Journal of Wound, Ostomy and Continence Nursing

The *Journal of Wound, Ostomy and Continence Nursing* is published by Mosby, Inc., and is the official journal of the Wound, Ostomy and Continence Nurses Society (WOCN), an Association of ET Nurses.

JOURNAL FOCUS/PURPOSE

The primary purpose of the journal is to address educational needs within the global community of wound ostomy and continence nurses and other health care professionals involved in wound, ostomy, and continence specialty practice nursing.

JOURNAL FACTS

Publication schedule: bimonthly
Circulation: approximately 5,000
Submitted papers per year: 45
Acceptance rate: 90%
Monetary honorarium: none
Average turnaround time: 3-4 months
Publishing timetable: 4-6 months after acceptance
Correspondence:

Journal of Wound, Ostomy and Continence Nursing
Mosby, Inc.
11830 Westline Industrial Drive
St. Louis, MO 63146-3318
Telephone: 1-800-453-4351
Fax: (314) 432-1158
E-mail: periodical.service@mosby.com
Internet Site: www.mosby.com or www.wocn.org

MANUSCRIPT SUBMISSION

The *Journal of Wound, Ostomy and Continence Nursing* welcomes original manuscripts concerning wound, ostomy, and continence specialty nursing care and related professional practice issues. Authors are encouraged to submit a letter of inquiry before submitting a literature review or when submitting a manuscript that is similar to one recently published in the journal. Manuscripts of original research, clinical series, or case studies may be submitted without a letter of inquiry.

Statements and opinions expressed in the *Journal of Wound, Ostomy and Continence Nursing* are those of the authors and do not necessarily reflect those of the editor, the publisher, or the WOCN. The editor, publisher, and the WOCN disclaim any responsibility for such materials. Neither the editor, the publisher, nor the WOCN guarantees, warrants, or endorses any product or service advertised in this publication, nor guarantees any claim made by the manufacturer of such product or service.

Submit three paper copies of the manuscript and supporting materials (figures, tables) to:

Mikel Gray, PhD, CUNP, CCCN, FAAN
Editor, *Journal of Wound, Ostomy and Continence Nursing*
1391 Delta Corners SW
Lawrenceville, GA 30045-5407

Telephone: (770) 978-0748
Fax: (770) 978-0748
E-mail: rgray@mindspring.com

As a result of the Copyright Act of 1976, which became effective on January 1, 1978, the following statement signed by all authors, must accompany all manuscripts submitted to the journal:

The undersigned author(s) transfer(s) to the Wound, Ostomy and Continence Nurses Society ownership and all rights to the manuscript entitled (title of manuscript), including those pertaining to traditional format, electronic formats and transmissions, and any other means that exist now or may exist in the future, under existing copyright laws, in the event the work is published. The undersigned author(s) warrant(s) that the article is original, is not under consideration by another journal, and has not been previously published.

Authors will be consulted, when possible, regarding publication of their materials. All manuscripts published in the *Journal of Wound, Ostomy and Continence Nursing* are the sole property of the WOCN. Permission to reproduce the material must be obtained from the publisher. A financial disclosure statement must be provided for any manuscript that represents work completed under a grant or any other financial support.

MANUSCRIPT PREPARATION GUIDELINES

If accepted, the manuscript must be submitted on a diskette in one of the following formats: Microsoft Word for Windows or DOS-based systems, WordPerfect for Windows or DOS, Word or WordPerfect for Macintosh computers, rich text format, or text only files.

The author accepts responsibility for ensuring that the diskette matches the manuscript exactly. Number pages, beginning with the title page, consecutively at the top right-hand corner of each page. A running title should not be included with the page numbers. Spell out all abbreviations the first time each is used. Use generic drug names; brand names may be provided in parentheses at first mention. Capitalize all trade name wound, ostomy, and continence products, and follow the first mention in the article with the manufacturer, city, and state. Generic product categories are not capitalized. The entire manuscript must be double-spaced.

Include the manuscript's title, name(s) of author(s), relevant degrees and certifications, each author's title and institutional affiliations. Provide the complete mailing address, including office and home telephone numbers, fax numbers, and e-mail address, of the primary or corresponding author. The title page composes page 1 of the manuscript.

All research reports require a structural abstract. The structured abstract contains the following sections: objective/purpose, design, setting and subjects, instruments, methods, main outcome measures, results, and conclusion. All other abstracts should contain a single paragraph briefly stating the scope of the issue to be addressed, two to three major points of the article, and the author's purpose in writing the article. The abstract should be placed on page 2, after the title page and separated from the introduction of the article, which is begun on page 3. (An abstract is not required for manuscripts submitted for Options in Practice.) Authors are referred to the following discussion of styles for each type of original manuscript or special feature of the journal.

The reference format must conform to that set forth in *Uniform Requirements for Manuscripts Submitted to Biomedical Journals* (Ann Intern Med 1997;126:36-47; http//www.acponline.

org/journal/annals/01jan97/unifreq.htm). Consider the following examples:

Journals:

1. Peiper B, Mikols C, Grant TRD. Comparing adjustment to an ostomy for three groups. J WOCN 1996;23:197-204.
2. Dallam L, Smyth C, Jackson BS, Krinsky R, O'Dell C, Rooney J et al. Pressure pain: assessment and quantification. J WOCN 1995;22:211-8.

Books and monographs (relevant pages may be indicated):

1. Palmer MH. Urinary continence: assessment and promotion. Gaithersburg (MD): Aspen; 1996.
2. Doughty DB, Broadwell-Jackson D. Gastrointestinal disorders. St. Louis: Mosby; 1993. p. 284-88, 298-302.

Chapters in an edited text (include chapter title, chapter author, and editors, as well as pages of the chapter):

1. Erwin-Toth P, Doughty DB. Principles and procedures of stomal management. In: Hampton BG, Bryant RA, editors. Ostomies and continent diversions: nursing management. St. Louis: Mosby; 1992. p. 29-103.

Publications by an organization:

1. Wound, Ostomy and Continence Nurses Society. Conservative sharp wound debridement. Costa Mesa (CA): WOCN; 1996.

Unpublished materials such as proceedings, theses, and lectures presented at meetings:

1. Gray M. Urinary incontinence grand rounds. 1996 WOCN Annual Conference; 1996 Jun 19; Seattle.

Personal communications should not be included in the references but may be cited in parentheses in the text.

Number figures, boxes, and tables as they appear in the text. Lightly pencil in the number of the figure and corresponding author's last name. Indicate the top of the figure when appropriate; do not mount illustrations. Include a diskette of all computer-generated figures, providing the name of the relevant file(s) and file type (TIF or EPS preferred). Do not send original artwork or X-ray films. Glossy print photographs 3″ × 4″ (minimum) to 5″ × 7″ (maximum) with good black-and-white contrast or color balance are preferred. Consistency in size within the article is strongly recommended. Color illustrations may be reproduced within the journal. The Editorial Board of the journal reserves the right to determine whether illustrations are published as black and white or color figures. Legends must be provided for all illustrations; these should be typed on a separate sheet and placed after the references for the manuscript. Data appearing in tables should supplement, not duplicate, the text of the manuscript. All tables, boxes, figures, or other special features must be mentioned in the text but placed at the end of the manuscript.

Figures may be submitted in electronic format. All images should be at least 5″ wide. Images should be provided as EPS or TIFF files on Zip disk, CD, floppy, Jaz, or 3.5 MO. Macintosh or PC is acceptable. Graphics software such as Photoshop and Illustrator, not presentation software such as PowerPoint, CorelDraw, or Harvard Graphics, should be used in the creation of the art. Color images need to be CMYK, at least 300 DPI, accompanied by a digital color proof, not a color laser print or color photocopy. Note: This proof will be used at press for color reproduction. Gray scale images should be at least 300 DPI with a proof. Combination of gray scale and line art should be at least 1,200 DPI with a proof. Line art (black and white or color) should be at least 1,200 DPI with a proof. Please include hardware and software information, in addition to the file names, with the disk.

The author is responsible for providing written permission for figures or tables borrowed from copyrighted materials (including the author's previous work) and for direct quotations longer than 75 words. Patient or guardian consent must accompany any photograph that shows a recognizable likeness.

REFEREED PUBLICATION

All original articles published in the journal will be reviewed by no fewer than three members of the Editorial Board, and special feature articles will be reviewed by no fewer than two Editorial Board members. The members of the Editorial Board are considered experts with specialty knowledge in wound, ostomy, and continence professional practice. Articles are reviewed and judged for publication on the basis of clarity, pertinence, accuracy, originality, and adherence to the journal's format. Revision of manuscripts is typically required before acceptance for publication. Authors of original manuscripts are provided the opportunity to review their accepted, edited manuscripts before publication. Authors cannot make extensive revisions or changes to edited manuscripts.

COPYRIGHT

Copyright by the Wound, Ostomy and Continence Nurses Society.

INDEXED

The *Journal of Wound, Ostomy and Continence Nursing* is indexed in the *Cumulative Index to Nursing and Allied Health Literature, International Nursing Index, Nursing Abstracts,* and *MEDLINE.*

SAMPLE JOURNAL ARTICLE TITLES

- "Development and Implementation of a Clinical Pathway for Radical Cystectomy and Urinary System Reconstruction"
- "Oral Care and Its Role in WOC Nursing"
- "Skin Integrity in Patients Undergoing Prolonged Operations"
- "The Development and Implementation of an Integrated Multidisciplinary Clinical Pathway"
- "The Pursuit of Colostomy Continence"

19

Specialty Practices

American Association of Occupational Health Nurses Journal

The *American Association of Occupational Health Nurses Journal (AAOHN Journal)* is published by SLACK Inc. and is the official journal of the American Association of Occupational Health Nurses, Inc.

JOURNAL FOCUS/PURPOSE

The primary purpose of the *AAOHN Journal* is to support and promote the practice of occupational and environmental health nursing by providing occupational and environmental health nurses with the most current research findings, clinical and technical data, and state-of-the-art information on issues which impact on the practice.

JOURNAL FACTS

Publication schedule: monthly
Circulation: 14,000
Submitted papers per year: 70
Acceptance rate: 80%
Monetary honorarium: none
Average turnaround time: 2 months
Publishing timetable: 6 months after acceptance

Correspondence:
AAOHN Journal
SLACK Incorporated
6900 Grove Road
Thorofare, NJ 08086-9447
Telephone: (856) 848-1000 or 1-800-257-8290
Fax: (856) 853-5991
E-mail: aaohn@slackinc.com

Internet site: www.slackinc.com/allied/aaohn/aaohhome.htm

MANUSCRIPT SUBMISSION

The *AAOHN Journal* welcomes the submission of original manuscripts of interest to occupational and environmental health professionals.

Manuscripts should be addressed to:
AAOHN Journal, SLACK, Inc.
6900 Grove Road
Thorofare, NJ 08086-9447

Manuscripts should include a self-addressed, postage-paid postcard with the title of the manuscript, to be returned to the author as acknowledgment of receipt. Manuscripts should not exceed 20 typewritten double-spaced pages. Submissions should contain only those tables or figures needed to clarify the presentation. The author has responsibility to obtain written permission to use tables, figures, forms, or any previously published material. Evidence of such permission must be submitted with the manuscript. Authors may submit articles in the following categories:

- Research study: A report of an original study, including methodology, results, and discussion and brief summary of practical applications/implications of the research for the reader. This will be highlighted in a sidebar "Practical Applications to Occupational Health."
- Survey article: A study that collects, describes, and critically analyzes survey data to aid in evaluating new concepts.
- Clinical article: A report of a clinical case affecting or involving occupational health nursing.
- Case report: A report of a clinical case affecting or involving occupational health nursing.
- Successful programs article: A report of the planning, implementation, and evaluation of successful programs in the workplace.

The Journal welcomes letters to the editor concerning either previously published articles or topics of interest to occupational and environmental health professionals.

Manuscripts should be written in the third person and five copies should be submitted. The author should retain a copy of the paper. If accepted for publication, the Journal reserves the right to edit, delete, and change titles to improve presentation of material without altering meaning. The Journal welcomes the submission of appropriate photographs illustrating the article. Photographs will be returned to the author. Each manuscript will be acknowledged and a copyright assignment will be required. Following review, the author will be notified of the decision of the Editorial Review Panel.

Manuscripts will be considered for publication on the condition that they are submitted solely to the *AAOHN Journal.* Manuscripts must include the following statements, signed and dated by all authors:

In consideration of the *AAOHN Journal* taking action in reviewing and editing my (our) submitted manuscript, the author(s) undersigned hereby transfers, assigns, or otherwise conveys copyright ownership to the American Association of Occupational Health Nurses, Inc. in the event that said work is published by the American Association of Occupational Health Nurses. The copyright so conveyed includes any and all subsidiary forms of publication, such as electronic media. The author(s) declares that the manuscript contains no matter that is, to the best of the author's knowledge, libelous or unlawful, or that infringes upon any U. S. copyright.

MANUSCRIPT PREPARATION GUIDELINES

The *AAOHN Journal* follows the *Publication Manual of the American Psychological Association,* 4th ed. (1994), for references. The author must assume responsibility for the accuracy and correct form of references.

The Journal processes accepted manuscripts on diskette or e-mail.

REFEREED PUBLICATION

AAOHN Journal is a scientific peer reviewed journal. Manuscripts are submitted to anonymous peer review by the Editorial Review Panel. The author's name, academic degree(s), present position, address, telephone number, and fax number should be provided on a separate sheet attached to the manuscript.

The author's name or place of employment should not appear on any manuscript page.

COPYRIGHT

AAOHN Journal is copyrighted by the American Association of Occupational Health Nurses, Inc.

INDEXED

The *AAOHN Journal* is indexed in the *Bibliographic Index of Health Education Periodicals, Combined Health Information Database, Cumulative Index to Nursing and Allied Health Literature, Current Contents/Health Sciences Administration, Excerpta Medica, International Nursing Index, MEDLINE, Nursing Abstracts, RNdex Top 100, Smoking and Health Database,* and *Work Related Abstracts.*

SAMPLE JOURNAL ARTICLE TITLES

- "Ambient Noise Levels in Mobile Audiometric Testing Facilities: Compliance With Industry Standards"
- "Form Follows Function: The Occupational Health Nurse as a Member of the Management Team"
- "Health Risks of Health Care Workers: Health Risk Appraisal Results From the Newly Independent Country of Georgia"
- "Occupational Health Surveillance: We're Making Progress, But Is It Enough?"
- "Orthopedic Problems of the Upper Extremities: Assessment and Diagnosis"

Computers in Nursing

Computers in Nursing is published by Lippincott Williams & Wilkins.

JOURNAL FOCUS/PURPOSE

The primary purpose of *Computers in Nursing* is designed as a forum for communication among nurses who use computers. As a refered journal, *Computers in Nursing* is a vehicle for the publication of high-quality, relevant, and timely articles on a variety of topics related to the use of computers in and application of computer technology to contemporary nursing practice, education, research, and administration. Articles in *Computers in Nursing* are selected to reflect the diversity of computer hardware, software, and applications that nurses use in their work to provide current and useful information to a broad audience of readers.

JOURNAL FACTS

Publication schedule: bimonthly

Circulation: approximately 4,000

Submitted papers per year: approximately 100

Acceptance rate: 42%

Monetary honorarium: none

Average turnaround time: 8-12 week

Publishing timetable: 6-9 months after acceptance

Correspondence:
    Lippincott Williams & Wilkins
    Business Offices
    227 East Washington Square

Telephone: (215) 238-4200

Or

12107 Insurance Way
Hagerstown, MD 21740
Telephone: (301) 714-2300
Fax: (301) 714-2398
Customer service: 1-800-638-3030

Internet site: www.nursingcenter.com/journals

MANUSCRIPT SUBMISSION

Although not required, authors are encouraged to submit query outlines of potential articles. Feedback and advice about the topic will be given.

Three copies of the manuscript should be sent to:

Leslie H. Nicoll, PhD, MBA, RN
Editor-in-Chief, *Computers in Nursing*
University of Southern Maine
P.O. Box 9300
Portland, ME 04104-9300
Telephone: (207) 780-4568
Fax: (207)780-4953
E-mail: LNICOLL@MAINE.MAINE.EDU

An Authorship Responsibility, Financial Disclosure, Copyright Transfer form must accompany the manuscript. The corresponding author will be notified by e-mail upon the receipt of the manuscript. If you wish to receive a hard copy letter, please enclose a stamped, self-addressed, business-sized envelope with sufficient postage affixed. In addition, enclose a stamped, self-addressed, manuscript-sized envelope with sufficient postage affixed to return two copies of the manuscript. This will be used to return the manuscript after the review process. In the event the manuscript is accepted for publication, the author will be asked to submit a copy of the manuscript on disk. Every effort will be made to notify the corresponding author of a decision regarding

the manuscript within 8 to 12 weeks after receipt.

All persons designated as authors should qualify for authorship. Each author should have participated significantly in the conception and design of the work and the writing of the manuscript and be willing to take public responsibility for it. The editor-in-chief may request justification of assignment authorship. Names of those who contributed general support or technical help may be listed in an acknowledgment.

MANUSCRIPT PREPARATION GUIDELINES

Manuscripts must be typewritten or printed on one side of good-quality, 8.5 × 11-inch paper with 1-inch margins. Dot matrix or draft printing of computer-prepared manuscripts is not acceptable. Double-space all pages, including the title page, abstract, text, acknowledgments, references, tables, and legends. Do not justify the text. Do not use proportional spacing. Do not hyphenate words at the end of lines. Number pages consecutively beginning with the abstract page. Include a running head (50 characters or less) at the top of each page to identify the manuscript. The running head must not contain any author names, initials, or other identifying information.

Each manuscript must contain the following elements: title page, biography, information, acknowledgments, abstract, text, and references.

The title page should include the title of the manuscript, author(s) name(s) and affiliation(s), and the running head. In addition, the title page should identify one author as the corresponding author and include the corresponding author's name, mailing address, preferred telephone number, fax number, and e-mail address. The title page will be removed from the manuscript prior to review.

The biography, information, acknowledgments page should include a brief biographic paragraph of each author (maximum 75 words); a paragraph providing information about the article, such as where the work was done, whether the work was supported by a grant or other source; and/or the meeting, if any, at which the paper was presented. Acknowledgments can also be included as separate paragraphs on this page. Include a running head, but do not number this page. This page will be removed from the manuscript before review.

Include a concise, 100- to 150-word summary of the article for the abstract. In addition, identify up to five key words that can be used to describe and index the article. Use MeSH® (*Index Medicus*) headings for key words whenever possible. Include a running head, and number the abstract as page 1.

Nonresearch papers should begin with a brief introduction followed by the body of the paper. Use headings and subheadings as appropriate to divide the text. Research papers should be in standard format. In both cases, use the *American Medical Association Manual of Style,* 8th edition, for references. Manuscripts should be 15 to 18 pages, including abstract, figures, tables, and references. As a general rule, an 18-page paper should have no more than four figures or tables. Tables must be numbered consecutively with arabic numbers, double-spaced, and have a title at the top. Figures and tables must be cited in numeric order in text.

Cite each reference numerically in the text in parentheses. A list of references is placed at the end of the manuscript and typed double-spaced. References are cited consecutively by number and listed in citation order in the reference list. Follow the guidelines in the *American Medical Association Manual of Style,* 8th edition, for format.

Examples:

Journal:

Minda S, Brundage DJ. Time differences in handwritten and computer documentation of nursing assessment. Comput Nurs. 1994;6:277-279.

Book:

Freedman A. The Computer Glossary: The Complete Illustrated Dictionary. 7th ed. New York, NY: Amacon; 1995:20-26.

The editor-in-chief reserves the right to edit all manuscripts for clarity, punctuation, spelling, grammar, and syntax. Substantive changes of any nature will be verified with the corresponding author before publication.

Written permission must be obtained from (1) the holder of copyrighted material used in the manuscript, (2) persons mentioned in the narrative or acknowledgment, and (3) the administrators of institutions mentioned in the narrative or acknowledgment. Where permission has been granted, the author should follow any special wording stipulated by the grantor. Letters of permission must be submitted before publication of the manuscript.

REFEREED PUBLICATION

Computers in Nursing is a refereed journal. Published manuscripts have been reviewed, selected, and developed with the guidance of our manuscript reviewers and the Editorial Board. Manuscript content is assessed for relevance, accuracy, and usefulness to nurses and their immediate associates. Manuscripts are reviewed with the understanding that neither the manuscript nor its essential content has been published nor is under consideration by others.

COPYRIGHT

Copyright by Lippincott Williams & Wilkins.

INDEXED

Computers in Nursing is indexed in the *Cumulative Index to Nursing and Allied Health Literature, Index Medicus, Information Science Abstracts, International Nursing Index,* and *Social Science Citation Index.*

SAMPLE JOURNAL ARTICLE TITLES

- "Cyber Solace: Gender Differences on Internet Cancer Support Groups"
- "Designing an Information Technology Application for Use in Community-Focused Nursing Education"
- "Patient Core Data Set: Standard for a Longitudinal Health/Medical Record"
- "The Copyright Quagmire on the Internet"
- "The Joint Commission on Accreditation of Healthcare Organizations' Indicator Measurement System: Health Care Outcomes Database"

Gastroenterology Nursing

Gastroenterology Nursing is published by Lippincott Williams & Wilkins and is the official journal of the Society of Gastroenterology Nurses and Associates.

JOURNAL FOCUS/PURPOSE

The primary purpose of *Gastroenterology Nursing* is to provide original contributions containing material of relevance to gastroenterology nurses with a focus on articles related to the practice of gastroenterology/endoscopy, including areas of clinical practice, education, administration, and research.

JOURNAL FACTS

Publication schedule: bimonthly
Circulation: 2,500
Submitted papers per year: 150
Acceptance rate: 90%

Monetary honorarium: none
Average turnaround time: 1 month
Publishing timetable: 2-3 months after acceptance
Correspondence:
    Lippincott Williams & Wilkins
    Business Offices
    227 East Washington Square
    Philadelphia, PA 19106-3780
    Telephone: (215) 238-4200
Or
    12107 Insurance Way
    Hagerstown, MD 21740
    Telephone: (301) 714-2300
    Fax: (301) 714-2398
    Customer service: 1-800-638-3030
Internet site: www.nursingcenter.com/journals

MANUSCRIPT SUBMISSION

The Journal seeks articles that are related to the practice of gastroenterology/endoscopy, including areas of clinical practice, education, administration, and research.

Unsolicited manuscripts are welcome. The editor invites authors to submit query letters in advance of manuscript. Telephone calls for feedback and advice about the topic and its development also are welcome. Manuscripts should be addressed to the editor. Include an original and two copies. Authors should retain one copy of their manuscript.

Send manuscripts to:

Kathy Wright, PhD (c), RN, CGRN, CS
Editor, *Gastroenterology Nursing*
University of Texas at Arlington School of
   Nursing
Box 19407
Arlington, TX 76019-0407
Telephone: (817) 272-2776
Fax: (817) 272-5006

Original manuscripts (research studies, case reports, and others) will be accepted with the understanding that they are contributed solely to *Gastroenterology Nursing.*

MANUSCRIPT PREPARATION GUIDELINES

Correct preparation of the manuscript will expedite the reviewing and publication process. Assistance in manuscript preparation is available from the editor.

Manuscripts must be typewritten, double-spaced, on $8\frac{1}{2} \times$ 11-inch white bond paper, with $1\frac{1}{2}$-inch margins. The title page, abstract, acknowledgments, references, individual tables, and legends each should appear on a separate page. Number pages consecutively.

All manuscript submissions must include the following.

Title of manuscript, name(s) of author(s) and degrees or certifications, authors' institutional affiliations and current status, and the complete mailing address and business phone number of the corresponding author should be given. If applicable, include a brief acknowledgment of grants or other assistance.

The abstract should contain 150 to 200 words stating the purpose and principal conclusions presented in the article. No abbreviations, footnotes, or references should be used.

The style for references is from the latest edition of the *Publication Manual of the American Psychological Association.* References used in the text should be cited by author's name and date of publication in parentheses (Smith, 1989), with page numbers cited for direct quotations. All references cited in the text must be included on the reference list.

The reference list should be double-spaced, should include only references cited in the text, and should be in alphabetical order. Examples of correct forms of references are given below.

Standard journal article (list all authors):

Roth, H. R., & Bennet, R. E. (1987). Nonsteroidal anti-inflammatory drug gastropathy: Recognition and response. *Archives of Internal Medicine, 147,* 2093-2097.

Complete book:

Sivak, M. V. (Ed.). (1987). *Gastroenterologic endoscopy.* Philadelphia: Saunders.

Chapter in a book:

Wurbs, D. F. W. (1987). Calculus disease of the bile ducts. In M. V. Sivak (Ed.), *Gastroenterologic endoscopy* (pp. 657-699). Philadelphia: Saunders.

Gastroenterology Nursing welcomes figures, illustrations, and good-quality photographs. Professionally prepared, camera-ready glossy prints should be sent with the manuscript.

A typed label on the back of each figure should include the arabic figure number, name of lead author, title of the manuscript, and designation of the "top" of the illustration. Type figure legends double-spaced on a separate page of paper.

Tables should be consecutively numbered, self-explanatory, typed (double-spaced) on a separate page, and headed by a brief, but descriptive, title.

Figures, tables, or quotations must be fully identified as to author and source. If text material totaling 75 words or more is borrowed, written permission must be obtained for use of the material. Letters granting this permission should be forwarded with the manuscript.

REFEREED PUBLICATION

Receipt of manuscripts is acknowledged. All manuscripts are reviewed by members of the Editorial Board. These reviews are anonymous; therefore, author identification should appear only on the title page of the manuscript. Do not include author information on any other manuscript pages.

Reviewers evaluate the accuracy and relevance of content, organization, style, clarity, originality, use of verifiable and current references, and the contribution of the manuscript to the specialty of gastroenterology/endoscopy. Authors will be notified of the results of the review of their manuscript.

COPYRIGHT

Copyright is by the Society of Gastroenterology Nurses and Associates.

INDEXED

Gastroenterology Nursing is indexed in *Biosciences Information Service, Cumulative Index to Nursing and Allied Health Literature, International Nursing Index, MEDLINE, Nursing Abstracts,* and *RNdex Top 100.*

SAMPLE JOURNAL ARTICLE TITLES

- "Development of the Conscious Sedation Scale: Establishing Content Validity and Reliability"
- "Keeping Current: Computer Basics for Gastroenterology Nurses"
- "Nasogastric Tubes: Insertion Placement, and Removal in Adult Patients"
- "Perspectives-Placement of a Wire-Mesh Stent: A Case Study"
- "Transjugular Intrahepatic Portosystemic Shunt (TIPS)"

Insight: The Journal of the American Society of Ophthalmic Registered Nurses

Insight: The Journal of the American Society of Ophthalmic Registered Nurses is published by Mosby, Inc. and is the official journal of the American Society of Ophthalmic Registered Nurses.

JOURNAL FOCUS/PURPOSE

The primary purpose of *Insight: The Journal of the American Society of Ophthalmic Registered Nurses* is to provide current and appropriate information to help ophthalmic nurses and nurses who deal with patient with eye problems. Also, the journal is a major source of news from the American Society of Ophthalmic Registered Nurses to its membership.

JOURNAL FACTS

Publication schedule: quarterly
Circulation: 1,400
Submitted papers per year: 18-25
Acceptance rate: 80%
Monetary honorarium: none
Average turnaround time: 1 month
Publishing timetable: 6 months after acceptance
Correspondence:
    Business Office
    Mosby, Inc.
    11830 Westline Industrial Drive
    St. Louis, MO 63146-3318
    Telephone: 1-800-453-4351
    Fax: (314) 432-1158
    E-mail: periodical.service@mosby.com
Internet site: www.mosby.com

MANUSCRIPT SUBMISSION

Insight: The Journal of the American Society of Ophthalmic Registered Nurses welcomes and encourages manuscript submission. Manuscripts must not have been published before or be under consideration by other publications. Papers should be pertinent to the specialty of ophthalmic nursing, professional issues, or subjects related to the practice of or of interest to ophthalmic nurses.

Completed manuscripts should be sent to the editor at:

    Sarah Smith, RN, MA, CRNO
    Editor, *Insight: The Journal of the American
        Society of Ophthalmic Registered Nurses*
    Department of Ophthalmology

University of Iowa Hospitals and Clinics
200 Hawkins Drive
Iowa City, IA 52242-1091
Telephone: (319) 356-7218
Fax: (319) 356-0363

Authors who have received financial support from a manufacturer or who have been given product free of charge to use in a study should acknowledge this support on a separate sheet.

Original articles, case studies, research articles, clinical technique discussions, and letters to the editor are accepted. Nonnurse authors should send a query letter to the editor before submitting.

One original and three copies of each manuscript must be submitted, including four copies of photographs, charts, and illustrations. If using a dot matrix printer, please submit all copies as originals because of inadequate ability to make clear copies from dot matrix printers. Once a manuscript is accepted, the final version may be submitted on diskette along with two copies of the printout. The author accepts responsibility for the submitted diskette's exactly matching the printout of the final version of the manuscript. Guidelines for submission of accepted manuscript on diskette will be sent to the author by the editor. Authors should retain a copy of the manuscript, photos, charts, and illustrations.

Manuscripts published in *Insight: The Journal of the American Society of Ophthalmic Registered Nurses* become the sole property of the American Society of Ophthalmic Registered Nurses. All manuscripts must be accompanied by the following written statement, signed by all authors:

The undersigned author(s) transfers all copyright ownership of authors: the manuscript entitled [title of article] to the American Society of Ophthalmic Nurses in the event the work is published. The undersigned author(s) warrants that he or she has participated sufficiently in the work described to justify authorship, that the article is original, that it does not infringe on any copyright or other proprietary right of any third party, that it is not under consideration by another publication, and that it has not been published previously. [type name(s) and signature(s) of author(s)]

MANUSCRIPT PREPARATION GUIDELINES

Papers must be typed double-spaced on 8 × 11-inch white paper with 1-inch margins on top, bottom, and sides and should not exceed 12 to 15 pages in length. Please proofread carefully for errors in grammar and spelling. It is advisable to have colleagues or mentors read the manuscript before submission (when possible) to avoid errors. All abbreviations and acronyms must be spelled out the first time they are used.

References should be numbered serially in the text and listed on a separate sheet double-spaced at the end of the manuscript in that order. Reference format should conform to that set forth in *Uniform Requirements for Manuscripts Submitted to Biomedical Journals* (Ann Intern Med 1997;126:36-47). Journal abbreviations should conform to the style used in the *Cumulated Index Medicus*. Each reference should include the following:

For journals: authors' names and two initials, title of article, journal name, date, volume number, and inclusive pages (list all authors when six or fewer; when seven or more, list three and add et al.). If the journal is paged sequentially throughout the volume, the issue number should not be cited; if the journal is not paged sequentially throughout the volume, then both the issue number and the volume number should be cited.

For books: authors' names, chapter title, editors' names, book title, edition, city, publisher, date, and pages.

Note the following examples:

Journal:

1. Servodidio CA, Abramson DH, Mendelsohn ME. Anterior ischemic optic neuropathy. Insight 1994;22(2):12-5.

Book:

2. Byrne SF, Green RL. Ultrasound of the eye and orbit. St. Louis: Mosby, 1992:195-6.

Chapter in a book:

3. Guyer DR, Yannuzzi LA, Slakter JS, Sorenson JA, Orlock DA. Indocyanine green videogiography and choroidal neovascularization. In: Lewis H, Ryan SJ, editors. Medical and surgical retina; advances, controversies, and management. St. Louis: Mosby, 1994:20-9.

For the title page, include manuscript title, author(s) name and credentials, professional position, and affiliations. Include correspondence address, work and home phone and fax numbers, and source of grant or financial support where appropriate.

For summary or abstract page, show manuscript title but omit author(s) name. This should be a concise summary or abstract not to exceed 100 words and should be numbered as page 1. A header stating manuscript title should appear at top of page.

The first text page should be numbered page 2 with subsequent pages numbered sequentially. A header stating manuscript title should appear at top of each page followed by page number. (Header example: Congenital Cataracts, page 10.) Author's name should not appear in header to facilitate blind review.

For references, type double-spaced on a new page, numbered in order of mention in text. A header stating manuscript title should appear at top of page followed by page number. See example in text section.

Figures include photographs, illustrations, line drawings, graphs, or diagrams. Photographs, clearly reproducible diagrams, and graphs should be numbered with an arabic numeral and labeled as Figure 1, Figure 2, and so on, corresponding with their sequence of appearance in the manuscript. A statement in the text should direct the reader to the appropriate figure: (Figure 1). All figure materials must have details large enough to withstand size reduction. Photographs (3×4 inches minimum to 5×7 inches maximum) may be color prints, black-and-white glossy prints, or slides. (Black-and-white glossies reproduce best.) Original drawings or graphs should be prepared in black India ink or typographic (press-apply) lettering. Typewritten or freehand lettering is unacceptable. All lettering must be professionally done and should be in proportion to the drawing, graph, or photograph. Do not send original drawings or X-ray films. Consistency in size within the article is strongly preferred. Figures should be marked on the back side with an arrow pointing to the top for orientation.

Illustrations are scanned electronically. For best reproduction, screening, shading, and lettering on a dark background should be avoided. Detailed instructions are available from the editor. Digitized electronic files for illustrations may be submitted along with four copies of the printout on high-quality laser printer paper. Special arrangements must be made with the editor for color illustrations.

The author's name must appear somewhere on only one set of the photos, charts, or illustrations for identification. Ballpoint pens and markers may distort the glossy surface; take care when writing on the back of photos. Package photos, charts, and illustrations in protective cardboard for mailing. Do not mar figures with staples, paper clips, or tape directly on the surface. When using figures adapted from another source, the author must obtain written permission from the original publisher.

A figure legend should be provided for each numbered figure. Legends should be clearly marked with the figure number to which they correspond. They should be typed double-spaced on a separate page. A header stating manuscript title should appear at top of the page.

Tables should be typed double-spaced on a separate page. Tables should be descriptively titled and numbered with a roman numeral (Table I, Table II, etc.). They should correspond with their sequence in the manuscript. A header stating manuscript title should appear at the top of the page.

REFEREED PUBLICATION

All manuscripts submitted undergo blind review by Peer Review Committee members. Reviewers will be rating applicability, clarity, value of contribution, accuracy, organization, and timeliness. If the manuscript is accepted for publication, editorial revisions may be made to improve presentation without altering meaning. If the manuscript needs major revision, it will be requested from authors before acceptance. Authors are responsible for all statements made in their work. In addition, the author is responsible for obtaining and providing written permission for the use of any materials, photos, charts, and illustrations previously published or copyrighted. The consent of persons photographed must be secured if the person is identifiable. All consents and written permissions must accompany the manuscript.

COPYRIGHT

Copyright by the American Society of Ophthalmic Registered Nurses.

INDEXED

Insight: The Journal of the American Society of Ophthalmic Registered Nurses is indexed in the *Cumulative Index to Nursing and Allied Health Literature, International Nursing Index*, and *MEDLINE.*

SAMPLE JOURNAL ARTICLE TITLES

- "Age-Related Macular Degeneration"
- "An Interunit Performance Improvement Program: Can You Get Me to the OR on Time?"
- "Retinopathy of Prematurity"
- "The ABCs of Visual Acuity Assessment"
- "The Mentor Commitment"

Journal of Addictions Nursing

The *Journal of Addictions Nursing* is published by Mary Ann Liebert, Inc., and is the official journal of the National Nurses Society on Addictions.

JOURNAL FOCUS/PURPOSE

The primary purpose of the *Journal of Addictions Nursing* is to provide practical information on identification and intervention in drug and alcohol abuse.

JOURNAL FACTS

Publication schedule: quarterly

Circulation: more than 2,500

Submitted papers per year: more than 150

Acceptance rate: 15%

Monetary honorarium: none

Average turnaround time: 4-8 weeks

Publishing timetable: 3-4 months after acceptance

Correspondence:
Mary Ann Liebert, Inc.
2 Madison Avenue
Larchmont, NY 10538
Telephone: (914) 834-3100
Fax: (914) 834-3688
E-mail: mliebert@liebertpub.com

Internet site: www.liebertpub.com

MANUSCRIPT SUBMISSION

The *Journal of Addictions Nursing* invites original manuscripts on current nursing issues, practices, and innovations as they relate to the field of addictions. Submissions are solicited from professional nurses and other health care professionals engaged in treatment, education, research, and consultation.

Send manuscripts and all correspondence to:
Audrey Shepard, Editorial Coordinator
Journal of Addictions Nursing
67-29 215th Street
Bayside, NY 11364
Telephone: (718) 224-0334
Fax: (718) 631-5218
E-mail: trjass@msn.com

Manuscripts should be original, never before published, and not submitted simultaneously to another publication. Submit four copies of the manuscript.

MANUSCRIPT PREPARATION GUIDELINES

Articles must be typed, double-spaced on $8\frac{1}{2} \times 11$-inch paper with at least 1-inch margins on all sides. Submissions must include a cover letter listing the authors' work and home telephone numbers and addresses, titles, affiliations, credentials, degrees, and small biographical sketches. Each article must contain an abstract.

Manuscripts should be no longer than 2,500 words; longer submissions should be cleared by the editor first. The article should have a main title, with subheads to indicate subdivisions in the text, and an abstract. Abbreviations and acronyms should be spelled out when first used unless common to the field. Generic names for drugs are preferred over brand names.

Type each table and its title on a separate sheet of paper. Use arabic numerals to number tables. Each table must stand alone—that is, contain all necessary information in the caption—and the table itself must be understood independently of the text.

Figures should be numbered with arabic numerals and mentioned consecutively in the text. Illustrations should be clearly lettered original line drawings (drawn and lettered in India ink), glossy photostats of drawings or graphs, or original glossy photographs. (Photocopies cannot be used for reproduction.) All illustrations should be identified on the back and bear the author's name. The top of the illustration should be indicated. A list of figure legends should be supplied at the end of the manuscript, double-spaced. A complete set of figures must be submitted with each copy of the manuscript.

Each manuscript submitted should include at least five references provided alphabetically and properly cited in the author/date system in the text. Manuscripts for Provider Pulse should include an annotated listing of suggested readings and resources for the practitioner as well as the consumer.

For a book:

> Kielhofner, G., *A Model of Human Occupation: Theory and Application.* Baltimore: Williams and Wilkins, 1986, 145-157.

For a journal:

> Ueno, R., Dextran sulphate. *Lancet* 240:646-649, 1988.

REFEREED PUBLICATION

Journal of Addictions Nursing is a peer-reviewed journal. Manuscripts are reviewed by the editor and members of the editorial board. Publication is at the discretion of the editor and editorial board.

COPYRIGHT

Copyright by Mary Ann Liebert, Inc.

INDEXED

The *Journal of Addictions Nursing* is indexed in the *Cumulative Index to Nursing & Allied Health Literature* and *RNdex.*

SAMPLE JOURNAL ARTICLE TITLES

- "A Comparison of Substance Use Rates Among Female Nurses, Clerical Workers, and Blue-Collar Workers"
- "Inside Russia: A Look at Alcohol and Opioid Withdrawal Management Strategies to Nursing Staff in a New Medical Center"
- "National Nurses Society on Addictions' Position Paper: Access to Therapeutic Cannabis"
- "New Findings Support Pharmacological Interventions in Addiction: Naltrexone and ReVia"
- "Treatment for Drugs and Alcohol Problems in the Small Island Nation of Malta"

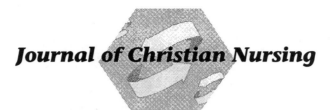

Journal of Christian Nursing

The *Journal of Christian Nursing* is published by Nurses Christian Fellowship and is the official journal of the Nurses Christian Fellowship, a branch of InterVarsity Christian Fellowship.

JOURNAL FOCUS/PURPOSE

The primary purpose of the *Journal of Christian Nursing* is to strive to help nurses view nursing practice through the eyes of faith.

JOURNAL FACTS

Publication schedule: quarterly

Circulation: 9,000-10,000

Submitted papers per year: approximately 100

Acceptance rate: 40%

Monetary honorarium: $25-$80/article

Average turnaround time: 1 month

Publishing timetable: 2 months to 2 years after acceptance

Correspondence:
Journal of Christian Nursing
430 E. Plaza Drive
Westmont, IL 60559
Telephone: (630) 734-4030
E-mail: jcn@ivpress.com

Internet site: www.ncf-jcn.org

MANUSCRIPT SUBMISSION

Topics covered include Christian concepts in nursing, professional issues, spiritual care, ethics, values, healing and wholeness, psychology and religion, personal and professional life, patient/client experiences that include a faith dimension (including case studies), and stories of nurses who have stepped out in faith to care for others in new or unusual ways in the United States or overseas. Articles must be relevant to Christian nursing and consistent with the purposes and statement of faith of Nurses Christian Fellowship (available on request). Priority will be given to nurse authors, although some articles by nonnurses will be considered.

If your article fits the guidelines, we prefer to receive the manuscript without a query letter. However, if you are uncertain about the suitability of your topic, please query either by e-mail letter or phone. Most articles by nonnurse freelance authors are rejected unless they have outstanding insights valuable to nurses. We will work with nurses who have significant information to communicate but need help with writing style.

Send one copy, typed double-spaced to:
Melodee Yohe, Managing Editor
Journal of Christian Nursing
Box 1650
Downers Grove, IL 60515-1650
Telephone: (630) 734-4030
Fax: (630) 734-4200
E-mail: jcn@ivpress.com

If your manuscript is accepted, we prefer to have a copy on disk. If you want your materials returned, enclose a self-addressed envelope with sufficient postage. Please keep a copy of the manuscript; we cannot guarantee safe return of your materials. Rejected manuscripts without return postage will be discarded.

MANUSCRIPT PREPARATION GUIDELINES

Scan a recent copy of *Journal of Christian Nursing.* You will see that the style is popular, not academic. Articles should be written to communicate clearly to staff nurses. Avoid (or define) technical jargon and abbreviations (these may differ in other clinical settings). Use lively illustrations. Give practical examples. Share; don't preach. Academic papers may have some good content, which *Journal of Christian Nursing* readers would appreciate, but they must be rewritten in article format. See "Avoiding the 'School Paper Style' Rejection," by Suzanne Hall Johnson, *Nurse Author & Editor,* Summer 1991, for help in revising an academic paper. Style is governed by *The Chicago Manual of Style,* 14th ed. (1993).

Limit your references to only those necessary to document your point. Avoid presenting a review of the literature. As the author of the article, you are the expert. Endnotes must contain the full name of authors (not just initials of first name) and be listed as they appear in article, not alphabetically. Be sure to include page numbers. See back issues of *Journal of Christian Nursing* for examples. You are responsible for accuracy in citation and interpretation of resources. Check spelling of authors' names carefully. If a reference has more than one author, list authors in the correct order.

Most articles range from 6 to 12 double-spaced, typewritten pages. Essays on "Why I Love Nursing" should be about 750 to 900 words. Use 1-inch margins.

Use letter-quality print and white paper. The review and editing processes require photocopying manuscripts. Manuscripts with light dot matrix print, or on colored paper, do not reproduce well. Number your pages and put your name on each page.

Good candid photos can bring an article to life. We can use diagrams and illustrations. Photos and illustrations will be used at the discretion of the editorial staff and art director. Do not write on photos or use paper clips. Include captions or explanatory material with each illustration. Place it in a labeled envelope and clip envelope to manuscript. Note: Identify all persons in photos and include a signed, written release for each. Suggested release format: I hereby give (author's name) permission to submit this photo of (subject's name) for possible use in the *Journal of Christian Nursing.*

Give a brief description of yourself, including your nursing credentials, where you work, your church and community involvement, and any other information you think readers might like to know—especially anything that would enhance your credibility in the topic covered in your article.

REFEREED PUBLICATION

Manuscripts with significant professional content will be sent to several review panel members for evaluation. If your manuscript is reviewed, you will receive copies of the reviewers' comments. We may ask you to revise an article based on reviewers' suggestions. Names of authors and reviewers are kept confidential in the review process.

COPYRIGHT

The *Journal of Christian Nursing* usually buys first rights. We occasionally purchase reprint rights. If your article has been published before, please indicate where and when. Never submit an article to two publications at the same time. We retain the right to grant permission to photocopy articles for educational purposes.

Copyright is by InterVarsity® Christian Fellowship.

INDEXED

The *Journal of Christian Nursing* is indexed in the *Christian Periodical Index, Cumulative Index to Nursing and Allied Health Literature, International Nursing Index, MEDLINE, Nursing Abstracts*, and *Uncover Company*.

SAMPLE JOURNAL ARTICLE TITLES

- "Claiming Our Heritage"
- "Documenting Congregational Nursing Care"
- "Miracles of Mercy"
- "Spiritual Care"
- "The Nursing Pin"

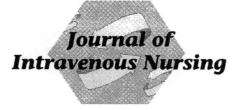

Journal of Intravenous Nursing

The *Journal of Intravenous Nursing* is published by the Intravenous Nurses Society through Lippincott Williams & Wilkins and is the official publication of the Intravenous Nurses Society.

JOURNAL FOCUS/PURPOSE

The primary purpose of the *Journal of Intravenous Nursing* is to provide and promote communication among all persons professionally involved in the field of intravenous therapy.

JOURNAL FACTS

Publication schedule: bimonthly

Circulation: 10,000 plus

Submitted papers per year: 80-100

Acceptance rate: 90%

Monetary honorarium: none

Average turnaround time: approximately 1-2 months

Publishing timetable: approximately 4 months after acceptance

Correspondence:
Lippincott Williams & Wilkins
Business Offices
227 East Washington Square
Philadelphia, PA 19106-3780
Telephone: (215) 238-4200

Or

12107 Insurance Way
Hagerstown, MD 21740
Telephone: (301) 714-2300
Fax: (301) 714-2398
Customer service: 1-800-638-3030
E-mail: ins@ins1.org

Internet site: www.ins1.org or www.nursingcenter.com/journals

MANUSCRIPT SUBMISSION

The *Journal of Intravenous Nursing* welcomes clinical and research articles for publication consideration. Manuscripts are accepted for consideration with the understanding that they are contributed solely to this journal, that the material is original and has not been previously published. If the work has multiple authors, it is reviewed on the assumption that all authors have granted approval for submission. Intravenous Nurses Society will respond to a query letter with proposed idea and outline.

Direct queries and manuscripts to:

Editor, *Journal of Intravenous Nursing*
Intravenous Nurses Society
Fresh Pond Square
10 Fawcett Street
Cambridge, MA 02138
Telephone: (617) 441-3008
Fax: (617) 441-3009

Four copies of the manuscript and the original will be submitted. A submitted manuscript should be accompanied by a letter that denotes one author as correspondent and includes his or her complete address and daytime telephone number. A signed statement of exclusive manuscript submission to the Intravenous Nurses Society and the following signed statement will also be included in this letter:

In compliance with the Copyright Revision Act of 1976, effective January 1,1978, the undersigned author(s), transfers all copy right ownership of the manuscript entitled . . . to INS in the event that material is published.

MANUSCRIPT PREPARATION GUIDELINES

Manuscripts will be typewritten, double-spaced on one side of good quality, $8\frac{1}{2} \times 11$-inch white paper with $1\frac{1}{2}$-inch margins. Preferably, an IBM compatible disk will accompany the hard copy. Manuscripts not meeting these specifications and those listed below will be returned to the author.

The cover sheet of the manuscript will include (1) title of the paper, (2) each author's name(s), (3) position title, and (4) institutional affiliation. The second page will contain a concise summary (50-100 words) of the article. On a separate page, a short biosketch for each author will include author's affiliation, academic degrees, and information of interest to peers in the field of intravenous therapy. Please submit this as it should appear in print.

Graphics: Illustrations, schematic diagrams, and drawings are generally published exactly as received. They must be clear and distinct, preferably in India ink on white paper, captioned and submitted unfolded. Photographs must be high-quality, glossy black-and-white prints. All illustrations or photographs should be plainly identified, with the top indicated. Captions or legends should be typed separately and attached to the associated material. Places in the text to which this material refers must be clearly identified.

Title should accurately and concisely describe content and/or significance of the manuscript. Intravenous Nurses Society reserves the right to create a title that is consistent with established editorial requirements.

Headings and subheadings will be used where appropriate to break the text. Pages will be numbered consecutively. Indicate, in the text, placement for tables and figures. Abbreviations will be explained the first time they are used. The generic name of a drug should be used instead of the proprietary name whenever possible. If it is necessary to use a trade name, it should be capitalized and inserted parenthetically after the generic name when first mentioned. Product names should be treated similarly and the manufacturer's full name, city, and state cited in a footnote or in parentheses in the text.

The numerical citations will appear at the end punctuation mark following the paraphrased or summarized reference. At the end of the article, the references will be listed numerically in order of citation in the text. Accuracy is the responsibility of the author. (For further details, consult *American Medical Association Manual of Style.*) In the case of multiple authors, include the first three authors followed by et al. For journal citations, include both volume and issue numbers. The reference list should be limited to published materials; personal communications should be inserted in the body of the text.

Examples of References:

Journal articles:

Larkin M. Intravenous therapy yesterday and today with a look to the future. NITA 1979;2:48-52.

Books:

Bennett JV, Bractiman PF, eds. Hospital Infections. Boston: Little, Brown and Co., 1979:50-52.

Intravenous Nurses Society reserves the right to edit all reader contributions for clarity, punctuation, spelling, grammar, and syntax. Substantive changes of any nature will be verified with the author before publication.

REFEREED PUBLICATION

Upon the receipt of a submitted manuscript, a letter will be sent to the corresponding author. The manuscript will then be reviewed by three or more referees. This "blind" process takes approximately 2 months. To protect anonymity in this process, authors' names should appear only on the title page, which is not sent to reviewers. The reviewers assess originality, validity, and significance to nursing practice. Authors will be updated as to the status of their manuscripts. All rejected manuscripts will be returned. Authors will have the opportunity to approve the final manuscript before publication.

COPYRIGHT

Copyright by the Intravenous Nurses Society.

INDEXED

The *Journal of Intravenous Nursing* is indexed in the *Cumulative Index to Nursing and Allied Health Literature* and *International Nursing Index.*

SAMPLE JOURNAL ARTICLE TITLES

- "Administering Continuous Vesicant Chemotherapy in the Ambulatory Setting"
- "Developing an Interactive Intravenous Education and Training Program"
- "Nurses Transition From Hospital to Home: Bridging the Gap"
- "The Registered Nurse's Role in Vascular Access Device Selection"
- "The Use of Unlicensed Assistive Personnel in the Delivery of Intravenous Therapy"

Journal of National Black Nurses Association

The *Journal of National Black Nurses Association* is published by the National Black Nurses Association.

Washington, DC 20013-1823
Internet site: www.nbna.org

JOURNAL FOCUS/PURPOSE

The primary purpose of the *Journal of National Black Nurses Association* is to (1) provide a forum for critical discussion of relevant issues relating to Black health and health care (these issues may include discussions of educational, social, economic, and legislative topics), (2) be a vehicle for the exchange of scholarly works of Black nurses, and (3) disseminate knowledge about critical practice, research, education, and health care management that affect the Black community.

JOURNAL FACTS

Publication schedule: biannually (Spring/Summer and Fall/Winter)

Circulation: 5,500

Submitted papers per year: 40-50

Acceptance rate: 50%

Monetary honorarium: none

Average turnaround time: 3 months

Publishing timetable: 6 months after acceptance

Correspondence:
Business Office
Executive Director
National Black Nurses Association
P.O. Box 1823

MANUSCRIPT SUBMISSION

Manuscripts submitted for publication, as well as correspondence on editorial matters, should be sent to:

Joyce Newman Giger, EDD, RN, FAAN
Editor, *Journal of National Black Nurses Association*
School of Nursing, University of Alabama, Birmingham
1701 University Boulevard, Room 213A
Birmingham, AL 35294-1210
Telephone: (205) 934-3960
E-mail: gigerj@uab.edu

Articles are considered on a continuing basis. Each paper is accepted with the understanding that it is to be published exclusively with the *Journal of National Black Nurses Association.*

The *Journal of National Black Nurses Association* publishes scholarly papers, research reports, critical essays, resource listings, documents, and reviews focusing on issues related to factors affecting Black health care and nurses.

Authors should submit an original and three copies of their manuscripts, retaining a copy for their files. Include an abstract of 150 words or less with the manuscript. Copies submitted will not be returned. The abstracts should summarize as completely as possible the objectives of the article and the facts and conclusions contained in the article.

MANUSCRIPT PREPARATION GUIDELINES

The manuscript (including references, tables, and appendices) should be double-spaced and typed on 8½ × 11-inch paper with margins of 1 inch on all edges. The name of the article should appear on the first page of the manuscript. A separate cover should indicate the title of the article, name, address, position, institutions, and should be made only on the cover page so that the manuscript may be reviewed confidentially. No more than a three-sentence biosketch should be included.

Although the importance of the article will in large part determine length, it is recommended that research articles, critical essays, and in-depth interviews should not exceed 3,000 words, or approximately 12 double-spaced, typewritten pages, including references, tables, and appendices. Reviews, resource listings, and documents should not exceed 6 typed, double-spaced pages.

The *Journal of National Black Nurses Association* utilizes the APA format. Therefore, authors should consult the *Publication Manual of the American Psychological Association,* 4th ed. (1994) for details as to format. These guidelines should be followed for all citations and references. Double-space references.

REFEREED PUBLICATION

A blind review process is used. Each manuscript is reviewed by at least two consulting editors. The *Journal of National Black Nurses*

Association reserves the right to edit as needed, in accordance with space limitations and guidelines, in consultation with the author.

The following are the criteria that reviewers use in judging the work submitted and are rated on the scale of 1 to 5: appropriateness of publication for *Journal of National Black Nurses Association*; the focus of the article; the relative importance of problems addressed in the paper; the adequacy of presentation (i.e., methodology/concept base, description of practice, etc.); and clarity of presentation (writing style, grammar, organization, conciseness, readability, etc.). Additionally, reviewers list the strengths and weaknesses of the paper. Comments will be shared with authors upon request.

COPYRIGHT

Copyright [year] by National Black Nurses Association. Nonprofit organizations or individuals may reproduce or quote from materials copyrighted by the *Journal of National Black Nurses Association* for noncommercial purposes on a one-time basis provided full credit is given.

No materials published in the *Journal of National Black Nurses Association* may be reprinted or published elsewhere without permission of the *Journal of National Black Nurses Association.*

INDEXED

The *Journal of National Black Nurses Association* is indexed in the *Bibliography of Agriculture, Cumulative Index to Nursing and Allied Health Literature,* and *Social Work Abstracts.*

SAMPLE JOURNAL ARTICLE TITLES

- "African American Women's Health Self-Assessment: Health Status and the Sense of Coherence"
- "Biological and Environmental Influences in Mental Health Care"
- "Breast Cancer Screening Among African American Women: Addressing the Needs of African American Women With Known and No Known Risk Factors"
- "Expanding Opportunities in Graduate Education for Minority Nurses"
- "Nursing Careers for the Homeless: A Curriculum for Success"

Journal of Neuroscience Nursing

The *Journal of Neuroscience Nursing* is published by the American Association of Neuroscience Nurses and is the official journal of the American Association of Neuroscience Nurses.

American Association of Neuroscience Nurses
4700 West Lake Avenue
Glenview, IL 60025-1485
Telephone: (847) 375-4733
Fax: (847) 375-6333
E-mail: INFO@AANN.ORG

Internet site: www.AANN.org

JOURNAL FOCUS/PURPOSE

The primary purpose of the *Journal of Neuroscience Nursing* is to publish original manuscripts pertinent to neurosurgical/neurological nursing standards, education, and practice, related paramedical fields, and clinical neurosurgical/neurological nursing research.

JOURNAL FACTS

Publication schedule: bimonthly

Circulation: over 5,300

Submitted papers per year: 75

Acceptance rate: 80-90%

Monetary honorarium: none

Average turnaround time: 3 months

Publishing timetable: 3 months after acceptance

Correspondence:

MANUSCRIPT SUBMISSION

Manuscripts are accepted for exclusive publication in the *Journal of Neuroscience Nursing*. The editor reserves the right to accept or reject manuscripts. Accepted manuscripts become the property of the *Journal of Neuroscience Nursing*. Rejected manuscripts will be returned to the author. Authors are not reimbursed for articles.

Submit one original and four copies of the manuscript to:

American Association of Neuroscience Nurses
4700 West Lake Avenue
Glenview, IL 60025-1485

Retain a copy for your use.

MANUSCRIPT PREPARATION GUIDELINES

Material should be double-spaced, including text, tables, references, and figure legends. Allow 1½-inch margins on all sides.

Use *Stedman's Medical Dictionary* for correct spellings. Abbreviate only after a term has been used in full with the abbreviation in parentheses. Use the metric system. Use the generic (nonproprietary) name of a drug with the trade (proprietary) name in parentheses after the first usage. Capitalize the first letter of trade, proprietary, or brand names. Do not use author name(s) anywhere in text.

On a separate sheet, list both work and home addresses and phone numbers, educational credentials, current position, and title. List any acknowledgments on a separate sheet. Number the pages.

Use of supplemental materials is encouraged to enhance the content and appearance. Tables, figures, drawings, or photos may be used.

A clean, clear image of any artwork should be submitted; photocopies are not acceptable. Photographs should be high-quality glossy prints, untrimmed and unmounted.

Submit one original and four copies, with the author's name and the illustration number on the top back of the photo. Indicate the top of the figure. Supply brief figure legends on a separate sheet of paper. Lettering must be professional quality. It is the author's reponsibility to obtain written permission from the copyright holder (usually the publisher) for use of artwork, illustrations, tables, or other figures not your original work. Supply the original of the permission letter and retain a copy for your records.

List references alphabetically by author. Cite by superior number in text. For abbreviations, use *Index Medicus* or the *Cumulative Index to Nursing and Allied Health*. Examples include the following:

Articles:

> White MB: Case studies in neuroscience nursing. *J Neurosurg Nurs* 1981; 13(4): 76-80.

Books:

> Edwards MP, Smith KN, Jones JS: *A Handbook for the Neuroscience Nurse*. Ohio Valley Publishers, 1980.

Chapters of portions of books:

> Hepp MR, Hardenbrook M: Pediatric head injuries and associated family traumas. Pages 319-347 in: *Pediatric Trauma Nursing*, Hoffman KP (editor). Adams Press, 1983.

Limit the number of references to only those that are necessary and cited in the text. A bibliography may be added if it enhances the content.

Authors are responsible for providing final manuscript corrections on request. Authors are required to read proofs and make only necessary corrections. Compliance with deadlines is essential.

REFEREED PUBLICATION

All manuscripts are subject to blind review by a minimum of two reviewers. Review criteria include scientific merit, relevance to neuroscience nursing and logical development of ideas. Average review time is 8 weeks. Accepted manuscripts are subject to editorial revision to enhance clarity and to conform to *Journal of Neuroscience Nursing* style.

COPYRIGHT

Copyright is by the American Association of Neuroscience Nurses.

INDEXED

The *Journal of Neuroscience Nursing* is indexed in the *Cumulative Index to Nursing and Allied Health Literature, Hospital Literature Index, Index Medicus, International Nursing Index,* and *RNdex Top 100.*

SAMPLE JOURNAL ARTICLE TITLES

- "A Case of Rapid Deterioration: Acute Multiple Sclerosis of the Marburg Type"
- "Building a Support Group for Parents of Children With Brain Tumors"
- "Neuroscience Nurses' Intentions to Care for Persons With HIV/AIDS"
- "Pathophysiology and Management of Idiopathic Parkinson's Disease"
- "Relating EEG Changes and I-Thou Feelings During Nursing Interview"

Journal of Ophthalmic Nursing and Technology

The *Journal of Ophthalmic Nursing and Technology* is published by SLACK Incorporated.

JOURNAL FOCUS/PURPOSE

The primary purpose of the *Journal of Ophthalmic Nursing and Technology* is to provide a forum for original articles that explore topics of interest to ophthalmic nurses and technicians.

JOURNAL FACTS

Publication schedule: bimonthly
Circulation: approximately 3,200
Submitted papers per year: approximately 40

Acceptance rate: approximately 85%
Monetary honorarium: none
Average turnaround time: 1-2 months
Publishing timetable: 3-6 months after acceptance
Correspondence:
SLACK Incorporated
6900 Grove Road
Thorofare, NJ 08086-9447
Telephone: (856) 848-1000 or 1-800-257-8290
Fax: (856) 853-5991
Internet site: www.slackinc.com/jont.htm or www.slackinc.com

MANUSCRIPT SUBMISSION

Send contributions to:
Heather Boyd-Monk, BSN, SRN, CRNO
Editor, *Journal of Ophthalmic Nursing and Technology*

6900 Grove Road
Thorofare, NJ 08086-9447
Telephone: (856) 848-1000 or 1-800-257-8290
Fax: (856) 853-5991
E-mail: jont@slackinc.com

All manuscripts for consideration should be submitted in quadruplicate (with quadruplicates of figures and tables). Manuscripts should include a self-addressed, postage-paid postcard with the title of the manuscript, to be returned to the author as acknowledgment of receipt. Manuscripts will not be returned to authors after review and will be destroyed in the editorial office. To have manuscripts returned, authors must request it in their submission letter and provide a postage-paid, self-addressed envelope.

All letters of transmittal to the *Journal of Ophthalmic Nursing and Technology* are required to contain the following language before manuscripts may be reviewed for possible publication:

In consideration of SLACK Incorporated taking action in reviewing and editing my (our) submitted manuscript, the author(s) undersigned hereby transfers, assigns, or otherwise conveys copyright ownership to SLACK Incorporated. The copyright so conveyed includes any and all subsidiary forms of publication, including electronic media. The author(s) declares that the manuscript contains no matter which is libelous, unlawful, or which infringes upon anyone's common law or statutory copyright.

Letters of transmittal must contain the title of the article and the foregoing statement signed and dated by all authors of the manuscript. Articles are accepted for review with the understanding that they are submitted solely to the *Journal of Ophthalmic Nursing and Technology* and have not been published previously except in abstract form.

MANUSCRIPT PREPARATION GUIDELINES

All manuscripts for consideration should be submitted typewritten on one side of $8\frac{1}{2} \times 11$-inch paper, double-spaced with 1-inch margins. Authors should retain a complete copy of the manuscript for their files. Manuscripts featuring a historical perspective or case study are also welcome.

The title page should be separate and include the following: title, author(s), institution of origin with city and state, acknowledgment of grant support, address, fax, and phone.

References are to be cited consecutively in the text in superscript numbers. References at the end of the text should be listed in numerical, not alphabetical, order. No more than six authors should be listed; authors after the third should be designated "et al." Abbreviations of journal names should follow *Index Medicus*. Following are examples.

Articles:

Stewart WC, Shields MB, Miller KN, Blasini M, Sutherland SE. Early postoperative prognostic indicators following trabeculectomy. *Ophthalmic Surg*. 1991; 22(1):23-26.

Books:

Spalton DJ. Systemic lupus erythematosus. In: Gold DH, Werngeist TA, eds. *The Eye in Systemic Disease*. Philadelphia: JB Lippincott; 1990:72-74.

Four sets of unmounted glossy prints or slides should be enclosed. Print lightly on the back of each figure the number, name of author, and top. The author should pay particular attention to quality and appropriateness of figures, and should be sure that each figure is cropped so as to provide maximum information in the given space.

Abbreviations should be kept to a minimum and preferably confined to tables. Periods are not used after abbreviations (eg, mm, mL). The proprietary name of a drug may be given only if it is preceded by the generic name the first time it is used.

REFEREED PUBLICATION

All manuscripts go through the classic peer review procedure common to the most respected professional journals. Your anonymous peers approve or disapprove your manuscripts based on merit and clarity of presentation. This process, we believe, reinforces not only the integrity of the *Journal of Ophthalmic Nursing and Technology* but also your profession through the dissemination of professional knowledge.

COPYRIGHT

Copyright by SLACK Incorporated.

INDEXED

The *Journal of Ophthalmic Nursing and Technology* is indexed in *the Cumulative Index to Nursing and Allied Health Literature, International Nursing Index, Nursing Abstracts,* and *Ocular Resources Review.*

SAMPLE JOURNAL ARTICLE TITLES

- "Iris and Pupil Evaluation: Key Considerations"
- "Fitting the Keratoconic Cornea"
- "Multifocal IOLS: Delivering Realistic Expectations to Patients"
- "The Foundation of Excellent Surgical Assisting"
- "Age-Related Macular Degeneration: New Treatments Show Promise"

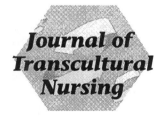

The *Journal of Transcultural Nursing* is published by Sage Publications and is the official journal of the Transcultural Nursing Society.

JOURNAL FOCUS/PURPOSE

The primary purpose of the *Journal of Transcultural Nursing* provides a forum for nurses, health care professionals and persons from other disciplines to discuss issues related to the advancement of knowledge in the area of culturally congruent health care delivery. *Journal of Transcultural Nursing* provides the mechanism for a dialogue by encouraging contributions from international researchers, practitioners, and theoreticians about the relationship between culture and health care. The journal's mission is to promote dissemination of research findings concerning the relationship among culture, nursing, and other disciplines, and the delivery of health care. Toward this end, the *Journal of Transcultural Nursing* seeks to foster the exchange of opinions from multiple perspectives on cultural topics that affect nursing and health care research, education, and practice throughout the world.

JOURNAL FACTS

Publication schedule: quarterly

Circulation: approximately 1,000

Submitted papers per year: approximately 100

Acceptance rate: 75%

Monetary honorarium: none

Average turnaround time: 3-4 months

Publishing timetable: 2-3 months after acceptance

Correspondence:
Transcultural Nursing Society Office
Madonna University
College of Nursing and Health
36600 Schoolcraft Road
Livonia, MI 48150
Telephone: (734) 432-5470
E-mail: 0007518450@mcimail.com

Internet site: tcns.org/journal

MANUSCRIPT SUBMISSION

Letters of inquiry are not required. Authors notified when the manuscripts are received. Manuscripts are examined by the editorial staff and peer-reviewed by at least two reviewers drawn from our Editorial Board and Panel of Peer Reviewers. Decisions for publication are made primarily on the basis of reviewers, but the manuscripts are not returned to the authors. The journal reserves the right to edit all manuscripts to its style and space requirements.

Do not send materials by means of mail services that require a signature. For example, if you are sending the manuscript via services such as FedEx or US Express mail, please waive the signature requirements as this will only delay receipt of the manuscript.

Submit the cover letter, five copies of the complete manuscript and accompanying materials, plus a diskette with IBM-compatible software, preferably in Microsoft Word for Windows format to:

Marty Douglas, Editor
Journal of Transcultural Nursing
360 Maclane Street
Palo Alto, CA 94306
Telephone: (877) 843-0508
Fax: (650) 843-0588
E-mail: martydoug@aol.com

A cover letter, stating that the material has not been published elsewhere and that it is not under consideration at any other journal, must accompany all manuscripts.

MANUSCRIPT PREPARATION GUIDELINES

Manuscripts should be prepared in accordance with the guidelines set forth in the *Publication Manual of the American Psychological Association,* 4th edition. Manuscripts, including abstracts and references, should be double-spaced using 12-point type, left justified margins, 1-inch margins on all sides, and should be printed on a letter-quality printer. All identifying information about the author(s) should be on the title page only. A short heading and page number should be typed on each page. Manuscripts should not exceed 20 pages, excluding references, tables, and figures. Each table, figure, graph, and so on should have their relative placement noted within the text. Tables should be typed one to a page with any notes/legends typed on the same page. Tables should be numbered, titled, typed double-spaced, tab delineated, and without use of lines. Label each figure on the back with its number and author name. Graphs and line drawings should be submitted as prints on matte-finished, heavyweight paper. Graphs or figures should not use gray scaling or shading but, rather, use hatch markings to demonstrate title and legend or caption typed on the same page. (Do not embed the number, title, or legend into the photographed print.) All tables, figures, graphs, and drawings should follow the reference list and not be placed within the text.

All manuscripts except letters to the editor or commentaries should be accompanied by an abstract of no more than 125 words. Abstract headings for research articles are purpose (include background and significance), design (include population, sample, setting), methods (include measures, intervention if applicable), findings/results, discussion and conclusions, and implications for practice.

A title page should accompany all manuscripts. Include the following for all authors: title, names of authors in the order to be listed, complete credentials, position titles, affiliations, and contact information (address, phone, fax, e-mail). Indicate the corresponding author with an asterisk (*). Author names should appear only on title page, not on any other page headings. A secondary title page listing only the title must also be included.

REFEREED PUBLICATION

When the manuscript is received, the editor chooses four or five peer reviewers. The reviewers are selected according to the author's major subject matter, the transcultural nursing area(s), theoretical insights, and research methods used by the author. It takes approximately 4-6 weeks for the reviews to be completed. The editor tries to inform the author of action taken by the reviewers within a 2- to 3-month period.

COPYRIGHT

Copyright by Sage Publications.

INDEXED

The *Journal of Transcultural Nursing* is indexed in the *Cumulative Index to Nursing and Allied Health Literature, Index Medicus, International Nursing Index, Nursing Abstracts, Nursing Citation Index,* and *RNdex Top 100.*

SAMPLE JOURNAL ARTICLE TITLES

- "An Ethnohistory of a Granny Midwife"
- "Community Assessment in a Suburban Hispanic Community: A Description of Method"
- "The Caring Needs of African American Male Juvenile Offenders"
- "The Construct of Culture Within the Transcultural Nursing Perspective"
- "Transcultural Nursing Administration: What Is It?"

Nursing Diagnosis: The International Journal of Nursing Language and Classification

Nursing Diagnosis: The International Journal of Nursing Language and Classification is published by Nursecom, Inc. and is the official journal of the North American Nursing Diagnosis Association (NANDA).

North American Nursing Diagnosis
  Association
Nursecom Inc.
1211 Locust Street
Philadelphia, PA 19107
Telephone: 1-800-242-6757
Fax: (215) 545-8107
E-mail: margon@compuserve.com
Internet site: www.nursecominc.com/html
  nd.html or www.nursecominc.com

JOURNAL FOCUS/PURPOSE

The primary purpose of *Nursing Diagnosis: The International Journal of Nursing Language and Classification* is to promote the development, refinement, and utilization of nursing language and classification. Manuscripts reflecting research on various aspects of existing and proposed diagnoses, utilization of nursing diagnoses in clinical practice, development of new knowledge related to nursing diagnoses, the process of diagnostic reasoning, and other aspects of nursing language and classification will be considered for publication. Papers submitted for consideration are assumed to be original, not previously published, and not under consideration by any other journal.

JOURNAL FACTS

Publication schedule: quarterly
Circulation: 1,300
Submitted papers per year: 40
Acceptance rate: 20%
Monetary honorarium: none
Average turnaround time: 3 months
Publishing timetable: 3-5 months after acceptance
Correspondence:

MANUSCRIPT SUBMISSION

Send the original and three copies of the entire manuscript to:

Rose Mary Carroll Johnson, MN, RN
Editor, *Nursing Diagnosis: The International Journal of Nursing Language and Classification*
1211 Locust St.
Philadelphia, PA 19107
Telephone: (661) 255-3805
Fax: (661) 255-3805
E-mail: Rose_Mary@earthlink.net

Each manuscript will be acknowledged on receipt. Manuscripts must be accompanied by a cover letter designating one author as correspondent with complete mailing address and home and work telephone numbers.

When a manuscript is submitted for review, please have the author(s) sign a letter of transfer of copyright to NANDA. The manuscript then becomes NANDA's property. Please include the statements:

I/we hereby transfer copyright ownership to NANDA if the work (include manuscript title) is published in *Nursing Diagnosis: The International Journal of Nursing Language and Classification.* I/we warrant that the article is original, has not been submitted to another journal, and has not been previously published.

MANUSCRIPT PREPARATION GUIDELINES

Type manuscripts double-space on 8½ × 11-inch paper, leaving margins of at least 1 inch. Number the pages consecutively beginning with the first page of text. Begin each element below on a new page.

1. Title page: Write a brief, specific, and descriptive title. Include the full names of all authors, their degrees, titles, affiliations, and any acknowledgments of financial support.
2. Abstract: Prepare a structured abstract. For research reports (100-120 words): problem, methods, findings, conclusions. For other articles (75-100 words): topic, purpose, sources used, conclusions. Identify three to five key words for indexing purposes.
3. Text: Prepare papers using standard manuscript form according to the *Publication Manual of the American Psychological Association* (APA), 4th ed. (1994). Length should be 12-15 pages inclusive of tables and figures. Use headings and subheadings as appropriate. Identify key sentences or points to help in selecting breakouts for the final manuscript.
4. Tables: Number tables consecutively. Cite each one in the text. Type each double-spaced on a separate page; place at end of the references.
5. Figures: Have figures professionally drawn and photographed; send a 5 × 7 glossy black-and-white photograph. Type a legend for each figure. On the back of each photograph indicate the name of the first author and figure number. Cite each figure in the text, following numbering/citations instructions given for tables.
6. References: Prepare in APA format. Cite all references in the text. Authors are responsible for accuracy of all reference citations.

7. If English is not your first language, manuscripts will need to be edited for English before submission.

At time of acceptance, send a copy of the manuscript on an IBM-compatible disk in Word or WordPerfect, or e-mail manuscript to margon@compuserve.com.

REFEREED PUBLICATION

All submitted papers are subject to blind peer review by a member of the Editorial Review Board and one or more expert reviewers.

COPYRIGHT

Copyright by the North American Nursing Diagnosis Association.

INDEXED

Nursing Diagnosis: The International Journal of Nursing Language and Classification is indexed in the *Cumulative Index to Nursing and Allied Health Literature, International Nursing Index,* and *RNdex Top 100.*

SAMPLE JOURNAL ARTICLE TITLES

- "A Multivariate Approach for the Validation of Anxiety and Fear"
- "Considerations in Diagnosing in the Spiritual Domain"
- "Development of Bilingual Tools to Assess Functional Health Patterns"
- "Stress Incontinence: Clinical Identification and Validation of Defining Characteristics"
- "You Make the Diagnosis: Case Study—The Family as Client in the School Setting"

Nursing History Review

Nursing History Review is published by Springer Publishing Company and is the official journal of the American Association for the History of Nursing (AAHN).

JOURNAL FOCUS/PURPOSE

The primary purpose of *Nursing History Review* is to trace new and developing work in the fields of nursing and health care history.

JOURNAL FACTS

Publication schedule: annually

Circulation: 900

Submitted papers per year: 15

Acceptance rate: 50%

Monetary honorarium: none

Average turnaround time: 6 months

Publishing timetable: annual journal

Correspondence:
Springer Publishing Company
536 Broadway
New York, NY 10012-9904
Telephone: (212) 431-4370
Fax: (212) 941-7842
E-mail: contactus@springerjournals.com or
editorial@springerpub.com

Internet site: www.aahn.org/nhr.html or
www.springerpub.com

MANUSCRIPT SUBMISSION

For solicited articles, length guidelines and submission deadlines will be specified in the solicitation letter. Unsolicited submissions are also welcome and will be acknowledged promptly; the length should be appropriate to the topic of the submission.

Submit the original copy of the typescript and six photocopies.

All correspondence concerning your submissions should be sent to:
Joan E. Lynaugh, PhD
Editor, *Nursing History Review*
University of Pennsylvania
420 Guardian Drive, Room 307
Philadelphia, PA 19104-6096
Telephone: (215) 898-4502
Fax: (215) 573-2168

MANUSCRIPT PREPARATION GUIDELINES

The entire manuscript must be typed fully double-spaced (including the bibliography, quoted or set-off text, lists, and any notes). All typescripts must be prepared with a typewriter or letter-quality computer printer. Draft-quality dot matrix printouts will not be accepted for publication. Margins of at least 1 inch on all sides must be used. Single-spaced typescripts will be returned to the author for retyping.

Pages should be numbered consecutively, including reference pages. The cover page for your article must include the following: article title (no more than two parts: title and subtitle); full names of the authors as they are meant to appear in print; a brief listing of the authors' major affiliations as they are meant to appear in print; an address, telephone number, and fax number for the corresponding author; brief acknowledgments of support or assistance (indicated in a note on the title page); and key words or phrases to use in subject indexing; with first submission, send photocopies of photographs or tables intended for publication.

Use up to three levels of text headings in your article, and differentiate the three levels clearly in your manuscript with distinct indentations and capitalizations.

References should be used solely to provide bibliographic citations to sources. For questions of style, follow the guidelines for numbered endnotes presented in the *Chicago Manual of Style* (14th ed.). In the typescript, all notes must be double-spaced and typed separately from the text (placed at the end of the article, not as footnotes).

Tables must be typed double-spaced, each on a separate sheet, and must be accompanied by a title and/or legend. Figures (line drawings, photographs, etc.) must be submitted as black-and-white, camera-ready glossy prints. All drawings, graphs, and charts must be professional-quality artwork. Illustrations prepared with computerized graphic programs will not be accepted unless they are indistinguishable from professional-quality artwork drawn by a graphic artist. Glossy prints must be labeled on the back with the name of the article, author(s), and figure number. Photographs must be accompanied by an appropriate source credit (name of photographer, archive, or collection). Captions or legends for all figures must be typed double-spaced and provided separate from the figures themselves. Be sure to make explicit reference to each table and figure within the text, but attach all tables and figures to the end of the typescript.

If a table or figure has been previously published, or if more than 500 words of text are quoted from a scholarly book (or 250 words from a scholarly article), the article manuscript must be accompanied by written permission from the copyright owner (who is not necessarily the author of the table, figure, or quote). It is the responsibility of the author to determine who owns the copyright and to provide the appropriate permissions letters. Final acceptance of the manuscript will be withheld until all necessary permissions letters are received.

REFEREED PUBLICATION

Nursing History Review is a refereed journal. All submitted papers are subject to blind peer review.

COPYRIGHT

Copyright by Springer Publishing Company.

INDEXED

Nursing History Review is indexed in *America: History and Life, Current Contents, Cumulative Index to Nursing and Allied Health Literature, Historical Abstracts, Index Medicus, MEDLINE, Research Alert, RNdex Top 100,* and *Social Science Citation Index.*

SAMPLE JOURNAL ARTICLE TITLES

- "Asylum Nursing and Institutional Service: A Case Study of the South of England, 1861-1881"
- "Entering the Professional Domain: The Making of the Modern Nurse in 17th Century France"
- "Full Circle: The Nurse-Midwifery Careers of Elizabeth Berryhill and Gabriela Olivera"
- "Nurse-Midwives, the Mass Media, and the Politics of Maternal Health Care in the United States, 1925-1955"
- "Refuge and Rescue: Jewish Nurse Refugees and the International Council of Nurses, 1947-1965"

Outcomes Management for Nursing Practice

Outcomes Management for Nursing Practice is published by Lippincott Williams & Wilkins.

JOURNAL FOCUS/PURPOSE

The primary purpose of *Outcomes Management for Nursing Practice* is to increase the knowledge and skills of nurses in evaluating and managing outcomes related to all aspects of patient care delivery across the continuum of care. Selected topics include identifying outcomes to evaluate; measuring and managing patient outcomes across the continuum of care; choosing and developing sound measurement instruments and tests; evaluating clinical protocols, programs, and critical pathways; planning and implementing outcomes initiatives; developing evidence-based nursing practice; and using outcomes data for performance improvement. From the latest measurement methods to strategies designed to improve the management of outcomes, *Outcomes Management for Nursing Practice* provides descriptions of outcomes initiatives in nursing and recent advances in outcomes management.

JOURNAL FACTS

Publication schedule: quarterly
Circulation: 1,000
Submitted papers per year: not available
Acceptance rate: not available
Monetary honorarium: none
Average turnaround time: 2 months

Publishing timetable: 6 months after acceptance
Correspondence:
   Lippincott Williams & Wilkins
   Business Offices
   227 East Washington Square
   Philadelphia, PA 19106-3780
Or
   12107 Insurance Way
   Hagerstown, MD 21740
   Telephone: (215) 238-4200
   Fax: (215) 238-4419
   Customer service: 1-800-638-3030
Internet site: www.nursingcenter.com/journals

MANUSCRIPT SUBMISSION

Submit four copies of the manuscript, along with a stamped, self-addressed, business size envelope if you want receipt of your manuscript acknowledged. If you want your original manuscript returned after the review process, enclose a self-addressed, manuscript-sized envelope with sufficient postage affixed.

Address correspondence to:
   Marilyn H. Oermann, PhD, RN, FAAN
   Editor, *Outcomes Management for Nursing Practice*
   168 North Cranbrook Cross Road
   Bloomfield Hills, MI 48301-2508
   Telephone: (248) 594-6933
   E-mail: moermann@msn.com

All persons designated as authors should qualify for authorship. Each author should have contributed significantly to the conception and design of the work and to the writing of the manuscript to take public responsibility for it. The editor may request justification of assignment of authorship. Names of those who contributed general support or technical help may be listed in an acknowledgment placed after the narrative and before the references.

Although not necessary, query letters allow the editor to indicate interest in, and provide developmental advice on, manuscript topics.

Authors will see only page proofs, not copyedited manuscript. Alterations to page proofs should be kept to a minimum and are subject to approval by the publisher.

MANUSCRIPT PREPARATION GUIDELINES

The maximum manuscript length is 15 pages including figures, tables, and references. As a general rule, a 15-page paper should have no more than three figures or tables.

Place tables and figures in the back of the manuscript after references. Number tables consecutively with arabic numbers, double-space them, and place a title at the top. Cite figures and tables in numeric order in the text.

Number pages consecutively in the upper right corner starting with the title/author biography page. Do not justify the right margin. Do not use running headers or footers. Use a 12-point font.

Divide the manuscript into main sections by inserting subheads in the text. Subheads should be succinct, meaningful, and similar in sense and tone. Relative weights of the subheads and their relation to one another should be clear.

Prepare references according to the style used in the *New England Journal of Medicine.* Sample references follow:

1. Parson LC. Delegation decision making: evaluation of a teaching strategy. J Nurs Adm 1997;27(2):47-52.
2. Uzych L. Transforming prenatal care. (Letter) Home Health Nurse 1996;25:554.

3. Nadzam DM. Nurses and the measurement of health care: an overview. In: Nursing practice and outcomes measurement. Oakbrook Terrace, IL: Joint Commission on Accreditation of Healthcare Organizations, 1997:1-15.
4. Schraut WH, Medich DS. Crohn's disease. In: Greenfield LJ, Mulholland M, Oldham KT, et al, eds. Surgery: scientific principles and practice, 2nd ed. Philadelphia: Lippincott-Raven, 1997:831-844.

Include journal issue number only when volume is not numbered consecutively throughout. Indicate when a letter, editorial, or abstract is being cited. Provide state of publication if not obvious. List up to three authors, then use "et al" to indicate the omission of others. Provide inclusive page numbers.

Place the references, typed double-spaced, at the end of the manuscript (before tables and figures). They should be cited consecutively by number and listed in citation order in the reference list. Whenever a reference is repeated in text, use the same reference number each time.

Place each of the following on a separate page: (1) a 50- to 75-word abstract that stimulates reader interest in the topic and states what readers will learn or how they will be better off after reading the article; (2) a title/author biography page. The author's biographic information includes name, credentials, position, place of employment, city, state, e-mail address (optional), phone and fax numbers; (3) reference list; (4) acknowledgments; (5) illustrations.

Written permission must be obtained from (1) the holder of copyrighted material used in the manuscript, (2) persons mentioned in the narrative or acknowledgment, and (3) the administrators of institutions mentioned in the narrative or acknowledgment. Where permission has been granted, the author should follow any special wording stipulated by the grantor. Letters of permission must be submitted before publication of the manuscript.

REFEREED PUBLICATION

Outcomes Management for Nursing Practice is a refereed journal. Published manuscripts have been reviewed, selected, and developed with the guidance of the Editorial Board. Manuscript content is assessed for relevance, accuracy, and usefulness to nurse managers and administrators, case managers, advanced practice nurses, staff development educators, and other nurses involved in outcomes evaluation and management.

Manuscripts are reviewed with the understanding that neither the manuscript nor its essential content has been published or is under consideration by others. The review process starts on the first day of every month. For example, February 1 is the start of the review process for all manuscripts received during January. Following review by the Editorial Board, authors will receive a letter notifying them of the manuscript's status.

COPYRIGHT

Copyright by Lippincott Williams & Wilkins.

INDEXED

Outcomes Management For Nursing Practice is indexed in the *International Nursing Index, MEDLINE,* and *Cumulative Index to Nursing and Allied Health Literature.*

SAMPLE JOURNAL ARTICLE TITLES

- "Client Satisfaction With Prenatal Care and Pregnancy Outcomes"
- "Nursing Outcomes Accountability Risk Adjustment in Nursing Effectiveness Research"
- "Patient Satisfaction With Nursing Care in Hospitals"
- "Report Cards: Tools for Managing Pathways and Outcomes"
- "Use of Serum Albumin Level in Studying Clinical Outcomes"

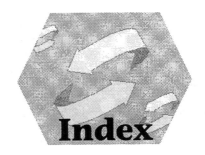

Index

About the Author

Jeanette M. Daly graduated from Northern Illinois University, DeKalb, Illinois, with a bachelor of science degree in nursing and a master of science in medical-surgical nursing. In 1992, she graduated from the University of Iowa with a PhD in nursing administration. Currently, she works as Geriatric Nurse Researcher in the Department of Family Medicine at the University of Iowa. Her research interests are care plan use in long-term care, elder abuse, nursing interventions, and geriatric functional assessment. Formerly, she was Chairperson at Marycrest College in Davenport, Iowa. She has been Patient Care Manager on an acute care surgical unit and Director of Nursing in long-term care.